S0-ABY-272

COMPUTERS
IN
MEDICINE

APPLICATIONS
AND
POSSIBILITIES

JONATHAN JAVITT, M.D., M.P.H.
Resident Surgeon
Wills Eye Hospital
Department of Ophthalmology
Jefferson Medical College of
    Thomas Jefferson University
Philadelphia, Pennsylvania

1986
W.B. SAUNDERS COMPANY
Philadelphia   London   Toronto   Mexico City
Rio de Janeiro   Sydney   Tokyo   Hong Kong

W. B. Saunders Company: West Washington Square
Philadelphia, PA   19105

Library of Congress Cataloging-in-Publication Data

Computers in medicine.

1. Medicine—Data processing.   I. Javitt, Jonathan. [DNLM:
1. Computers. 2. Practice Management, Medical. W 26.5
C7458]

R858.C656 1986   610'.28'5   86–1777

ISBN 0–7216–1578–3

Illustrated by Dan Reeves

Editor: Dana Dreibelbis
Designer: Terri Siegel
Manuscript Editor: Lee Walters
Production Manager: Laura Tarves and Bob Butler
Illustration Coordinator: Walt Verbitski

Computers in Medicine: Applications and Possibilities   ISBN   0–7216–1578–3

© 1986 by W. B. Saunders Company. Copyright under the Uniform Copyright Conven-
tion. Simultaneously published in Canada. All rights reserved. This book is protected
by copyright. No part of it may be reproduced, stored in a retrieval system, or transmitted
in any form or by any means, electronic, mechanical, photocopying, recording, or otherwise,
without written permission from the publisher. Made in the United States of Amer-
ica. Press of W. B. Saunders Company. Library of Congress catalog card number 86–
1777.

Last digit is the print number: 9   8   7   6   5   4   3   2   1

To my grandmothers,
who continue to wonder
why a doctor should be interested in computers.

PREFACE

My interest in computers began during medical school when I began to combine my interests in epidemiology and ophthalmology. At that time most people identified an Apple as a type of fruit and related computers to engineers and mathematicians. Being neither of these, I sought a basic book that would introduce physicians to computers. That search, which proved fruitless, led me to far more involvement with computers than I ever expected. While the journey has been enjoyable, there is still a need for the introductory book I sought in the first place.

Many individuals have offered the support and asked the questions that caused this book to be written, and I would like to acknowledge their contributions. To the people who pointed me in the right direction: Mr. William Bowen, Dr. B. H. Kean, Dr. Walter Riker, Dr. Michael Bruno, Dr. Robert Ellsworth, Dr. Alfred Sommer, and Sir John and Lady Wilson. To the people who asked the important questions along the way: Dr. Geoffrey Galbraith, Dr. Fernando Flores, Mr. Chauncy Bell, and Mr. and Mrs. Arthur Wellman. Most of all, I thank my colleagues and mentors at Wills Eye Hospital, in particular Dr. William Tasman, Dr. George Spaeth, Dr. William Annesley, Dr. Jerry Shields, and Dr. James Augsburger for their support and teaching.

Jonathan Jacott M.D.

CONTRIBUTORS

ERNEST BEUTLER, M.D.
Chairman, Department of Basic and Clinical Research, Scripps Clinic and Research Foundation, 10666 N. Torrey Pines Road, La Jolla, CA 92037; Clinical Professor of Medicine, University of California, San Diego School of Medicine, La Jolla, CA 92093

ROBERT S. BLACKLOW, M.D.
Senior Associate Dean, Jefferson Medical College of Thomas Jefferson University, 1025 Walnut Street, Philadelphia, PA 19107

MR. DAVID BROUSSEAU
Medical Student, University of Pennsylvania, 36th and Hamilton Walk, Philadelphia, PA 19104-6015

THOMAS CHALMERS, M.D.
Distinguished Service Professor, Mount Sinai School of Medicine, One Gustave L. Levy Place, New York, NY 10029; Visiting Professor at Harvard School of Public Health, Boston, Massachusetts

JAMES FATTU, M.D., Ph.D.
Clinical Associate Professor of Medicine, Indiana University School of Medicine, 3841 Bellemeade Avenue—Suite 230, Evansville, IN 47710

JONATHAN JAVITT, M.D., M.P.H.
Resident Surgeon, Wills Eye Hospital, Jefferson Medical College of Thomas Jefferson University, 9th and Walnut Streets, Philadelphia, PA 19107

FREDERICK JELOVSEK, M.D.
Associate Professor, Department of Obstetrics and Gynecology, University of Arkansas College of Medicine, 4301 West Markham Street, Little Rock, AR 72207

CHESTER KING
Product Manager for Medical Information Systems Division of Clinical Data, Inc., 1172 Commonwealth Avenue, Boston, MA 02134

PAUL MARINO, M.D.
Clinical Assistant Professor of Medicine, University of Pennsylvania School of Medicine, 36th and Hamilton Walk, Philadelphia, PA 19104-6015; Director, Medical Intensive Care Unit, The Graduate Hospital, 19th and Lombard Streets, Pepper Pavilion, Suite 501, Philadelphia, PA 19146

EDMUND MESSINA, M.D.
Associate Neurologist, Michigan Headache and Neurological Institute, 3120 Professional Drive, Ann Arbor, MI 48104; Clinical Assistant Professor of Medicine (Neurology), Michigan State University, East Lansing, MI 48824

EDWARD A. PATRICK, M.D., Ph.D.
Professor of Engineering and Computer Science, University of Cincinnati College of Medicine, 231 Bethesda Avenue, Cincinnati, OH 45267

WILLIAM STEAD, M.D.
Associate Professor of Medicine, Director of Medical Center Information Systems, Duke University Medical Center, Box 3900, Durham, NC 27710

CHARLES E. STEWART, M.D.
Director, Emergency Services, Saint Mary Corwyn, Pueblo, CO

J. JON VELOSKI, M.S.
Assistant Director, Center for Research in Medical Education and Health Care, Jefferson Medical College of Thomas Jefferson University, 1025 Walnut Street, Philadelphia, PA 19107

CONTENTS

ELEVEN

Computer-Aided Diagnosis and Decision Making 201

James M. Fattu, M.D., and Edward A. Patrick, M.D.

TWELVE

Computerized Medical Records 234

Frederick R. Jelovsek, M.D., and William W. Stead, M.D.

THIRTEEN

Data Management Systems in Clinical Research................. 256

Chester King

Introduction

This is a book about possibilities—the possibilities that computers open for the practice of medicine today and in the future. There is a plethora of information available today about specific products for use with computers both in medicine and elsewhere. There is an almost total lack of information that enables the thinking person to interpret that information in its proper context and to make intelligent assessments and decisions regarding computer use.

Perhaps the most important distinction that this book can offer is in resolving the question of what you want a computer for in the first place. I assert that it is generally not to assist you in *computing* but rather to assist you in *working*, and thus to enable new possibilities and levels of effectiveness. One does not buy a refrigerator in order to have an electric motor that can power a compressor but rather in order to store food. Similarly, computers for us are information storage machines, information analysis machines, and information retrieval machines. Most important, however, may be their role as machines that can transmit not only information but commitment for action. As a simple example, interns in many hospitals write periodic lists of all medications being administered to a patient in order to keep track of frequent additions and deletions. Anyone reading the chart since the last list was compiled must scan the orders for any further changes. In hospitals in which medication orders are written only via the hospital-wide computer system, a physician's request for a new medication triggers an automatic search for allergies or drug incompatibilities, a request to the pharmacy for the substance, a request back to the physician to order blood levels when appropriate, and an updating of that patient's medication list. This analogy can be extended to any other request for treatment, diagnostic procedure, or consultation. We as physicians have access to up-to-the-minute information on disease and its treatment in unprecedented ways. This book is dedicated to exploring these possibilities for practicing medicine that were unavailable prior to the advent of computers. To a large extent, this book focuses on microcomputers because this is the level at which you are most likely to enter the computer age.

As with any book, you are reading these words at least 2 years after the inception of the project. During the period of time the leading edge of technology has advanced exponentially. Although every effort has been made to assure currency of material at the time of publication, there is no question but that enormous advances will have been made before this book reaches your hands. For this reason, a book about specific products and programs is not feasible and is of limited value. Fortunately, the advertising needs of the computer industry have spawned a healthy industry in magazines specifically devoted to computers in medicine. This is always where the most current product information will be found.

Part I of this book provides an overview of what computers are, how they can maximize personal productivity, and how they may be incorporated into the mainstream of medical practice and education. Part II focuses on current applications of computers to patient care.

In the opening chapter, *Dr. Thomas Chalmers* draws upon many years of experience as a physician, educator, and dean to point to some of the shifts that computers will bring about in our practice of medicine and even in the qualities that we associate with physician excellence. I have followed this opening with three chapters designed to introduce you to computers, especially microcomputers, and their uses. Chapter 2 is an overview of the basics of computer hardware and software. It presumes no technical understanding of either and serves as a gentle introduction to these topics. Chapter 3 is a comparison of the capabilities of microcomputers and mainframes. Although most of this book is devoted to microcomputers and their capabilities, hospitals are installing large computer systems with which the physician must interact directly. A basic understanding of the "machine in the basement" that lives behind the video screen is thus extremely useful.

Chapter 4 serves as a critical overview of basic software tools for everyday work and introduces the reader to word processors, spreadsheets, and data base programs. In Chapter 5, *Dr. Charles Stewart* offers an overview of the electronic network of medical data that is now available to anyone with a computer and offers an approach to accessing it effectively. *Dr. Ernest Beutler* amplifies that theme in Chapter 6 by discussing the enormously powerful role that computers can play in effective management and updating of personal reference data bases.

In Chapter 7, I have drawn upon my consulting experience in computerizing medical offices in order to offer an approach that saves large amounts of time and money and simultaneously circumvents many of the most dangerous pitfalls in the process. It is interesting to note that, at press time, the only books on computers in medicine to be found focused upon office computerization. The explosion in technology and products since those books were written has made office computerization, billing, and accounting systems an increasingly smaller, although vital, part of the medical computer industry.

Part I concludes with an overview of the integration of computer knowledge into the medical school curriculum. In the past year, the Association of American Medical Colleges has formed a task force to develop effective programs and guidelines to fill this pressing need in the education of physicians for the 1990s. *Mr. John Velosky* and *Dr.*

Joseph Gronella of Thomas Jefferson University discuss the strides that are being made in their institution and elsewhere in the United States.

Part II focuses upon major applications that are available today to assist us in caring for patients. In Chapter 9, *Dr. Edmund Messina* discusses the utility of computerized history-taking in the physician's office and the systems available for that purpose. Although computer-driven history-taking is one of the first areas to which computers have been applied, only in the past year has this technology been easily affordable to the practitioner. In this chapter and its successors, the focus is upon programs that can operate on affordable microcomputer hardware both in the hospital and the office setting.

Chapter 10 provides an overview of some of the products that have recently been introduced for clinical management of patients. In discussing these packages, *Dr. Paul Marino* succeeds in presenting what is possible today. New approaches and products enter the market monthly, but his discussion of existing products can be used as a basis for evaluating new products with which you come into contact.

In Chapter 11 *Dr. James Fattu* and *Dr. Edward Patrick* succeed in making the highly complex field of computer-aided diagnosis intelligible to those of us who do not routinely think in terms of probability theory. The chapter focuses upon experience-based diagnostic systems in which hard clinical data from previous patients feed the decision-making process on an ongoing basis. In contrast, an expert-based system relies upon rules generated by a panel of experts in a field, and those rules are only as good as the collective opinions assembled. Although the data base needed to drive an experience-based system is far more extensive, the system ultimately draws upon a much larger knowledge base and is more rapidly updated than the best expert system.

In Chapter 12, *Dr. William Stead* and *Dr. Frederick Jelovsek* draw upon their experience as pioneers in the area of medical record systems to provide an overview of this field. During the past 10 years, the computerized medical record has evolved from a single electronically stored list to an intelligent system that includes its own checks and counterchecks to ensure optimal patient care. The approach described has been applied in many of the clinical services at Duke University and continues to prove and expand its power and flexibility.

Chapter 13 is a comparative survey of the major products available today for the management of clinical data. An in-depth survey of these products is appropriate in this case for two reasons: They are not adequately discussed either in the medical or nonmedical computer journals, and they are extensive and stable programs that have taken years to develop and are unlikely to change significantly by the time you read this book. *Chester King,* of Clinical Data Incorporated, has done an admirable and impartial job of reviewing this field.

The largest challenge in preparing this book has been in forcing myself to stop collecting material and send it to press. I am certain that between now and tomorrow morning, when the last page of manuscript hits the publisher's desk, I will discover at least one more topic or application that absolutely must be included. I am equally certain that you will be equally quick to find areas that should be included, covered more extensively, or reported differently. A large part of the satisfaction that I anticipate in having compiled this book is in hearing from you about what I have left out. Only through this form of partnership can I hope to keep this book a current reflection of the possibilities provided by computers in medicine.

JONATHAN JAVITT, M.D.

COMPUTERS AS TOOLS FOR PERSONAL PRODUCTIVITY

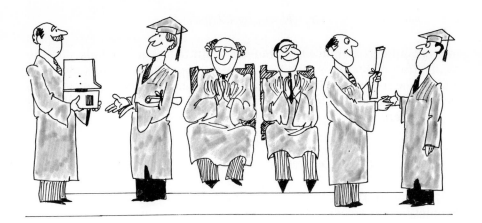

O N E

A Computer-Driven Shift in the Practice of Medicine

Thomas Chalmers, M.D.

Part of the reason for the slowness with which computers have caught on in the practice of medicine lies in the fact that many computers, programming, and available software have been too complex for practicing physicians to have time or interest enough to grasp. The advent of the microcomputers, and especially the development of software for all possible professional uses, will literally revolutionize the practice of medicine. The latest innovations that will make computers indispensable to physicians are the truly portable machines with an easy interface with microcomputers in office or home and mainframes in hospitals, and the availability of the laser disk for storage of enormous amounts of words and data and high fidelity pictures. There has also been and will continue to be an explosion in software related directly to the day-to-day activities of physicians.

THE HISTORY OF COMPUTER USE BY PHYSICIANS

Financial Transactions. As in most fields, the computer has been adopted rapidly when it has facilitated directly the collection of money. Although operations of laboratories, scheduling of patients, and record keeping could be considered the most important aspects of patient care in the use of computers in hospitals, the patient account section was the first to be adequately equipped and operational. In addition, the first software on the market for physicians' offices has to do with the collection of bills. There are now good enough systems available, and the manufacturers can devote their attention to the more substantive and important parts of the practice of medicine.

Scheduling and Appointment Keeping. This also has been a quickly adopted application because of its simplicity and obvious advantages. Numerous commercial software products are now available to facilitate keeping track of patient visits and sending letters reminding patients to return for follow-up. The last is also likely to catch on quickly because it is a source of additional income as well as good practice.

Cognitive Processes. Primitive software programs are now available to help physicians with their decision making. Programs such as "Internist" are examples of the knowledge and experience of the good clinician put on the computer so that those memories and thought processes can be made available to other practitioners. There are many other such systems available as well.

Medical Education. Finally, undergraduate and graduate medical schools have been interested for a long time in computer-assisted instruction. As in most fields in medicine, there are very few randomized control trials comparing computer-assisted instruction with the classic kinds. A few have indicated that there is no greater efficacy in the case of students who can grasp things quickly, but computer-assisted and programmed instruction may help in getting across difficult concepts to ordinary students and in aiding those with language or other background problems. In the next few years there should be continuing advances in the software and hardware of computer-assisted instructions such that medical education will in part become more efficient. However, there is still much skepticism as to whether computers have aided the education process other than through facilitating the examination process. Even in that case, there is some reason to mourn the death of the essay question.

Artificial intelligence, however, will give a big boost to advanced education. Extra time will be required for the faculty to prepare the basics, but in the long run, faculty time will be freed for more one-on-one teaching of students.

Accessing the Literature. One of the most important advances in the application of the computer to improving the practice of medicine has already reached its fulfillment: on-line access to the medical literature. The ability of physicians at almost any time of the day or night to access titles and abstracts of pertinent articles is a major contribution to the quality of care. The process is constantly being simplified, and the physician who does not use it directly is getting behind the times. Although at present most physicians still have to go through their local library for on-line searches, one day's training will soon allow the physician or one of the office staff to access numerous on-line data bases, including the National Library of Medicine, at very low cost, and this process has infinite applications to the daily thinking processes that physicians must go through.

THE FUTURE OF COMPUTERS IN MEDICINE

What follows is a rough outline of what is bound to happen; different scripts could be written by physicians with more or less first-hand knowledge of the applications of computers. Much of this will be covered in the following chapters in this book. However, certain basics might be reviewed here. The future daily usage of computers by physicians can be best summarized by the case method.

The Chief Complaint and History of the Present Illness. The ideal scenario of a physician-patient encounter in an office will begin with the doctor or receptionist making the patient feel at home in front of a computer console. A competent medical history should evolve as result of friendly interaction between patient and computer.

Vital Signs and Initial Laboratory Work-up. The office nurse will draw blood and obtain urine for routine multichannel automated determinations and will measure the temperature, pulse, and blood pressure of the patient. The data should be available on the console of the physician's desk by the time he or she is halfway through the physical examination.

The Encounter of Physician and Patient. The results of the physical examination can be placed quickly in an interactive computer. The physician can then recheck physical signs based on additional information from the history or laboratory data or can ask additional questions based on the other kinds of data. Either way, the process is rapid and efficient. This could allow the physician time to see more patients in a single day, or preferably would allow the physician more time to spend with each patient. Because in the eye of the average patient, time to chat is the major determinant of the good physician, and because in the next 5 to 10 years there will be a surfeit of physicians competing for patients, one of the ways in which the computer can lead to better patient care will be by freeing up physicians from time now spent on routine record keeping chores and allowing more time for conversing with the patient.

Making the Diagnosis. Here we are entering a phase not yet developed well enough for routine application. The good clinician makes diagnoses by fitting the findings about the patient in with the various possible diagnoses. The process easily can be applied to the computer and will be as time goes on. One scenario has the physician inserting the findings, which indicate various possibilities, and responding to queries from the computer about other possibilities. Accurate diagnoses in the computer age will result from accessible data on the sensitivity, specificity, and receiver-operating characteristics of various tests and useful probability estimates.

Therapy. Now the physician has nailed down the diagnosis sufficiently to warrant a trial of therapy. Care may require merely reassurance or reassurance plus some nonspecific sedative or pain-relieving medication. A more serious diagnosis might require a specific therapy, or the situation might still be obscure and some specific therapy might be indicated as a diagnostic maneuver. In the latter case, it is very important that the data be carefully recorded before start of the medication, and that a placebo or standard therapy be randomly assigned so that the physician can determine as rapidly as possible the long-term benefits to be expected from persistent treatment with the potentially active agent. The computer can perform the randomization and call for the essential response data.

New Methods of Diagnosis and Therapy. In thinking about whether or not a more complex and expensive laboratory procedure should be ordered, the physician should have access on-line through the computer to the latest data on sensitivity, specificity, predictive values, and the operating characteristics of each of the expensive available technologies. The patient might have just been discharged from the hospital after an acute myocardial infarction, and the physician may need to decide whether he or she should receive long-term beta blockade, antiplatelet drugs, anticoagulants, or an antiarrhythmic drug. Most randomized control trials (RCTs) of these drugs are undersized and of variable quality so that the data must be combined. The physician's office or home computer will allow on-line access to the latest meta-analyses of the completed RCTs of these drugs for particular groups of patients or, in the case of equivocal data, will allow access to the opinions of experts. Proper therapy can then be based on the best available evidence instead of what the latest drug salesman has advised or what the latest journal article, which might already be out of date, has concluded.

Record Keeping. The most inefficient and ineffective activity of physicians has traditionally been the accurate keeping of detailed patient records. Progress notes, analyses of laboratory data, and reasons for ordering various procedures have traditionally been written in haphazard and unreadable form and are either often overly wordy because they are disorganized or useless because they are too brief.

Although there are no randomized control trials showing that good record keeping is better for patient care, that is, that outcome is improved by adequate record keeping, it does stand to reason that physicians can make better decisions when they know what has happened before. Attempts by the various accrediting bodies to inspect hospital records have not really worked because visits are routinely announced in advance, allowing staff time to improve the situation and put on a good show, and the previously used procedures are often resumed as soon as the inspection is over. Furthermore, there is no inspection by an accrediting body of the doctor's office records.

Two rapidly changing aspects of medical care are bound to increase the use of computers in record keeping. Of foremost importance is the fact that malpractice suits are becoming more common, and the physician is almost always better defended when the records are adequate. Thus, this fear should lead to greater attention to the details of record keeping. Equally important, however, will be the need for greater documentation of thoughts and procedures for payment purposes. In the effort to facilitate this, systems are being worked out for ordering and recording data in logical ways that will make data readily available to the doctors, accountants, and lawyers who deal with it. Software systems can be developed for pointing out omissions. Most important of all, the hardware and software manufacturers will make it more convenient and easier, and even more enjoyable, for doctors to record what they are doing in the office, home, or hospital. Truly portable computers will allow the writing of quick notes at the time of each office visit and while making rounds in the hospital. Electronic interchanges can easily make those notes available to the hospital or office record, as indicated. Laboratory data can be transmitted directly from the hospital to the doctor's office so that the doctor can review the information before arriving at the hospital to see the patient. Hopefully, the efficiency of record keeping will be a potent factor in leading doctors to get over their antipathy to computers as an integral part of the practice of medicine.

THE TEACHING OF CLINICAL MEDICINE

This aspect is considered separately because it is the one that will change the most in the next few years. The great medical teacher has always been the one who can gather facts rapidly, put them together with speed, and talk about the most likely diagnosis with authority. The great clinician has an enormous memory of past patients and articles. Adequate use of the computer will make the average clinician good and the great clinician superb.

Visualize a scenario of rounds in a teaching hospital. Consider a patient who has had a myocardial infarction and is about to go home but has some persistent arrhythmias. Someone suggests that the patient be sent home on one of the newer anti-arrhythmic drugs. Someone else has read a report of a randomized control trial published a month before in which the patients on antiarrhythmic drugs had a higher mortality rate than those on placebos. The doctors on rounds turn to the computer consoles on which they have been looking at the patient's record. With a few key strokes, they are connected with an outside on-line source of published journals. The article in question is quickly recovered, and a summary of other data on the subject is reviewed. The physicians ask if there is a meta-analysis of all the randomized trials in this field, and one is quickly found by typing in "meta-analysis" and "anti-arrhythmic agents." When data from all the published RCTs are placed on the screen it is clear that chronic therapy does not prolong life and may even shorten it. The meta-analysis has been kept up to date as each new RCT is published, and unpublished data are made available for peer review.

It is obvious that this method of teaching and learning is far superior to the present one in which groups of doctors talk on rounds about what they remember, visit the library to review literature that night, and resume the conversation the next day when they have refreshed their minds. However, it does require that the research accessed through computers be exemplary in its design and in its reporting. Most clinical trials fall far short of the ideal at present. The ultimate and most important impact of computers on the practice of medicine will be the revelation of the defects of clinical trials of new diagnoses and therapies and the improvement that is bound to result from popular discussion of those defects. As is so often said regarding computers: garbage in, garbage out. Thus, superb clinical experiments in, and highly useful information out. Everyone benefits. The microcomputer is in the physician's life to stay.

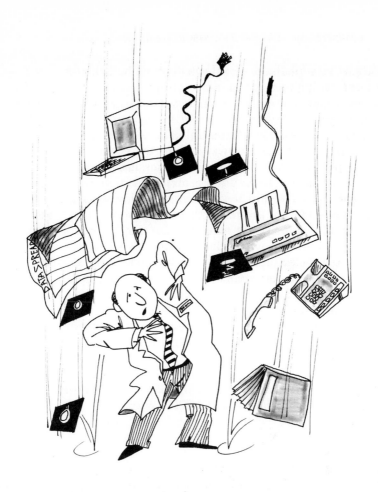

T W O

Understanding Microcomputer Hardware and Software

Jonathan Javitt, M.D.

There is a plethora of information in both books and magazines about purchasing microcomputers, telling what, where, and how. At the same time, microcomputers are being purchased in increasing numbers, and only after the purchase does it become apparent that the task for which they are slated is infeasible. Because microcomputers fit into department budgets, grant awards, and the economic capability of the average practice, organizations are witnessing a proliferation of microcomputer hardware with little central direction and much attendant waste. Although I would never advocate allowing a computer services department to control all microcomputer products purchased within an organization, I assert that it behooves the purchaser of a microcomputer to have some sense of where the machine fits within the technology and culture of computers. It is essential to understand the relative capabilities of small and large computers and what tasks might be best performed on each rather than assuming that mainframe computers are the dinosaurs of the 1980s. For this reason this chapter focuses not on how to buy a microcomputer, or its components, but on understanding microcomputers within the context of a much larger industry and culture.

THE TWO ESSENTIAL FEATURES OF A COMPUTER— HARDWARE VERSUS SOFTWARE

All computers—microcomputers and mainframes alike—use both hardware and software interactively to achieve the tasks that they are expected to perform. It is unfortunate that these two terms are discussed so matter-of-factly in advertisements on commercial television and radio, because many physicians (and indeed the lay public) do not actually understand the difference between the two. Constant exposure to the more basic computer terms has made professionals more familiar with the jargon (which allows one to be a more effective consumer), yet many do not really understand what this jargon means, and therefore they place unrealistic expectations on the products that are bought.

Software

With the purchase of a new computer, the medical professional acquires a machine that has the ability to perform almost any complex or simple thought process that a human being can perform, and much more. However, the key word here is "ability." A computer does not have the "capability" to perform complex or simple tasks on its own or even upon simple commands from the user without a set of guidelines to follow. A computer must be taught to perform the tasks expected of it, but it does have the ability to communicate in a common and specific language. Because of this capability, the computer can be rapidly taught to perform tasks through a set of instructions called software. The computer needs software to perform every task, no matter how basic, and its performance is limited by the extent of the instructions in the software.

The Operating System

A computer can be used at three different levels, and thus the software can be divided into three levels as well. The first and most basic level is known as the operating system. Typically, the operating system software is capable only of controlling the flow of information into and out of the computer's main memory area so that the micropro-cessor (the computer's brain) may have access to it. For example, the operating system controls the loading of programs from long-term storage devices and their subsequent execution, as well as information storage onto these devices. The best-known operating systems in the microcom-puter world today are CP/M, for many eight-bit computers, Apple-DOS for Apple computers, PC-DOS and MS-DOS for IBM and IBM-compatible computers, and UNIX for newer 16- and 32-bit computers.

The operating system is the basic link between the computer and most programs that run on it. In theory, a program that runs in a particular operating system will run on any computer that has that operating system. For this reason, many computers may be compatible with each other, even though they contain different circuits. Rather than addressing the computer directly, a program merely addresses the standardized operating system.

Although an essential link, the operating system has limited func-tional capacity. It may be likened to a traffic signal that controls the flow of information along common and heavily traveled pathways to various parts of the computer. Thus, the operating system is responsible only for the generic functions of the computer, which include running and operating storage devices such as tape drives and disk drives, allocating memory for tasks, and allowing the loading and execution of other previously stored instructions from these devices. Most computers come with an operating system as a standard feature when the computer is purchased, just as one can expect that a new car will be delivered with tires. More advanced operating systems may also be purchased separately as they are desired.

The Program Language

A more advanced level of software is the programming language. There are many available today, such as BASIC, FORTRAN, COBOL, and

APL. These languages serve as interpreters between the user and the computer. They contain simple instructions that allow the user to tell the computer to add numbers, to store and retrieve information, and how to display such information, thus allowing the user to customize the machine to a specific application (such as text or data processing). It is important to realize that a computer without a programming language or other language-independent software does not have the capability to perform any of these functions. In fact, the computer does not have the capability to perform any task other than the loading and execution of previously stored instructions with the operating system. Notice that the computer has the ability to perform these tasks; however, without a set of instructions that tell it how, it is unable to do so. The operating system merely provides an environment in which the programming language performs; in essence, it directs the traffic that is created by the language.

The Program

The third level of software complexity is the "program." The program is a set of instructions that allows the user to perform a task or series of tasks such as word processing, bookkeeping, or data analysis. When a computer is directed to perform such a task, it is given all the necessary instructions (the program) in advance. Thus, there is no such thing as improvising with a computer. In most cases, the computer knows exactly what it is going to do, and in what order, from the very beginning. A complete set of instructions imparts additional power to the computer over and beyond that which is associated with the sum of the individual instructions. Hence, instructions can be combined to create more powerful instructions. This creates different levels of programming power. Likewise, multiple programs working together can also be combined to increase their capabilities beyond the sum of their individual powers. All these factors acting together impart the tremendous power and capabilities that are associated with computers.

With some programs, the instruction set of a programming language may be needed to act as an interpreter between the program and the computer before it can be executed; with others, this may not be necessary. Programs lend variability to a computer. They prevent it from being dedicated to one task. By simply changing the software or by programming the computer, one can have it perform several tasks instead of having to buy several individual instruments such as a calculator for data analysis and a typewriter for word processing. In such an arrangement, each separate device would occupy office space; most would be less powerful than the use of an undedicated computer with the proper software.

How do all three levels of software fit in with one another? To answer this question it is easiest to consider a real-life situation: you are speaking on the telephone when you are asked to hold the line for a minute. Consider what you do when this occurs. You quickly realize that relatively little is being done in the interim, however, your brain is executing a specific series of instructions in a loop-like fashion. First, you listen. If you hear anything, you must then determine if the sound is pertinent to the situation or simply noise which should be ignored, and finally whether it is an acknowledgment from the person on the other end to continue. If you determine that the conversation should be resumed, then another set of instructions is executed to allow you to respond to the information that is received. If, however, it is determined that the sound should be ignored, you then start all over by listening again.

This process is analogous to the workings of the operating system. Like the person waiting on the telephone, when the computer is turned on, it executes the instructions of the operating system; the instructions tell it to wait for some recognizable command from the user. If the user instructs the operating system to load a specific program into the computer's memory and then to execute the instructions, the computer will cease execution of the operating system instructions and begin to execute the program's instructions. Thus, the operating system acts as a link between programs and between programs and their programming languages. It performs all the necessary housekeeping functions of the computer, including the transferral of data into and out of the programs themselves.

THE MAINFRAME VERSUS THE MICROCOMPUTER

The first mainframe computer was built of vacuum tubes and filled a large room. The advent of transistors, otherwise known as solid state electronics, decreased the size, power requirements, and heat dissipated by an equally powerful vacuum tube computer by many orders of magnitude. The invention of integrated circuits allowed us to etch hundreds of thousands of transistors onto a single wafer of silicon less than a half square inch in area. When this silicon wafer is enclosed in a plastic shell and equipped with metal contacts for its input and output, it becomes the chip that we know today. This chip requires little power, dissipates little heat, can be switched on and off at will, and has minimal likelihood of failure given normal usage.

The technologic revolution represented by microcomputers is that much of the processing power that was available to the user of a powerful large computer 10 years ago can now be packed onto a single silicon wafer. In fact, the remainder of the microcomputer box that we are familiar with is filled with the power supply to feed that wafer, the memory it must address, and the ancillary circuits that allow it to receive and return information. The largest component of that box, in fact, is air, which is essential for dissipating heat from the circuitry.

Even as this book is being written, the distinction between microcomputers and their larger cousins, known as mainframes, is becoming less and less distinct. Both the IBM 370 and the DEC VAX, two of the best known university and corporate mainframe computers, are available as desk-top microcomputers that fit in familiar microcomputer-sized cases. Today's distinction between microcomputers and mainframes, then, cannot be one of processor power or software power. It is a distinction that is both technologic and cultural. The desk-top IBM 370 may be able to run all the software of the room-sized version. It may even appear to the user of this machine that it is running as fast as the mainframe IBM 370 used the day before. It lacks, however, the ability to serve hundreds of users with that speed, to churn out thousands of pages of text each day, and to process massive amounts of information. The desk-top IBM 370 also lacks the need for a full-time staff of system operators and service personnel, a dust-free air-conditioned room, and a massive maintenance budget.

The foregoing example illustrates how close the technology of microcomputers and mainframes has come in 10 years since the introduction of the Apple computer. For the purposes of this discussion, a microcomputer will be defined as a machine that does not need a system operator to maintain it, that can be turned on and off at will, and that does not require special support facilities except for an electrical outlet.

The largest difference between microcomputers and mainframes is cultural. Microcomputers are generally purchased to perform a specific task. With increasing frequency they are packaged with their software to be an office management machine, or a patient diagnosis machine, or a patient history-taking machine. The fact that there is a computer inside it becomes incidental. Similarly, one buys a refrigerator to cool food and not because it contains an electric motor. The users of microcomputers are mostly interested in buying their capabilities.

The culture of mainframe computers is entirely different. Computers are generally centralized within an organization or institution, and programs that run on those computers can be purchased or written only under the control of the computer services department. The machines are generally purchased in order to offer a certain amount of computing power, not to do a specific job. The emphasis is clearly on the machine, rather than on what it can do. Marketing companies have found out, often the hard way, that microcomputer owners have less interest in computing power. They buy a machine to do a particular job.

Relative Costs and Benefits

For the physician, a microcomputer is a more beneficial and practical investment than either buying time on a mainframe computer or buying a mainframe itself. A cost-benefit analysis indicates why. Currently, microcomputers that have the ability to handle the requirements of a medical practice or laboratory cost between $2000 and $6000 initially. Most mainframe computers, on the other hand, start with initial costs in the range of $200,000. Obviously, no physician or group practice can afford to obtain a mainframe computer, nor would they want to. The yearly costs to simply support a mainframe computer would easily exceed the start-up costs of even the most expensive microcomputers available. Moreover, microcomputers continue to drop in cost yearly. This is because the cost to produce a given chip in a computer system continues to drop. The initial buyers bear the brunt of the cost for design and development. As more chips are sold, this cost disappears, and chip costs decline, as do the relative costs of the computer in general. Integrated circuits (chips) are almost the sole reason for the existence of microcomputers because their small size permits tremendous power to be packed into a small area.

Many people will ask why they need to buy a microcomputer when they can simply pay for time on a mainframe that will perform the same function. Although sharing time on a mainframe at first seems to be a good idea, the total expenditures of this type of service can be staggering. One of my colleagues reported being charged over $100,000 for entry and compilation of data that was ultimately successfully analyzed on a microcomputer system costing $4000. Storing even a reasonable amount of information on a common mainframe computer can run up costs of at least $50 per month. Without considering printer time, or use of any other device, this cost adds up to $600 per year. In addition, terminal time on most systems costs at least $3 to $4 per hour. Consider that most secretaries would spend at least 2 hours per day on the terminal performing whatever tasks were necessary (such as word processing), causing an office to incur yearly costs of more than $1600. Thus, without considering processor time and other associated costs, terminal and storage costs alone add up to $2200 per year. Within 2 years, perhaps 3, most physicians and group practices would have paid for their own microcomputer system at least once, and this is a conservative estimate.

Service and Support

Having established that the microcomputer is a fiscally more sound investment than paying for time on a mainframe, consider other aspects of the cost-benefit analysis; for example, the servicing of a computer.

Mainframes tend to be quite convenient in this aspect. Most mainframe centers maintain ongoing service contracts with the corporations that have supplied them with their hardware. This means that these computers are regularly serviced and tend to have very little down time (time when they cannot be used because of failure). On the other hand, with a microcomputer it is the owner's responsibility to conduct the regular servicing of the computer, either by the owner or through some other means. In addition, when a major failure occurs, it can, in some instances, cost as much as the piece of equipment itself. This is not to say that it is not wise to buy a microcomputer. Although these machines do have a definite time until obsolescence, their usefulness will usually far exceed the investment over their lifetime. With a mainframe, peripheral devices can be expected to last a minimum of 20 years. On a microcomputer, however, a good peripheral may be expected to last only 8 to 10 years. With a mainframe, repairs are performed relatively quickly, and there is very little time until service arrives because there is a repair contract. However, with a microcomputer owners are dealing in a free market in which the demand for repair far exceeds the supply; thus, it may take 6 to 8 weeks just for a simple chip replacement.

Software Availability

For the computer user whose needs cannot be met with a few well-chosen software products, use of a mainframe computer may have a built-in advantage. Because the users on a mainframe tend not to be commercially oriented (particularly in the university and government settings), there is a large volume of software that is available free of charge. This means the odds are good that someone has already written a software package to perform the needed task. In most cases, it also means that the user does not have to pay for the privilege of using this software. With a microcomputer, software distribution is dominated by the commercial market. Most packages cost between $50 and $300. Although there is a wider range of software on the microcomputer market, the consumer has to be more selective because it is not financially feasible to obtain a large software base. Fortunately, because one pays for the software from the commercial market, the consumer can expect better documentation of the programs and also that they will be more user friendly than the software that might be acquired free of charge in a mainframe facility. In addition, commercial software can be expected to be free of errors (although this is not always the case). With the free software that is acquired on a mainframe, a user has very little recourse when a program error is encountered. You can't look a gift horse in the mouth. The user usually must "debug" the program personally. With commercial software, support personnel are usually available to troubleshoot and fix the errors their software has created, saving the user time and effort.

It becomes evident that all-in-all the cost-benefit ratio comes out on the side of a microcomputer. Not only is it cheaper to operate, but it is also easier to use. With careful selection of software, one can perform all the required end tasks at a reasonable cost. With regular maintenance and acceptance of the fact that microcomputers and peripheral devices have a limited lifetime, service and repair can be dealt with as necessary.

Why Mainframes Cost So Much

The key factor in the enormous price gap is one that is applicable to all areas of the computer industry. Developing any product costs a certain amount of money, and the costs of that development must be recouped in the sales of that product before the producer can make a profit. An enormous amount of development technology goes into selling relatively few mainframe computers. Their price in part reflects their complexity and the cost of the materials used, but it also reflects the numbers in which they are sold. Before the reader writes them off as obsolete dinosaurs, it is important to understand what the buyer of a mainframe does get for this money.

Although they perform similar tasks, mainframes are much more expensive than microcomputers. One reason for this is the sturdiness of the mainframe. Just as a shovel is not used to clear a highway after a snowstorm, a microcomputer is not expected to nor can it effectively handle the time-sharing tasks that are required of a mainframe. At best, a microcomputer may have a fan in its central processing unit which acts as a cooling device. Mainframes, however, require a wide variety of support systems such as air-conditioned rooms and liquid-cooled hardware. This allows the hardware to be more efficient in that it is able to run at higher temperature because it is being cooled. In computers, higher temperatures typically translate into faster processing times, and thus, more information can be processed per unit of time than can be expected from any microcomputer.

There are several other reasons why mainframes cost more and can do more. With most microcomputers, one processor performs all the functions of the computer. However, although it is true that most mainframes do have one dedicated processor that does all the calculations required in a program, it is also true that mainframes have many different processors that perform ancillary tasks for the computer. There are processors that take care of storing information on the disk drives, processors that take care of printing information on the printer, and processors that take care of communication between the operator and the computer. Each piece of hardware increases the price and performance of a mainframe system. For many tasks the increased price that is incurred pays off in the long run.

Not only are a mainframe's processors and memory banks capable of a greater work load than a microprocessor's, but its peripherals can also be expected to produce more and withstand more activity. For example, a mainframe's line printer is usually an order of magnitude faster than even the fastest dot matrix printers that are commercially available. Like the processor and memory banks, the mainframe's line printer also has special cooling systems that allow it to run at faster speeds and increase the time until breakdown. This means that the user can expect a much greater production of information from a mainframe's line printer in its lifetime than it can from a microprocessor's. On inspection it also becomes readily apparent that the size and complexity of a mainframe's peripherals are very different from those of the microprocessor's. Whereas most microprocessor disk drives may occupy 300 cubic inches, a mainframe's disk facilities may occupy 300,000 cubic inches. The same analogy holds true for the line printer. In fact, the processor units themselves may be 8 to 10 feet long in a mainframe. Fortunately, for most of us, a microcomputer's output is sufficient for our needs.

Support Features

Hardware Support. In reviewing hardware features, it is important to note that a mainframe's hardware is usually supported by the corporation that has supplied it. Once again, this means that repair contracts usually have been initiated and that the company that supplies the computer will be attentive toward its repair. When you pay for time on a mainframe, it is the burden of the facility to see to it that repairs are made in a timely manner. This becomes your responsibility when you become a microcomputer owner.

Another important feature of mainframe facilities is that they maintain a full-time staff of paid engineers and programmers. It is the duty of these individuals to perform daily routine maintenance in order to prevent unexpected problems. Although problems do occur on these systems, daily mantenance keeps them to a minimum. This is an important lesson for the microcomputer owner. Because the owner does not hire a staff or trained individuals to maintain a microcomputer system, the microcomputer user needs to be more cautious than the mainframe user. Unexpected data should be rechecked, and files should always be backed up. On a mainframe, the facility's staff takes care of backing up diskettes and system information. Obviously, this is the user's responsibility with a microcomputer.

Because it is the owner's responsibility to perform routine maintenance on a microcomputer, manufacturers usually specify guidelines for assessing components of the system. Fortunately, microcomputers also have the capability to diagnose themselves. All computer suppliers provide commercially available programming that can go through the microcomputer system and check each electrical component to determine if it is working correctly. These programs will alert the owner of potentially faulty chips and circuits. Unfortunately, these programs are not a panacea for many of the ailments that afflict microcomputers. Many errors are detected through experience. Although mainframe facilities maintain a staff to provide computer support, it is not necessary and indeed is unwanted for the microcomputer owner. No physician or group practice can afford to hire a full-time staff to maintain a small computer system. This cost can easily add $20,000 to $30,000 per year to operating costs and defeats the purpose of the microcomputer.

It is a generally accepted tenet that there is less hardware support for the microcomputer owner than there is for the mainframe user; thus, microcomputer owners have traditionally accepted the role of technician/trouble-shooter when problems occurred. The potential benefits of the microcomputer to the physician far outweigh the few headaches that may be incurred with hardware errors over the life of a microcomputer system.

Software Support. Unlike hardware support, software support is usually much more extensive with respect to microcomputers than it is with mainframes. As was stated earlier, most mainframe facilities have a very large software base that is available free of charge. This useful attribute, however, is not without its disadvantages. One of the biggest drawbacks is that there is very little user support for this software other than the computer manuals (read "Greek"), if they are even available. Much of this software base is written by independent users who have specific tasks in mind and are very familiar with the software because they programmed it themselves. These individuals are not going to be very receptive toward teaching an uninitiated user about the prospective software package. Another distinct disadvantage is that except for the software that is developed at the facility, most of the mainframe software is provided by very few sources. Quite often, the main source of software is the mainframe manufacturer. This means that there is not the intense commercial competition to generate diverse and better software as there is in the microcomputer market. Quite often, the software tends to be mediocre, it is not very user friendly, and usually it does not perform all the tasks one might want.

There are still other disadvantages to the mainframe software base. Although there may be a large staff to provide hardware support and answer short, specific questions about the software, this staff is generally uninterested in teaching a customer how to use a specific program and quite often does not have very much time to do so. Many of these systems will have from 20 to 100 users sharing the facilities of the computer at the same time. It is impractical for a staff member to spend much time with any specific user. Therefore, mainframe facilities do not provide a useful tool for the manipulation of information to the uninitiated computer user. Although there is a large software base, quite often individuals will be expected to modify programs to suit their specific needs. Normally, this requires that mainframe users know how to program. This is obviously not a practical requirement for the physician. Likewise, it is impractical for most of the lay public as well. Fortunately, the commercial software that is available on the microcomputer market does not assume that the user knows how to program and is well suited to the needs of the average physician.

A Revolution in Software. Until the advent of microcomputers, the software market was dominated by a few very large corporations that stimulated little diversity. With the proliferation of microcomputers in the home and office, the software industry turned from a vendor's market to a buyer's market.

Microcomputer software is being written with several key assumptions that shape the industry. The first is that the computer has essentially no other tasks while running this program. Programs that can take over the entire processor of a computer allow for all the sophisticated screen displays, such as windows, spreadsheets, and graphics, that are commonplace to microcomputer users. Mainframe computers still expect to receive and to return most of their information one line at a time, just as they once read a single punch card at a time. Although a microcomputer user expects to be able to move around the entire display screen, to open several documents at once, and to display large spreadsheets, these functions would paralyze the ability of a mainframe to serve its multiple users.

The second assumption by which microcomputer software is produced, priced, and marketed is that each machine using that software will pay a license fee to do so. The courts have so far upheld this as a valid application of copyright law. In fact, several corporations have paid large settlements after being sued for sharing software from one machine to another within a single office. This assumption of licensing allows the producers of microcomputer software to distribute their costs over an enormously large number of users. For this reason, a $20,000 mainframe word processing package and a $75 microcomputer version may be of equal power and complexity and have cost a similar amount to produce.

The strategy of programs being written without considering the competence of the user was abandoned with the introduction of mass market microcomputer software. Commercial software vendors soon realized that they needed to write programs that did not require computer knowledge to use. Therefore, user-friendly programming was developed. The definition of "user-friendly" varies from vendor to vendor. At one extreme, there are fortunately few products that require the user to have a programmer's knowledge. At the other end of the spectrum, there are user-friendly programs that would more aptly be called "idiot-proofed." As expected, there is a whole continuum in between. Finding a level at which the user is comfortable is of major importance in selecting a package.

Strangely enough, it was not the large corporations that led the industry toward user-friendly software. Relatively young software companies, which were started by recently graduated software engineers, have pioneered the directions into which microcomputer software has delved. These individuals were not constrained by iron-clad corporate structure or policies and therefore were allowed to be innovative.

Major Benefits of Microcomputers: Integrated and User-Integrated and User-Friendly Software. Friendly Software. One of the most significant developments to evolve from microcomputer software is the concept of integrated software. Integrated software evolved because consumers had a need to mix text, numerical data from spreadsheets, and information that could be received via modem from external data bases. Integrated software allows this information to be stored in a common manner. Thus, in forming a report, results from an analysis completed on a spreadsheet program may be incorporated into the text of a document being made in a word processing program, at the touch of a button. These data never need be typed in again. In addition, if there is information (such as epidemiologic data) from a data base to be incorporated into a report, it too may be incorporated via simple commands without ever having to type in the data. Prior to integrated software, if data from an external data base needed to be incorporated into a word processing program, the user had either to write or purchase a program that would convert the data to a file format that would be compatible with the word processing program. Thus, mixing data among programs was tedious and not very practical.

There are several distinct advantages for the microcomputer user that are not available to the mainframe user. The most distinct benefit, as we have mentioned, is the tremendous diversity of the available software. Not only is software being written for specific applications such as word processing and spreadsheet analysis, but there are even software companies that write software that is being used specifically to write more software. At first, this sounds rather extreme. However, some of the currently available software is so complex that it can be written only with the aid of programs that provide basic utility functions to the programmer. For example, consider programs that divide the computer monitor into two separate screens. If a programmer is writing a program that will allow word processing to be viewed on half of the screen and a spreadsheet analysis to be viewed on the other half, it is much easier to have that part of the software that performs these screen-splitting functions already designed by a commercial software package. This means that the software engineer can spend more time designing the word processing and data analysis programs and less time on simple housekeeping functions, such as dividing the screen. In the long run, this means that the software package ends up costing less to the consumer, and it also allows the programmer to begin generating another software package and thereby to increase the already tremendous diversity of commercially available programming. The software market in the United States is one business arena in which economic principles work in textbook style: Competition stimulated diversity. Diversity created consumer interest. Consumer interest created a greater demand and thereby increased the size of the market. New software companies seem to appear every day, and the market has continued to grow.

Fortunately, the commercial software market for microcomputers is a buyer's market. Software companies soon realized that consumers were dictating the type and style of software that was being sold. Unlike the mainframe market, hardware sales were dependent upon the amount and type of software available and not the other way around. This is important for the physician. It means that specific consumer groups can cause the industry to move in directions of mutual interest. For example, if physicians express a need for a program that will generate chart notes, some corporation is going to write the software. On the other hand, if physicians do not make their needs known, software will continue to be developed in a business-oriented manner. Software companies are no longer willing to speculate on what the needs of the market may be. Thus, unlike the publishing industry, which might speculate on how well a book might sell, software companies do not take a chance on developing application software. This type of attitude has evolved owing to the demise of many corporations that speculated on the needs of the market and were wrong.

User-friendly software was a key element in the widespread acceptance of microcomputers. To understand why, consider the qualities of a program that make it user-friendly. One of the first criteria of user-friendly software is that it ask questions in a specific and direct manner without the use of computer jargon. The most user-friendly programs are either menu-driven or provide a limited list of possibilities to the user when performing a task. They did not assume that the user is familiar with all the possible answers to any question. Instead, most programs offer the uninitiated user the ability to see a list of possible options at all times. In addition, as the user becomes more familiar with the possible options, the user is allowed the opportunity to restrict the amount of help the computer gives it. In this way, the program will not hinder an experienced user.

With the advent of integrated software, the definition of user-friendly has begun to include the ability to easily integrate many tasks with one software package. This makes the overall task easier to perform and greatly simplifies the movement of information from one medium to another. An example of this is integrating information from a data base to a personal bibliography, a task which, without integrated software, would entail uploading information from a data base, printing it, and then retyping it into the appropriate format. With an integrated software package, the information is simply uploaded, merged with an existing bibliography file from the word processing package, for example, and subsequently alphabetized appropriately, perhaps with data base routines. Currently available integrated software packages routinely integrate filing, analyzing, communications, text entry, and graphing into one simple package. For most scientists and physicians, almost every possible function that is necessary to generate a manuscript is available in one simple package.

Enhanced Support and Documentation

Stimulated competition among commercial software companies has also increased the amount of software support that the user can expect from a company. (Recall that on a mainframe this type of support is virtually nonexistent.) High-quality microcomputer software and software support have directly resulted from this intense competition. Whenever a new software package dominated the market for any length of time, it was not long before competing software packages began to flood the market. In order to entice consumers to purchase their products, software companies began to offer useful services such as toll-free telephone numbers a consumer could call about specific problems with a program and receive assistance. In addition, many of the more popular computer corporations such as Apple, Commodore, Hewlett-Packard, IBM, and Digital Equipment Corporation started user support groups. These groups, which exist apart from the computer company itself, consist of individuals who own the same type of computer systems and can offer assistance to one another. Quite often, user support groups offer additional programming to their members free of charge. In fact, there are usually individuals in the user support groups who can be of more help with simple questions about a program than the engineers who designed the program themselves.

Increased competition among companies has also resulted in more comprehensive manuals to accompany the software. This makes the software easier to learn and means that a user will spend less time learning how to use the software and more time using it in the appropriate applications. In addition, commercial microcomputer software companies also appear to be more interested in specific consumer complaints and questions than companies that deal mainly in mainframe software. The major difference here is that the user is the consumer. Although large corporations that deal with mainframe software will respond to questions and problems if the mainframe facility itself requests such assistance, these companies are unlikely to be very responsive to any particular user because the users are not the consumers of the software (the facility is).

Frequent updating of programs is another advantage of microcomputer software. Because most of the software packages that run on mainframes are extensive detailed packages, they are updated only occasionally, perhaps every 5 to 7 years. Microcomputer software, however, is usually updated on a regular basis several times per year. Many companies offer these updates free of charge. Others offer updates for a nominal fee.

Unlike the software available on mainframe systems, commercial software is not available free of charge. This effectively prevents the accumulation of a large software base. It means that software consumers need to be more selective about these purchases. They cannot afford to try several different software packages, finding the one that suits them best, as they would on a mainframe. Although this is a slight detriment to the microcomputer user, it simply means that the microcomputer user's goals need to be more clearly defined from the onset when purchasing software. The consumer must know what the program is expected to do, what the size of the task will be, and the level of competence of those who will be performing the task. For example, will manuscripts be written with the word-processing software, or will it be used only to generate memos? Also, does a secretary need to attend a workshop to learn how to use the program, or does the person have enough experience to learn from a manual? Maybe an in-house tutorial is needed if many individuals need training. If training is needed, perhaps a program that is more expensive but easier to learn would be more economical. By determining the answers to these questions before the physician purchases a software package, the proper choices are more likely to be made and a waste of money will be avoided. An important point to note is that most software companies will not allow software to be returned once the sealed packages have been opened (presumably this is because copies of the disks could have been made).

The Bottom Line

Comparing and contrasting microcomputers and mainframes can get confusing. What's the bottom line? As has been noted, mainframe systems offer a lot of technical and hardware support. In addition, mainframes also seem to remove the burden of responsibility for the product's performance from the user and place this burden on the facility's shoulders. With a microcomputer, product performance becomes the responsibility of the owner. It is also true that mainframes offer a larger but not necessarily more diverse software base than microcomputers. Fortunately, all of these attributes are details that most microcomputer owners do not have to deal with. The truth of the matter is that microcomputers rarely break down, and the number of applications that the computer will be involved in is so limited that a small software base is all that is necessary. Also, diagnostic programs are able to substitute, in most cases, for a well-trained staff in detecting hardware failure. Microcomputer software is better documented and more comprehensible than mainframe software. In addition, microcomputers are more integrated and virtually fool-proof. In general, microcomputer software has much better support. It is also easier to learn how to use.

Which is more important: hardware or software? For the average physician, the answer is simple. The software is much more important. Because the end task is what the physician is most interested in, the hardware that gets the results is relatively unimportant. Microcomputers offer the consumer the ability to strike a balance between the best of both worlds. Because the consumer is in the microcomputer market, one can take advantage of the large software base available. At the same time, even though the average consumer cannot afford to acquire hardware of the quality found at most mainframe facilities, he can be relatively sure that the hardware that is purchased will exceed its investment lifetime and provide quality service if he chooses carefully and does not simply buy the cheapest equipment available.

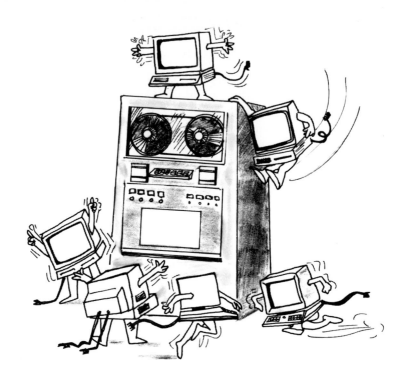

T H R E E

The Capabilities of Microcomputers Versus Mainframes

Jonathan Javitt, M.D.

David Brousseau

RESOURCES AND TASKING CAPABILITIES

Although microcomputers are not without their drawbacks, it should be clear that, all in all, microcomputers are the wisest choice for the physician who is considering enlisting a computer in practice. Although it appears that the resources of both the microcomputer and the mainframe are similar, what about the capabilities? Consider the differences and similarities.

It should be obvious from the preceding discussions that both microcomputers and mainframes have access to the same hardware resources. It follows, therefore, that both types of computers are capable of performing the same tasks. However, each type of computer is suited for a different need. In addition, although each computer has the same essential hardware, the mainframe has more of the "essential" pieces of equipment. For example, it is not uncommon for a mainframe facility to have as many as five or six disk drives and three tape drives. On the other hand, most microcomputer systems have no more than two disk drives, and few have a tape drive. Many mainframe facilities have approximately 60 or more modem lines for users who phone in to have access to the computer. It is rare for a microcomputer to support more than one modem.

Memory-Intensive Applications

Computer tasks that require large amounts of memory are known as memory-intensive applications. Memory-intensive applications are best served by the mainframe because these facilities have very large memory capacities. An average mainframe system will contain between 4 million and 12 million units of memory. On the other hand, even some of the best microcomputer systems currently available are just approaching the 1 million unit level (a megabyte). The main deterrents to large memories in microcomputers are cost and size. As the industry accumulates experience, the total price per unit of memory is dropping steadily. For example, in 1973, the cost per unit of memory was approximately 0.5 cent. By 1983, however, the cost per unit memory had dropped by a factor of more than 20 to less than 0.02 cent. Cost is not the only parameter that has dropped over the years. The same phenomenon has been observed with the amount of space required per unit of memory. As an example, in the Apple computer, 64,000 units of memory required a total space of approximately 64 square inches. On the other hand, recently released memory chips with the total capacity of approximately 256,000 units of memory use no more than approximately 4 square inches. Even with the rapidly advancing technology, however, it does not seem likely that microcomputers that can compete with mainframe systems with regard to the amount of available memory will be commonplace in the next 5 to 10 years. However, this possibility holds promise for the future.

If a microcomputer runs out of memory when performing a task, why can't it simply use its disk drive as an added scratch pad? Certainly, it has been noted that by simply replacing disks, an unlimited amount of long-term storage memory can be made available. Actually, the system could indeed be used in such a manner. However, such an arrangement can decrease the speed at which the computer is able to complete the task by a factor of one or two orders of magnitude. It takes much longer to access information on a disk drive than it does to randomly access information in memory. Whereas information in memory is readily accessible without a delay, information that must be retrieved or stored on a disk drive gets bottlenecked at the electronic line that feeds information into and out of the disk drive. Thus, although both microcomputers and mainframes have the capability to perform memory-intensive applications, the mainframe usually does so with much greater speed. This ability makes the mainframe well suited for tasks such as organizing data in a data base. In addition, a mainframe is almost always necessary to efficiently complete large sorting tasks such as those required in a census or a national poll. In tasks such as these, its large memory base allows the computer to have a large area for use as a "scratch pad."

Typically, memory-intensive tasks are endogenous to such applications as strategic defense, aerospace, weather prediction, and monitoring public utilities. Each of these tasks requires that the computer hold large volumes of reference data so that the computer may make decisions based on previous knowledge. These tasks also tend to require very long, complex programming that in itself requires large amounts of memory storage. For example, both weather forecasting and the monitoring of public utilities need the computer's ability to supply large volumes of reference data when making predictions. The complexity of their programming is probably on a level that would be able to be executed on a large microcomputer. At the other end of the spectrum, the programs used in both aerospace and defense are on such a complex level that their implementation would not be easy on a microcomputer. In addition, these applications quite often require large volumes of reference data as well.

Speed-Intensive Applications

Speed-intensive applications are tasks that require an enormous number of computations and usually a nominal amount of storage space. An example of such an application would be trying to calculate prime numbers. If such an operation were performed in a conventional manner, it would take several million calculations just to find the first 100 prime numbers (starting with the number 2). Fortunately for microcomputer owners, speed-intensive applications can be done just about as fast on a microcomputer with the proper combination of hardware and software as on a mainframe system. Technology has advanced microprocessors to the point at which their instruction execution speed is almost as fast (and, indeed, sometimes faster) than the processors that are used in many mainframes. Many of today's simplest microprocessors can execute instructions faster than most of the processors used in mainframes 10 years ago. Although the mainframe processors are slightly faster overall, the proper microprocessor software package can overcome these limitations in speed.

One of the main differences between mainframes and microcomputers is that mainframes can achieve faster effective processor speeds because they are not limited by the amount and speed of random access memory. Sometimes, microprocessors are incapable of attaining their top speeds because they are slowed down by multiple disk accesses or because they cannot access information in memory as fast as the processor can execute instructions. Microprocessor speed is not limited by current technology, per se, and processor speeds can be equivalent to the fastest mainframe processors. However, computer designs are limited by the amount of heat the chips are capable of dissipating. The faster a chip runs, the more heat it produces. Most mainframe systems, which rely on extrinsic cooling systems such as air conditioning, are capable of dissipating more heat and can therefore run at higher speeds. Fortunately, even this limitation is beginning to be overcome by engineers with innnovative designs for heat dissipation. For the physician, faster processor times means less time waiting for decisions to be made and more time spent implementing those decisions.

Intelligent Peripherals

Although the processor itself is a major element in determining the speed at which a task can be performed, there are other devices in a computer system that are capable of significantly increasing the speed of performance. One of these is the use of intelligent peripherals. This type of peripheral can significantly increase processor speed because it is capable of acting independently of the central processing unit. In essence, intelligent devices are dedicated computers. They usually contain their own microprocessors and a small amount of random access memory. The small amount of memory in these devices is usually referred to as a buffer. The size of a buffer in an intelligent peripheral is usually the key to how much an intelligent peripheral can speed up a task. This is important because peripherals cannot perform their tasks (data storage, printing, communications) as fast as they can receive data.

When the computer sends information to a peripheral, one of two things can happen. Either the peripheral processes the information appropriately, or the information is placed into a buffer until the peripheral is capable of processing it. As an example, consider what happens when a line of characters is sent to a line printer for printing. If there is an intelligent device with a buffer, it will receive all the information as fast as the computer is capable of sending it. Each character or piece of information is stored in a temporary buffer. As long as the amount of information does not exceed the buffer capacity, the peripheral is capable of receiving all the information at the maximum rate of transferral. If you are word processing, this means that you can continue to type a document while it is being printed. The on-board intelligence of the printer is capable of keeping track of information in the buffer and printing that information independent of guidance from the central processing unit.

What would happen if the buffer was too small to store the complete document or the printer was unintelligent? In that situation the user would not be able to print the document and type information into the word processor in an efficient manner at the same time. In the case of a full buffer (such as one that was too small to handle the complete document), the central processing unit would be constantly interrupted by the printer to send information. While the computer was sending information to the printer, it would not be able to receive information from the typist. In the case of the unintelligent printer, the processor of the central processing unit would have to oversee all the functions of the printer mechanism. This would completely monopolize the computer's time during the period in which the document was being printed. This is often a problem in "notebook" type computers that have a built-in printer.

Fortunately, almost all printers have some degree of intelligence. The biggest differences are found in the sizes of their buffers. The size of the buffer can be one of the most important specifications of any peripheral. If the buffer is large, the user will not have to spend a lot of time waiting for ancillary tasks such as printing to be performed. Essentially, this means that two tasks can be performed at the same time. Intelligent peripherals speed things up because they distribute the amount of work among several processors as opposed to having only one processor in the central processing unit performing all the tasks. The major drawback of intelligent peripherals is their cost. For example, the buffer for the Epson printer series, with 64,000 units of buffer, can add 50 per cent to the total price of the printer. However, in an office with a potentially large amount of printing, such an investment will easily pay for itself in the amount of typist time it saves. By assessing the needs of the office, professionals should be able to strike a balance between the amount of peripheral intelligence needed and the extra initial investment to be made.

Although microcomputers may be slower than mainframe systems in certain tasks, microcomputers can be quite fast. Naturally, a major factor is the intelligence of the peripherals in the system. However, this is not the only factor. The speed of the task depends not only upon the processor speed and types of peripherals but also upon the amount of available memory and, most important, the efficiency of the software. The difference in task performance speed between microcomputers and mainframes may often be invisible to the user. For example, to put a character on the screen may take a microcomputer one millisecond. It may take a mainframe only half a millisecond. The user is not likely to notice the difference. Increases in speed become important only if they are noticeable—quite often they are not. When analyzing the needs of an office, it will be important to realize where potential bottlenecks in the processing of information are most likely to occur in the various applications. If the system is expected to generate a lot of printed information, then a print buffer with intelligence is a necessity. Likewise, if receiving large volumes of information from a data base is a prime use, then an intelligent modem with a sizable buffering capacity can significantly decrease the amount of money spent on time to connect to the host mainframe.

Tools That Affect Processing Time

In the last couple of years, the efficiency of microprocessors in performing mathematical computations has increased by more than an order of magnitude. This ability is due mainly to the evolution of coprocessing chips. A mathematical coprocessing chip (some manipulate text as well) acts as a slave to the main microprocessor in the computer. It usually has limited capabilities, which perform addition, subtraction, and multiplication. A coprocessor speeds things up tremendously because it can perform these functions with 64-digit precision (perhaps more by the time you read this) in the execution speed of a single instruction. This type of speed and precision can compete effectively with many mainframes. As was the case with intelligent peripherals, the major drawback of coprocessor chips is price. Again, this type of investment can pay off if the tasks that the microcomputer is expected to perform involve a large number of mathematical computations. By using a coprocessing chip, a microcomputer will have the capability to perform tasks that otherwise would be delegated to a mainframe owing to significant processing time.

Hardware advances are not solely responsible for the decreasing differences in processing time for a given task between microcomputers and mainframes in the last few years. Recent advances in the type and availability of high-level software (see Glossary) have also played a significant role in narrowing the differences between the two types of computers. In particular, the current availability of language compilers has played a key role. Compilers are software tools that digest the program and break it down into smaller, more manageable pieces for the central processor. This allows the program to run faster. All programs on a mainframe are sent through a compiler before they are actually executed. Because compilers are capable of finding errors, faulty programs do not waste valuable processor time. On a mainframe system, it is important that processor time not be wasted because many users are waiting to have access to the same processor. With a microcomputer this is obviously less important.

This brings up an important difference between mainframes and microcomputers. Although a microcomputer may take more processing time to perform a given task, the operator is actually waiting while the task is being processed. With a mainframe, however, it may take just as long to get the same answer even though less processing time is required. This is because the operator actually has to wait to receive processing time on the computer. In this regard, microcomputers can be much more convenient. For example, if a microcomputer is directed to solve an equation, it may take 3 seconds. On a mainframe, however, the same problem may take only one half second. Unfortunately, with the mainframe, the user may have to wait a minute or two just to get access to the processor. Thus, for small tasks that require a minimal amount of processor time, microcomputers can actually be faster even though they take longer to perform the computations.

It must be emphasized that microcomputers are capable of being (apparently) just as fast as a mainframe for any given task. If this is true, why do some things still seem to run faster on a mainframe? The main reason is that mainframes are designed to handle the most rigorous conditions possible. The engineers made no assumptions about the potential uses of the machine as a professional would when selecting a microcomputer. Thus, every peripheral in a mainframe has both intelligence and a large buffer capacity. When selecting a microcomputer, however, it is unlikely that you will need every peripheral to have intelligence. In addition, mainframes are intrinsically designed to handle mathematical computations quickly. If a physician chooses to have such an ability on a microcomputer, then a computer with coprocessing power must be selected. In summary, if the consumer is willing to spend the money for the best available printers, processors, and other peripherals, almost all tasks that would be performed on that microcomputer system would compete with processing times on a mainframe. In fact, with the evolution of text coprocessors, certain text applications may run faster on current microcomputers than most mainframes.

The computing systems most physicians will purchase are more likely to be dedicated to a few tasks. Parts of the system that will have little effect on overall productivity should be purchased in a more frugal manner with the appropriate selection of hardware and software. For example, if one intends to use the computer mainly for word processing and not for filing or some other disk-oriented task, then it is unlikely that a very high-speed disk drive is going to affect productivity. Such a peripheral would be a necessity if the computer were being used as a data base and needed access to large volumes of information or long-term storage. Similarly, a math coprocessing chip with its supportive software is unlikely to help very much in office-oriented tasks. However, in the laboratory setting, it would be of significant service in monitoring feedback loops and in data processing. It should be evident that although decreases in productivity should be carefully avoided by not underestimating the requirements which will be placed on the system, it is really of no advantage to spend money on hardware or software that is not going to speed up specific applications.

The Changing Roles of Computers in Society

Because microcomputers are rapidly becoming the workhorses in offices and laboratories, the role of the mainframe computer in society is changing. No longer are mainframes the first machines that come to mind when a computer is mentioned. To most of the lay public, the word "computer" has become synonymous with the microcomputer. More and more commonly, mainframes are being put to use in the tasks they handle best and with which microcomputers are incapable of competing: memory-intensive applications. Most notably, users will find that at the heart of almost every public data base is a mainframe which is providing the information to the microcomputer. One of the main reasons that mainframes have accepted this role is because they are the only machines that can efficiently handle many users. It is not uncommon to find a data base service that is providing information to as many as a hundred users simultaneously. This means that all users are vying for the same resources. Because mainframes are supported by a host of intelligent peripherals, they are at present the only machines whose systems are distributed enough to handle the large volumes of information that must flow in and out.

The "Virtual Machine"

Although a mainframe handles a large number of users simultaneously, each user thinks that he or she is the only one using the machine at any one time. Each user is in control of a "virtual machine." Thus, the mainframe presents a virtual machine to every user who signs onto the system. Because the mainframe is capable of performing over a million instructions per second, it is able to attend to the needs of each user (sometimes hundreds) without delay. Thus, although the computer is actually receiving information from each user in a round-robin fashion, the operator is never aware that the computer was unavailable for a split second.

By presenting virtual machines to each user, the mainframe is capable of being very efficient with its time. Unfortunately, one of the biggest problems with this type of system is that it can often be inefficient with the user's time. This is because the mainframe has one or perhaps two main processors that actually perform the instructions of any program being executed. Consider what happens if there are 100 users on the system simultaneously. If there is only one processor and one user sends in a program that requires 5 minutes to be executed, other users will have to wait until that task is completed before they can run their programs. At this point, programs start to line up, one behind the other, in order to be executed when the processor is ready. A user would certainly not want to be the 100th person in line. In this worst-case scenario, a user may end up waiting several hours just for the program to be run. This type of problem does not tend to occur when only a few users are on the mainframe at any one time. Thus, the speed of a virtual machine is directly dependent on the number of users connected to the system.

Another problem with virtual machines is that any one user does not have access to the full power of the mainframe. As the number of users on a system continues to increase, the amount of available memory per user continues to decrease. In addition, items such as the line printer or the plotter also tend to get overloaded with information. This means that individual users have to wait longer to receive the results from a task. Another problem with parceling the machine into small pieces is that large memory-intensive applications may not be able to run until full access is available. Typically, a mainframe system with 12 million units of memory will be broken up into three segments of 4 million units each. If the machine were set up for one user, there would be 12 million units of memory available, but because the machine is broken up into three parts, no task that needs more than 4 million units of memory can be performed (unless disk space is used).

Mainframes are quite capable of handling data base arrangements because a virtual machine will work very well in this setting. Even though a large number of users need to be accommodated, no particular user is going to be doing much computation on the system. Essentially, the mainframe is used as a switching station by simply routing information in the proper directions. In addition, its large memory base is capable of providing instantaneous access to large volumes of information.

The Front versus the Back End

To handle many users, mainframes are essentially divided into two machines. Each machine is intimately related to the other (and each is actually just a part of one larger machine). One part of the computer, known as the "front end," is user-oriented. The other part of the machine, the "back end" of the mainframe, is code(program instructions)-oriented. When users connect to a mainframe system, they are actually communicating with the front end. The front end has its own processor and a small amount of random access memory. It is responsible for receiving commands from the user and sending information back to the user or to other peripherals in the system. The back end of the mainframe does all the computation required by the programs that are executed in the processor. When one speaks of processor time on a mainframe, the amount of time that the program spends in the back end of the mainframe is actually what is being referred to. The back end has large fields of memory available to the processor when performing its task. Conversely, the front end has a rather limited amount of memory, and it is responsible for creating the virtual machine that is presented to each user.

A major operational difference between mainframes and microcomputers is that microcomputers have only one processor. The microcomputer is both the front end and the back end in one package. The microcomputer is capable of performing both tasks with one processor because there is only one user. Mainframes have traditionally been divided into front and back ends because it is very inefficient for the main processor to handle filling and the creation of new programs that are being typed in by slow programmers. For a single-user microcomputer, efficiency is less of a problem. Either the user is executing a program or the user is typing in a program. It would be very unlikely for someone to have the need to do both at the same time.

Although microcomputers today tend to be single-user–oriented, pressure is being applied from medium-sized firms and small businesses to develop limited multi-user systems on microcomputers. A connected system of microcomputers allows hardware and software resources to be shared among many users. Although some configurations require that additional hardware be purchased in order to support a multi-user system, the difference between a multi- and a single-user microcomputer system depends mostly on the software that is running the operating system. A microcomputer in a multi-user environment can show great flexibility. By using the appropriate operating system (multi- versus single-user system), it can participate in a multi-user network, sharing the resources of a common system, and yet maintain its autonomy. Moreover, with a single-user-oriented operating system, network users have the capability of isolating themselves when performing tasks that they would prefer were unshared with the rest of the system. Thus, microcomputer owners can have the best of both worlds.

Page- versus Line-Oriented Machines

Aside from the way in which information is processed inside the machine, information is presented to the user in two vastly different manners when comparing the microcomputers to most mainframes. The mainframe tends to be a line-oriented machine. This means that if a command is being sent to the mainframe, the user will type information on one line and hit the "return key" to send that information to the computer. Likewise, information is sent back to the user, from the mainframe, one line at a time. Although the mainframe is capable of presenting information on the screen in specific columns or rows, it is usually incapable of highlighting specific information or utilizing graphics functions without significant delays. It turns out that presenting information in a complicated (that is, customized and distributed) manner on the video screen requires a significant amount of processor time. Americans are page-oriented. Their educational process relies upon the printed page when learning or reviewing information. People are used to seeing information highlighted, and pictures used to present difficult concepts. A microcomputer is well suited for presenting page-oriented information. Page-oriented presentation of information makes the computer easier to use and allows people to retain a dependence on the printed page. This is probably one of the main reasons that microcomputers, in particular, have been accepted so well in society: They reduce many of the barriers that have existed between computers and traditional thinking.

When the benefits of presenting information in a page-oriented manner were realized, computer manufacturers initiated fundamental changes in their approaches to hardware design. The increased possibilities offered by these new hardware devices stimulated changes in the way programmers designed their programs to communicate with the user. This meant that hardware like the mouse was combined with user-friendly programming that allowed the user to point to selections on the screen, making the use of a computer child's play. Page-oriented machines allow professionals to view larger amounts of information at any one time, highlight important points, make decisions without memorizing a large number of commands, and be neater. In fact, becoming page-oriented directed microcomputers toward user-friendly programming. By being able to control the contents of the entire screen, the programmer can "idiot-proof" certain tasks by showing the user the directions that are allowed in a program. In a word processing program, for example, the typist no longer has to remember every command in order to perform a specific function. Because the screen can be controlled easily, the programmer can put a menu of possible directions on the screen, the user can select an option, and the menu can be removed—without affecting the layout of the text—and the task performed. Thus, even the inexperienced user is capable of making decisions within this type of program.

Split-Screen Capabilities—"Windowing"

Initially, the evolution of page-oriented microcomputers made such things as spreadsheets and word processing possible. However, until recently, the user was limited to performing one task or another at any one time. With the evolution of "windows," software engineers have allowed more than one program to be run at the same time (a process called multi-tasking) and information from each program to be presented on the screen at the same time. "Windowing" performs the familiar split-screen functions that most people have seen on television, especially in sporting events. Essentially, "windowing" creates another monitor for viewing information. In fact, some programs allow the monitor to be broken up into four or more screens at one time. The convenience of such a device is obvious. If a complex manuscript is being generated, information from a spreadsheet could be brought up to be viewed in one window and then incorporated into the document being synthesized with a word processing program in another window on the monitor.

Windows allow many tasks to be performed at once, and thus, they increase the user's productivity. More important, microcomputers are the only machines that can offer this feature. Mainframes are incapable of effectively offering this type of programming because they need to support a large number of users. The mainframe processor would be incapable of keeping up with the demands of the system if each user had page-oriented, multi-tasking software being executed.

Efficiency of Microcomputers versus Mainframes

Having considered the resources and capabilities of microcomputers and mainframes, we can now review the efficiency of each system. In terms of the efficient use of resources, the mainframe is clearly a better system. The hardware per person ratio is much lower on the mainframe than on the microcomputer. For instance, on a mainframe, five disk drives may be used by more than 100 users; however, on a microcomputer, there is normally at least one disk drive per user. In addition, the amount of time that the resources of a mainframe are being used is greater, and thus, there is a more efficient use of them. Because mainframe resources are used 24 hours a day, there is very little idle time. A microcomputer, on the other hand, is normally idle at least half the day. Therefore, for society as a whole, time-sharing systems are a more practical approach for providing computer service. The apparent waste of resources incurred with a large number of microcomputers in our society may be overcome by the fact that individuals will tend to be more productive with microcomputers than they would with a main-frame. In the long run, distribution of tasks to many small computers may end up being more beneficial to our society.

Microcomputers make more efficient use of the operator's time because the user will not have to wait for processor time. This is especially apparent in tasks that involve interactive use between the processor and the operator. The microcomputer is more convenient in this aspect because it is capable of carrying out instructions immediately. Remember that the efficiency of a microcomputer system depends not just on the hardware but also on the software, the operating system, and the task. Most office and managerial tasks tend not to be computation-intensive; thus, a microcomputer is really a much wiser choice than time sharing for the physician intending to computerize.

Security of Electronic Information

In addition to achieving increases in productivity and efficiency, an electronic office can also provide increases in security and privacy that rival the best conventional office protocols. It is unfortunate that the local and national media inflate the stories about "computer hackers" who gain access to sensitive information. The information they access is rarely important, and the frequency of such instances is low. Fortunately, these "hackers" do not have access to microcomputer systems unless the system is capable of receiving incoming phone calls and servicing them appropriately. Computer enthusiasts who gain access to information are doing so by contacting large commercial mainframe systems that are intended for use by large corporations. Unless they get very lucky, they do not get past the stringent security measures that protect important information. Actually, electronic information provides more restricted access by being stored on a microcomputer than if the sensitive infor-mation were locked in a filing cabinet.

The techniques for electronic security on microcomputers were borrowed from those used in mainframe systems for many years. Main-frames provide security on many levels. To gain access to particular information, a user must know not only that information's access number but also its password. Even if it were possible for someone else to find out a user's access number and password, the user could prevent them from having access to private information by giving that particular file additional security measures. A user who wanted access to a particular program or file that was specially restricted would also have to know the password to that particular file. In addition, different levels of access hierarchy can prevent the disk drive from reading a file or writing over it without the proper password.

Security on a microcomputer is provided in much the same way. Most of these computers are not part of large time-sharing systems, so the initial access code and password are usually not necessary in order to gain access to a particular filing system. However, on microcomputers the operating system can allow different levels of access. For example, in a hospital setting, by giving the medical staff and the general public a different access code to a particular file, the computer can restrict or allow access to different parts of a patient's file. The general public could have access to a patient's name and room number, but the interns and residents could have access to laboratory results and chart notes by using the more permissive access code. Computers allow us to establish an access hierarchy that allows information to be both available and restricted at the same time. In addition, because microcomputers are usually not capable of receiving incoming phone calls, they are not subject to illegal access.

The Essential Features of All Microcomputers

To be able to effectively use a microcomputer in a laboratory or office, there are four absolutely essential pieces of hardware that must be purchased. First, the central processing unit (CPU), which is at the heart and brain of the system, is necessary to run all the programs. The CPU usually comes with a keyboard for input of information; however, a means of information output such as a monitor also must be purchased. In addition, the system will be relatively useless unless there is a means of outputting information on paper. Thus, a printer is the third essential element. Finally, because the user will not want to type in every file each time the machine is turned on, some form of mass storage will also be necessary. Thus, either a disk drive or a tape drive is the fourth essential element. Many people find that a modem is also quite useful. This should not be considered an essential piece of equipment because not everyone is going to have a need to send and retrieve information to other computers. An office management system that is intended to do billing and accounting and generate letters for the physician is not going to need the ability for computer-to-computer communication. However, a laboratory engaged in multicenter collaborative efforts would do well to purchase such a device because it will provide for the sharing of information among centers.

In terms of software, there are also four essential packages that are necessary for a complete basic system. First, some operating system software is absolutely essential for the proper storage and retrieval of information on peripheral storage devices. A good operating system that automatically backs up files and updates appropriately can save several work hours per week. Many programs also require that a programming language be available for their proper execution. Therefore, the acquisition of a programming language of the type that will be used by most of the system's programs is also a necessity. The third essential element that is necessary is text editing or word processing capabilities. Word processing software can be used to generate not only original manuscripts and letters but also form letters and billing forms. Finally, most medical offices will find that some type of spreadsheet or accounting software can also be quite useful.

Another key factor that led to the acceptance of microcomputers, aside from the advances in hardware and software, was the ease with which one can learn to operate a personal computer. One of the joys of using a personal computer is the feeling of complete control the user gets by having the on/off switch so close at hand. The user is in charge. Nothing is going to happen unless it is allowed to happen. And if the operator becomes confused in the beginning, the machine can simply be turned off, and the user may start the task once again. Once the computer is set up, the operator is unable to damage it in any way from the keyboard. Copies of programs or data may be lost, but as long as the correct procedures are followed, there is little chance of doing irreparable damage to the machine.

Because the microcomputer is smaller and more manageable than a mainframe system, the user feels more in control, and in fact, the user is in more control. With the advent of user-friendly software, the programs themselves prompt the user to go in the proper directions. In fact, most word processing and spreadsheet programs can be learned with some degree of competence in a few hours. Compare that to the amount of time that it might take an uninitiated user on a mainframe system just to learn how to log in. With personal computers, the manuals tend to be self-explanatory, and there are also plenty of sales people willing to help with a problem.

Features Offered Only by Microcomputers

Microcomputers are the only type of computer that is portable. This has led computer enthusiasts to speculate on the evolution of electronic note pads and electronic briefcases. Today, there are computers available that are no larger than the size of a loose-leaf binder. Typically, these so-called "note-pad" computers come with built-in programs. Many contain word processing, appointment schedulers, address and phone directories, and even telephone auto-dialers with a built-in modem. In addition to these features, most note-pad computers can be hooked up to cassette recorders for mass storage. The beauty of these systems is that they allow the user to generate letters and notes while out of the office, and they can be printed when back in the office. Because most of the note-pad computers weigh less than 5 or 10 pounds, carrying them around is no more of a hassle than carrying around a notebook or tape recorder.

Computers that fall into the category of the electronic briefcase are slightly larger and have even better capabilities. These computers, which weigh between 15 and 30 pounds, are slightly larger or smaller than a briefcase, thus accounting for their name. Not only can they contain a full keyboard with a numeric keypad, but they may have the capability for high-resolution graphics, dual disk drives, modems, and a variety of other functions. Many professionals, especially psychologists, have complained about the intrusion of devices like the electronic note pad and briefcase on the life-style of the workers in the United States, claiming that the work place is intruding on even our time spent in traveling to and from work. Whatever the complaints, it is clear that these machines have taken a permanent position in the lives of many professionals.

Besides being useful as office tools, these computers hold great promise for use in the emergency setting. For example, paramedic teams could use a small computer (remember, these are capable of running on batteries) to monitor vital signs, alert them to specific problems, and transmit information via two-way radio. In fact, programs are being written to allow a computer to be able to analyze an ECG and suggest appropriate treatment. This could remove the need for a physician to be on stand-by for consultation; it could be especially important in situations in which consultation was unavailable.

Small size is also a feature offered by microcomputers alone. Even the nonportable microcomputers such as those made by Apple, IBM, and Digital Equipment Corporation are easily capable of being stored on a small desk. Microcomputer systems are capable of being integrated into an office without major disruption. They are small enough to be stored almost anywhere, and in the long run they make room in an office by eliminating the need for typewriters, filing cabinets, calculators, and other common office equipment.

Another unique feature of microcomputers is their versatility. Before the electronic age, a typewriter was required to generate documents, a calculator was necessary to do accounting (along with a ledger sheet), and an answering machine may have been necessary to receive phone calls. With the proper selection of hardware and software, a microcomputer can perform all these tasks. The microcomputer is capable of being configured for many tasks in very little time with a minimum of effort. Fortunately, products are commercially available that can perform all these tasks. And, unlike a mainframe, the microcomputer does not require expert attention and support. Luckily for the personal computer owner, microcomputers are subject to little hardware failure, and even when this does occur, it can be easily diagnosed.

To prevent hardware failure and to diagnose it before the microcomputer's warranty expires, there is a simple procedure that consumers should be aware of. When the equipment is set up, leave it turned on for a few weeks. If the computer has cooling fans, they are likely failure points in the system. If the disk drives are going to fail, they will probably do so in the first 20 to 30 hours of use. When the computer is running, it gets warm. The circuits inside will be stressed as they change shape in response to heat. A well-designed computer will dissipate heat quickly. If it is going to fail, it is better that it happen sooner than later. The point of this exercise, called burning in, is to force the machine to fail under warranty. If it doesn't fail during the first couple of weeks of continuous use, it is unlikely to fail until it reaches its expected lifetime. The computer retailer will probably suggest that it is not necessary to leave the computer on, but do so anyway. The retailer is more interested in saving the store's time and effort than in saving the buyer's money. (A word of caution: be sure to turn the intensity on the video monitor down so that the screen is barely visible during this period. This prevents damage to the screen from a single image being displayed on the monitor for a long time!)

Microcomputers also offer the ability to be easily expandable. Microcomputers are designed to be open systems. The owner can usually add as many disk drives, printers, and other essential features as necessary within reasonable limits. Mainframe systems, on the other hand, tend to be somewhat closed. Not that they are incapable of being expanded, but they are usually designed with a specific goal in mind and are aimed at serving a specific number of users. If you have ever bought time on a time-sharing system, it is unlikely that the available equipment was expanded during the period that you were a user. However, it is not uncommon for a microcomputer system to continually expand as the needs of the office or laboratory increase.

APPROACHES TO SHARING OF RESOURCES: SUPERMICROS VERSUS NETWORKS

Until this point, it has been convenient to contrast microcomputers with mainframe computers and to view them as distinctly different machines. Most people think of microcomputers as single user machines, and in fact most microcomputers serve one user. As I have already described, mainframe computers exist in a completely different culture that involves many users, skilled support staffs, and expensive hardware and software.

As more tasks are computerized, there is an increasing need to allow users to share information and resources without resorting to a mainframe computer. Two solutions that have evolved to meet this need within the microcomputer world are multiuser microcomputers (supermicros) and local area networks (LANs). The goal of each is to allow groups of computer users to share access to common files and to exchange information while minimizing the amount of hardware that must be purchased and maintained. Each approach has distinct advantages and disadvantages.

The Multiuser Microcomputer, or Supermicro

When microcomputers were first introduced into common use, they were single user machines whose processors could just manage to keep up with the demands placed upon them by that user. Over the past five years we have seen the introduction of much larger and faster integrated circuits. Many of these single chips are as powerful as the entire processing section of some small mainframes. At the same time, they can be used as the central processor in a microcomputer that needs no system operator, no support staff, and is relatively inexpensive. At this time, a supermicro computer system with terminals for three users is only three times the price of an IBM-AT single user system.

One way for a group of individuals to share computer resources is for them all to work on the same supermicro computer. This allows them to share any and all files and programs. At the same time, each user may restrict access to his own files if he chooses. The system may be configured in a way that permits each user access to only certain programs, files, or devices.

The essential ingredient in this development is the growth of multiuser operating systems to operate the computer. At the present time, UNIX and its derivatives are rapidly dominating the marketplace in this area. The operating system on a supermicro must enable the users to share the resources of the processor and the disk drives in an equitable manner. Although the processor is actually handling many tasks at once, the speed with which it is able to do so makes its performance comparable to that of most single user microcomputers.

The operating system is also responsible for system security and communications. By virtue of the user name given at sign-on time, the system is instructed as to the permissions given that user with respect to file, program, and device access. The operating system takes care of sending files from one user to another and even includes a mail program that allows users to send each other memos and similar documents.

Because each terminal in a supermicro system is a simple serial device that can run over the telephone, it is easy for an individual to work on a supermicro system by modem. It is possible to link two offices in this way. Furthermore, if several terminals, printers, and similar devices are in a remote location, the information flow between them and the supermicro computer can be channeled over a single phone line using a device called a multiplexer.

This description may sound suspiciously like the description of the mainframe computer of five years ago. There are several major differences, however. These systems cost $10,000 to $20,000 rather than $100,000 and up. Because they are built of far fewer components, often with the entire CPU on a single chip, there is very little maintenance compared to a mainfarame system. Although there must be one person to set up the system initially and assign passwords and permissions, the system is essentially self-tending. Even functions such as file backup can be set to happen automatically at convenient intervals. Last, the popularity of the UNIX operating system has generated a large installed base of supermicros, driving software prices down to the same range as comparable software for microcomputers. In the last year, the UNIX software market has matured to the point where excellent versions of most basic software tools are available at reasonable cost.

The Local Area Networks

Local area networks (LANs) are a solution to this problem. LANs comprise a series of microcomputers that share a common communication line and each other's peripherals. They permit a user to have the power of a mainframe and the convenient attributes of the microcomputer. The big advantage of an LAN over a modem-based mainframe network (actually, it would be possible, although impractical, for an extensive interactive network to be set up on a mainframe) is that it can communicate data among different stations at least 100 times faster than the fastest available modem-based phone lines. With a modem-based system, the user often keeps the amount of data that is transmitted to a minimum. Large amounts of information are still transmitted to and from the user in a modem-based set-up; however, page-oriented software with screen-based editing is usually avoided by necessity. It would be too slow. On the other hand, LANs are capable of supporting page-oriented systems because they can maintain the data rates that are necessary to prevent the system from being very slow, and also because there are a large number of processors in the system to handle the tasks.

Important Aspects of the LAN. Today's local networking products allow simultaneous interconnection between hundreds of users and devices and offer much better transmission-error rates than dial-up phone lines. In a nutshell, LANs differ significantly from phone line–based networks in four main areas: geographic scope, the hardware devices that support the network, data rate supported, and the type of information transmitted (page-oriented information). Local area networks are constrained in the end-to-end distances that they support. LANs are considered "local" in contrast with the "long haul" nature of the telephone network. Although a modem-based network is capable of connecting a user in New York to a user in Hong Kong, maximum distances between user devices in the LAN are much shorter. Therefore, local networks are oriented toward single buildings or a university-type environment.

Dial-up phone line services connect only two parties, resulting in a point-to-point physical connection. Local networks, in contrast, connect many stations in a point-to-many-points pattern. To send a message to another user on a mainframe system, the message would be sent to the computer, processed, and then sent to the other user. Local networks, however, allow information to be sent directly to another user without processing. Each functioning device on the local network may generally access any other device, or any group of devices, at any time.

Because all LAN users share a common transmission channel at the same time, the network requires a high transmission speed. LANs usually operate with data transmission rates at or above 1 million units of information per second. This is necessary because each of the users in the network needs a portion of the overall data-carrying capacity. By contrast, only two users need to share the data-carrying capacity of a phone-line circuit: the user and the host computer. In addition, phone lines are capable of maintaining data rates of only approximately 2400 (perhaps as high as 9600) pieces of information per second.

LANs usually employ a single coaxial cable that connects each user in the entire network. At the end of the network, there is some hardware device that controls the use of the transmission line. To support this type of data transmission, each personal computer in the network needs a special operating system in order to communicate with other computers and devices in the system. Instead of using personal computers that are networked, some LANs use a relatively small minicomputer (a small version of a mainframe) with many terminals. Although this set-up allows each user to interact with one another and provides similar computing power as compared to a normal LAN, it does not allow the autonomy that is gained by having a series of networked personal computers. A multi-terminal microcomputer LAN has many of the time-sharing drawbacks of a mainframe system. Therefore, the industry is tending to lean toward the networking of many autonomous personal computers.

In an LAN system, each user can have a separate disk drive and printer, or all users can share a common resource. If each user has his or her own disk drive, then the amount of available mass storage increases with reference to each individual user but stays the same with reference to all users collectively. More commonly, LAN participants get together and share powerful intelligent peripherals. In an LAN, the machines that oversee the use of peripherals are known as "servers." The sharing of resources among many users allows the acquisition of more advanced equipment. For example, a local area network might be able to afford a high-quality, large-capacity laser printer, whereas a single personal computer owner could not. With the sharing of common resources, the actual cost to each user can actually be less than if each user bought his or her own peripherals. This is mainly due to the fact that the CPU is rapidly becoming the least expensive part of any system.

The LAN Environment—Servers and Virtual Peripherals. Recall that in a mainframe each user was presented with a virtual machine. In an LAN each user actually has a real machine. Each machine is capable of performing its own programs without being dependent on the networking system. Instead of a virtual machine, in an LAN with several servers overseeing the use of peripherals, each user has access to a "virtual peripheral." Although information may be sent from one user to a peripheral, it may not be acted upon until that peripheral is available. In order to make the transmission line available during this waiting period, the server places the information in a temporary buffer. As long as the system is not overloaded with users trying to use the same peripherals at once, the back-up time is relatively small and usually unnoticeable. In addition, each user does not have to wait for a chosen program to be processed because each computer has its own processor. Therefore, this problem, which is common in mainframe, is avoided.

The elimination of phone line circuits in LANs not only increases the spread of communication but eliminates the need for a modem. Being directly connected to all users means that costly phone charges can be avoided. Also, the information on each user's personal computer is always available to the entire network even when a particular user is not using a machine (if it is turned on). Although direct connection means elimination of modems, additional hardware must be purchased in order to connect the CPU to the network. Usually a control group and some type of internal communications device are necessary in conjunction with the operating system in order to make use of the network. Thus, the money saved by eliminating the modem is usually spent on this equipment. In addition, each network participant also bears part of the cost for the hardware that oversees the use of the transmission cable by each computer.

Drawbacks of LANs. LANs are not without their drawbacks. One problem is the constrained distance of communication. Because most networks do not allow communication beyond approximately 30 miles,

LANs are not effective at connecting the offices of national corporations spread out over many cities or for providing data base access to users across the country. Another problem with LANs is their lack of standardization. Because this is a relatively new field that has not fully developed, computer manufacturers have not settled on hardware and software standards that will be used in these systems. In the United States, there are perhaps 40 manufacturers of personal computer local networks in the computer industry. None of these systems is fully compatible with the others. Most of these networks were introduced in 1983, and many are from "me-too" vendors that have jumped on the bandwagon.

It should not be surprising that every vendor claims that it has the best technology and the best software. Each hardware manufacturer makes slight modifications in the accepted standards, and thus, not all systems are compatible. In addition, most of the microcomputer local networks tend to be highly proprietary, leaving the end user at the mercy of the vendor. Unless the need for an LAN system is immediate, microcomputer owners would do best to wait and see which standards and vendors come out on top.

Other problems with shared resources in LANs include bottlenecking and single-point failure. Obviously, if many users are sharing a common printer through a server and that mechanism fails, all users in the network are without that device. Therefore, single-point failure becomes a problem for everyone in the network. Also, if too many users in a very large system try to use the same peripheral device at the same time, bottlenecking can occur. In general, these situation will occur only in systems with low capacity servers (not much buffer space) and a large number of users. Nonetheless, it remains a significant problem.

LANs can present additional problems. Quite often in large systems, expertise is needed in day-to-day operations to maintain and administer these systems. Fortunately, many manufacturers provide diagnostic tools to help maintain the network. These are typically software programs that do a variety of tests, such as testing each computer and all the servers within the network. If most of the users within the network have a reasonable amount of computer experience, then a full-time operator to maintain the network may not be necessary. On the other hand, if a full-time employee is necessary, this adds to the yearly operating costs of the system. Another financial problem with LANs is that some software vendors charge for the software by the number of users connected to the network. If a word processing program normally costs $200 for a single personal computer, the software vendor might charge as much as $4000 for a 20-station network. The rationale for this is that each user has access to a common program base, and therefore the vendor should be entitled to charge for each user. Clearly, this is unfair to the users who do not intend to use specific software packages or who prefer others. The aforementioned limitation tends to offset the practicality of an LAN from a software standpoint. Undoubtedly, increased competition, standardization, and buyer dissatisfaction will cause the industry to set fair policies and make these systems affordable and enticing.

For a multi-physician practice, it might be wise to consider purchasing a personal computer that has the capability of being incorporated into the LAN. In this way, should LAN systems become attractive after the initial computerization of the office, the system can simply be upgraded. All in all, LANs conserve the software and hardware features of a microcomputer and allow users to share resources as they would in a mainframe. Although the LANs that have been discussed were intended for offices in which information was meant to be shared, it should be noted that these systems also allowed password and security measures to protect sensitive information that a user does not want shared. This possibility, combined with the relatively low cost of an LAN, makes them particularly well suited for applications such as a hospital filing system and data base.

LANs are constrained in the distances they can cover by the fact that a single cable has to be maintained for the entire distance. Even within a city, if two hospitals wanted to connect to each other a LAN would be a rather impractical solution owing to the amount of cable that would have to be laid down. A number of companies have paid up to $1000 per foot for cable installation. Thus, distance is minimized and kept as local as possible.

Supermicros Versus Local Area Networks for Multiuser Systems

In brief, the supermicro is best in a situation where many people must share the same files on an ongoing basis, and the tasks that they perform are oriented around data entry and recall rather than intensive analysis of data. Any program that demands large amounts of calculation or graphic output will slow the performance of a supermicro system. Easy access to files and economy of hardware are maximized in this environment.

The LAN is ideal in situations where individuals work primarily with their own information but must frequently exchange files and must have access to common files. The LAN also allows a number of individuals to share printers, modems, and other hardware devices. The primary advantage of a network is that each user has his own microcomputer, dedicated to him. This ensures that programs requiring large amounts of computing time, graphic displays, or other processor-intensive functions will run with maximum speed. In addition, users may use whatever software they wish on their own machines. They have the choice of the full range of software available for microcomputers.

The chief disadvantages of LANs are that they are significantly more expensive in terms of hardware that must be purchased per user, and file exchanges are slower and more hazardous than in the supermicro environment. By this I mean that complex safeguards are needed to ensure that two individuals do not attempt to modify the same file at the same time. It this were to happen, the data would be damaged or lost entirely. There are a number of programs designed to accomplish this "file-locking" function, but none has been accepted as standard. This means that in order to operate properly on a network, rather than on an individual machine within that network, a piece of software must not only operate successfully on the individual machines but must interact successfully with a third party's file-locking protocols.

Supermicros, on the other hand, are not networks. They are true multiuser computers in which all the users share the capabilities of a single microprocessor. Several years ago, this capability was available only on minicomputers costing $60,000 and up. Multiuser capability can now be had on microcomputers costing as little as $6000. The operating systems that support this sort of work have evolved in the large computer environment over the last 15 years and are now mature products with few ongoing problems. Perhaps the best known and most standardized of these is UNIX, originally invented by Bell Labs and commonly used within the academic community. Because all users are sharing the same processor and disk drives, common files are accessed very quickly. The protocols for protecting against two people's modifying a file simultaneously are built into the operating system so that any program running within that system recognizes them. Because there is only one processor, one set of drives, one power supply, and so forth, hardware costs for this type of system are much lower than for a network. The only software available to each user, however, is that which is installed in the supermicro itself. At present, software that runs under the multiuser operating systems has a smaller market demand than single user microcomputer software. Hence it is a bit more expensive and sometimes not as user-friendly.

It is difficult if not impossible to successfully computerize a medical practice with a local area network approach. File exchanges have inherent problems and are slow. Since it is impossible to extend a network over a telephone line, a second office cannot participate easily in the network. On the other hand, supermicro computers are ideal in situations where patient records must be accessed and modified by many people on an ongoing basis. In contrast, the local area network is ideal in departments that primarily share each other's documents or datasets, but in which the primary work of the individual is oriented toward writing and editing documents or analyzing those datasets.

Information received from public data bases, such as bibliographies and article search results, can be transferred to a local data base for easy immediate access. For commonly used information, local storage of public data base information is preferred over continually re-accessing the information through the phone lines. Local maintenance of such information reduces the connect time charges and high phone bills that can be associated with this practice. Obviously, local data base programs may be used to manage information other than that acquired from public data bases. The ability of data base software to manage all types of information is what makes it a useful tool for the physician.

Local data bases are easier to use than public data bases or even private data bases on time-sharing mainframes. Microcomputer data management systems are more user-friendly because they are screen-oriented and may provide a significant amount of help to the user. Alternatively, public data bases are usually command-driven and provide little help to the user. Local data bases seem to respond faster to commands. This is probably due to the reduced size of the files in a local setting as well as the interactive nature of the program, which is not vying for time on a time-sharing computer. Local data bases allow more information to be extracted from a data set because more limited and defined associations between pieces of information can be searched.

The use of both public and local data base management systems from a microcomputer requires different types of hardware. For example, access to a public data base requires only a modem and telecommunications software. The microcomputer simply acts as a terminal and the host computer performs all the computations. In contrast, local data base management requires a significant amount of mass storage in order to be efficient. In addition, because the computer itself performs all of the computations, a coprocesser may be useful for increasing response time. The utilization of devices such as hard disks and optical storage media is also providing distinct increases in power to microcomputer-based systems. It is now foreseeable that local data base systems might be able to compete with their mainframe counterparts.

Text Versus Regular Data Bases

Two main types of data base management systems have appeared in the microcomputer software market. Each has different capabilities. One approach uses a data base management program to store and catalogue information. This is the traditional data base program in which each piece of information is labeled and associated with other types of information. In this way, searching the data for a common association yields a list of associated facts. For example, searching a data file using the phrase "peripheral vascular disease" to associate information could yield a list of names corresponding to patients who had that disease.

In recent months, several text management systems have been introduced as an alternative type of data base management. These programs utilize text editing and data retrieval shortcuts to rapidly locate fragments of information and allow them to be incorporated into longer documents. Each stored fragment in the system behaves like an index card of information, which can be quickly reviewed, edited, and manipulated. In this manner, text data base systems act as a bridge between word processing and data base management. Text data bases allow the user to construct a skeleton of levels, topics, and subtopics (an outline), each part of which may be expanded to incorporate manageable chunks of text. The user then has the option of reviewing the text as a complete document or reviewing only the headings of each subsection. The collapsing feature allows the user to shrink the report to a size that is easy to comprehend at a glance. Naturally, a useful feature of the programs is their ability to move text around within a document by simply moving a heading within the outline.

Free-form databases, as they have been named, have different needs than typical data base management systems. Instead of computational or associative coprocesser power, these programs benefit from coprocessers that can rapidly move information from one section of memory to another. These data bases are also more memory-intensive than traditional data bases. Because an important feature is the assembly of documents, constant disk storage and access slow the system down considerably; this is avoided whenever possible. Finally, be aware that there is also major discrepancy within the text data base field as to the way in which programs should be designed. Certain programs impose a structure such as an outline on the data entry process. This can inhibit spontaneity. Other "free-form" text data bases allow a block of text to be assigned one or more identifying key words and then stored in the data base. With these programs, assembly of the document is more difficult because an outline structure does not exist. Instead of the automatic assembly that an outline program permits, each block of text must be assembled individually into the complete document.

Attributes of All Traditional Data Bases

Most traditional data bases utilize three levels of file management to organize and control information. In order of decreasing complexity, these levels are the file, the record, and the field. A data field contains a single piece of information, which can consist of any combination of letters or numbers. A field might contain an address or the name of a patient. It may also be used to categorize information. For example, "yes/no" fields may be used to answer questions about the data. If the data base were being used to track accounts receivable, two fields would be necessary to determine which patients should be billed and which should not. The first data field would contain a patient's name. The second data field would be a "yes/no" field that answers the question: Did the patient have an office visit this week?" By associating a patient's name with a "yes" response, the data base could establish a list of patients' names who should be billed. From this point, the data base could be used to assemble billing information about procedures that were performed by association of the patient name list with other fields. "Yes/no" fields are an efficient means of storage because they use only one unit of storage space and take up very little area on a disk.

The intermediate level of organization in an information management system is the record. A record is composed of a number of fields, each containing information about one defined category, such as a patient. To segregate information, the user specifies the length and type of data to be stored in each field of the record. For example, a record might contain the following: a 50-character field reserved for a name, a 50-character field for an address, a 10-character field for the date of admission, a 10-character field for the room number, and a 50-character field for the attending physician's name. This record, which might appear in a hospital data base, could also contain fields about treatment and diagnosis, laboratory values, chart notes, and so on. Obviously, the sequence of the fields must be the same in every record of a file so that the proper information is searched in a review of all records. When establishing the data base, the program allows the user to label each of the fields in the record. This is a necessary feature when establishing "yes/no" fields or when managing numerical data. In addition, most user-friendly programs control the input and manipulation of data to prevent information from being placed in the wrong field of a record. Obviously, such mistakes can be disastrous.

The most severe restriction placed on a record is a limitation on the number of characters in it. At one end of the spectrum, the best programs allow approximately 65,000 characters per record. At the other end, there are programs that allow only 600 characters per record. A 600-character record is clearly not long enough if notes and other types of text are being stored in the data base. Such a record would hold an average of only 100 words. Generally, at least several thousand characters per record will be needed to adequately handle the needs of a physician. Likewise, for maximum flexibility, an ideal data base program should be able to manage more than 100 fields per record. In addition, most good software allows at least 254 characters per field with the option to create a memo field, which can be as long as the length of an entire record.

The highest level of organization in a data base is the file. A file is a collection of records, each with the same format. A file contains all the information associated with one category in the data base—for instance, all cancer patients. Programs that place unusually small limitations on the maximum number of records per file will not be very useful. Some programs only allow as few as 1000 records per file. As a general rule, most physicians will need the capability for at least 10,000 records per file. Other bothersome limitations on file structure may include a restriction on the number of files opened at one time (the number of files which may be searched at one time) and restrictions on the total number of files in the data base. Naturally, all these limitations are important factors in selecting a package; many are trade-offs on each other.

All data base software utilizes one of two storage strategies: they store data in either variable or fixed length form. With a fixed length strategy, the program determines the length of an individual record by multiplying the number of fields by the specified field length. The program asks the user for the maximum number of records that will be used and then automatically assigns disk space for this theoretical amount of data. In contrast, programs using variable length storage utilize only as much disk space as there is information. These programs do not waste disk space on blank records. Also, some programs utilize a little of both strategies. These programs utilize a variable length file structure with a fixed length record structure. Thus, if just one field of a record is filled with information, space is made for the entire record on disk. However, the program does not utilize disk space for records containing no information.

A variable length storage structure requires fewer disks and therefore is cheaper to maintain. However, the programming architecture must be more complicated in order to manage this type of storage. Also, program performance may not be as good in software that uses variable instead of fixed length storage because the additional data manipulation of this storage strategy requires extra processing time. On the other hand, programs using variable length storage can be easily expanded to include extra records and fields within the data base. Fixed length storage prevents this because disk space has already been allocated. Changes in the characteristics of the data base would require complete recopying of all the information in it (on disk). Both types of storage have good and bad qualities; thus, selection of a software package in this regard is often based upon user preference.

Another major difference between software packages is variable versus fixed screen formatting. A program that uses fixed screen formatting inputs and displays data by some standard and unchangeable format. In contrast, some programs allow the user to manipulate the display of information on the screen so that it may be customized to the application. Customized screens allow the user to feel more at ease with the software and can be used to make a program more user-friendly. A drawback of variable screen programs is that manipulation of the data and features on the screen requires the use of an instruction set very similar to a programming language. Quite often, efficient use of this instruction set may require prior programming experience. Because the screen has to be set up only once, this problem can be avoided in normal use, but, nevertheless, it may require an experienced computer operator for the initial setup. Fixed screen programs have a different problem. They may display unwanted information that can clutter up the screen and make it difficult to read. With simple records or small quantities of data, this is less of a problem.

Like electronic spreadsheets, data base packages tend to be machine specific, much more so than word processing software. Data base software also suffers from the incompatibility of file structures between different programs, which plagues all other software. Although no universal file format exists, some semblance of compatibility has begun to emerge in many programs. Several programs are starting to support the ASCII and DIF formats. Consumers should consider purchasing a program that supports one of these common file structures (there are others), especially if compatibility of the data files with other software such as spreadsheets and word processors is an important consideration. In this situation, the buyer should consider integrated software packages with data base management or those that work closely with an associated package. Owing to compatibility problems, it is absolutely imperative to make a wise software selection with an initial purchase. Because the data base management system is likely to control more information than both the word processing and spreadsheet programs combined, a transfer of information from one data base to another can be extremely time-consuming should the wrong software package be selected.

Types of Data Bases

Currently, there are five distinct types of data base management systems available on the market. The most basic and limited data base management programs are called file management systems. A file management system is analogous to an index card file. However, a card file may be searched by only one field (such as a name), but a file management system can search any of the fields in the records, for example, by disease as well as by name.

In a file management system, an example of a record in one file might be "patient name, disease, age." A record in a second file in the same system might be "patient name, address." A limitation of file management systems is that they will not combine information from one file with information from another file. In other words, the information from the "disease" file could not be merged with the information from the "address" file. Although it is true that the information in the two files originally could have been combined into one file, this luxury is usually not attainable in real life because associated data are being continually added to a data base system.

A better type of information management system is the relational data base. Like a file management system, it is made up of records and fields. However, a relational data base may combine records from different files as long as the records in the different files have one field in common. Typically, commands such as "project" and "join" are used to merge the appropriate sections of the different files. For example, "project" could create a file of records that contained "patient name, disease," from a file with the records "patient name, disease, patient age." The "join" command could then take this new file and merge it with an address file to create a patient name and address file that is associated with disease. This final file could ultimately be stored on disk or printed.

Relational data bases are convenient because data can be entered without much regard for the way in which it will be used. In other words, records do not have to be planned so that every field that will ever be needed must be thought up in advance. However, if no planning of file structure is done before entering data, the user will spend a lot of time retrieving the information from the data base.

The hierarchical data base is another way to manage data. Like the relational data base, this system is made up of records, but the records do not have to be broken up into fields. The hierarchical system doesn't search the contents of a record the way a relational system does. Hierarchical data bases impose specific associations between files; these connections are called "hooks." Because the connections between files do not depend on the information within the files, the connections are defined at the start and are fixed for the life of the data base.

The advantage of a hierarchical data base system is its speed. The computer does not have to search through the data fields in order to establish relationships. For example, a file of records with patients' names and addresses could be definitively associated with a file that maintained history and physical findings and at the same time be associated with a file that contained laboratory values and chart notes. (Remember that files are associated record for record.) With the data base formatted in this way, all information centers around a common file, such as patients' names and addresses. In addition, further associations could branch from any of these files.

In the hierarchical system, a search of the patients' names file will then allow the user to search either the chart note file or the history and physical examination file. After entering and reviewing the information in one of those files, further search options would be presented to the user. In a good system, an update of the records in the patients' names file automatically updates any information it affects in the other two files and any other files connected to them. The architecture of this data base is similar to an upside-down tree. A single file is connected to several files which in turn are connected to many more files. In schematic form, the data base does indeed look like an upside-down family tree.

Two other types of data base software available are the free-format data base and the multi-user data base. The free-format data base was discussed earlier in the chapter. This text processing data base allows data to be retrieved by means of key words, which are used to tag the information. A multiuser data base may have any of the structures previously discussed. The defining feature of multiuser data bases is the ability to provide access to several people at the same time. However, a good program will allow only one person to change a particular record at any one time. In this way, other users are "locked out" of the record until that user is finished. This type of data base is used in the transportation industry to assign seats on airplanes or trains. The critical feature to evaluate in studying a multiuser data base is whether this record locking feature can adequately protect against two users writing to a file simultaneously. If not, that file could be severely damaged.

Traps and Problems

The biggest problem most professionals encounter with data base software is nonexpandability of the system once it is established. This occurs particularly often in programs using fixed-length storage strategies. Typically, nonexpandability is a problem when the user fails to reasonably anticipate the amount of growth the data base will undergo. Another familiar problem occurs when professionals have unrealistic expectations about the capabilities of the software. Quite often, programs are not used to their fullest potential, as, for example, when a relational data base is used more as a file management system than as an associative tool to link pieces of information.

A lack of storage space plagues most microcomputer-based information management systems. Unfortunately, it is a problem not easily solved. Hopefully, the introduction of optical storage devices and widespread use of hard disks will obviate this problem. An accurate estimation of the amount of necessary data storage when a computer is purchased can prevent a storage problem from occurring early in the life of a data base system. A good estimate can determine whether a hard disk will be necessary and if additional random access memory should be purchased.

The extent of user-friendliness varies even to a greater extent with data base management than with the previous two types of software mentioned. Menu-driven programs quickly become tedious, and command-driven programs can be difficult to learn. A few programs have found a middle ground, and others have survived in the market because of their powerful capabilities. As with spreadsheets, documentation can be vitally important, especially in command-driven programs. Assessment of program performance is also another problem with data base systems. Most systems can perform simple searches rapidly and thus appear decent in a demonstration. Unlike other software types, the user's ultimate application cannot be adequately tested in the showroom. Perhaps the best way to select a program in this field is to compare software vendors' specification sheets, which list the qualities and capabilities of the different software packages.

GRAPHICS SOFTWARE

Computer graphics can handle a large number of tasks that currently are performed by the professional artist. With the use of graphics software, the high cost associated with having an artist draw simple charts and graphs can be avoided. Also, the turnaround time is drastically reduced because the computer can instantly create the material and print it. Freeing artists from producing these simple charts and graphs gives them extra time to work on projects that truly need their talents. Thus, this software is beneficial to everyone.

Graphics programs are particularly useful when used in conjunction with spreadsheets. With integrated spreadsheet and graphics software, information is easily funneled between the two programs. Lotus 1 2 3 is one program noted for its outstanding spreadsheet and graphics capabilities. Even VisiCalc, the most basic of all spreadsheets, can work in conjunction with other Visi series programs to generate graphics.

Spreadsheet-associated graphics programs are not the only type of graphics packages available. There are many high-quality stand-alone graphics programs as well. In fact, stand-alone graphics packages tend to be more sophisticated and have more power than those associated with spreadsheets. Of course, a problem with these stand-alone packages is that the data must be typed in manually unless a common file structure is used. The better packages are able to capture data from several spreadsheet types.

Spreadsheet-associated graphics programs usually contain only the basics: bar graphs, pie charts, line graphs, and tabular data. These four capabilities usually fit the needs of most professionals. Users who need more extensive capabilities such as histograms and line-fitting usually need to seek assistance from a stand-alone graphics package. Especially when working with plotted data, be sure to consider whether or not a spreadsheet's file format is compatible with the graphics program. Typing in x,y coordinate pairs is very time-consuming. If your analyses are going to call for a significant amount of plotting, it is imperative that the spreadsheet be compatible with the graphics program.

Split-screen operation or "windowing" can be a useful feature of graphics packages. This ability allows the user to compare two different graphs on the screen at the same time. This can be important in the analysis and comparison of data. However, one drawback may be that the entire portion of each graph may not be viewable when the screen is split. If the program reduces to fit the entire graph in the window, resolution problems may obscure subtle differences. In addition, the creation and elimination of windows on the screen can be an awkward process with certain software packages. In many situations, it may not be worth the trouble it creates.

Software Considerations

With graphics software, the most important characteristics to look for are the number of different graphing formats and the amount of data the program can effectively work with. In addition to the basic four graphing options (bar graphs, pie charts, line graphs, tabular data), several other useful formats can be used to display data, including stacked bar charts, scattergrams, histograms, and trend analysis. With regard to restrictions on the amount of data, be aware that some programs either don't allow or don't work well with very large sets of data because of problems in resolution or decreased computation speed (especially in trend analyses). A program's ability to work with a mouse or other drawing device may also be a very important aspect of the software. Such a device allows the user to draw figures and symbols that can be inserted into the output. Not all programs can support this type of hardware; therefore, the need for this capability may serve to initially define a limited set of packages from which to choose.

The ability of a program to label and distinguish between individual parts of a graph is also of prime importance in choosing a graphics package. Proper labeling of the axes and graphs make the material more immediately understandable. The number and type of symbols used to distinguish between bars on a bar graph should not be so limited that duplication of symbols on the same graph is necessary. By estimating one's needs based on previous experience, the minimum number of different symbols needed can be estimated.

Some packages will allow the user to put in floating labels at any position, even near the data points or lines. It is important to assess whether or not there are limits on the way the graphs can be labeled. Also, find out whether custom symbols can be generated and added to the program. These are often needed in technical writing.

Particularly in medicine, results center around comparative and analytical graphs. The ability to superimpose graphs and overlay several different types of graphs on one another can also be a useful option of some programs. In addition, the ability to scale graphs in a prescribed manner is equally important. Functions that can make a graph larger or smaller while retaining the same proportions can be desirable in the superimposition process. For example, such features allow control graphs to be reduced and placed in uncluttered portions, usually the corners, of experimental graphs. Such abilities help to poignantly point out information from experiments.

Like all software, user-friendliness is essential. Graphics programs can be either command-driven, menu-driven, or both. On-screen help with either type of program is a plus for the new graphics user. It prevents continuous referral to the documentation. Ideally, a program should offer several levels of on-screen help in order to accommodate experienced as well as inexperienced users. In general, an interactive program such as a graphics package is more convenient when it is command-driven; however, it also requires more time to learn. Software developers can usually put more power into a command-driven program because they can worry less about the user-friendly interface. As with all programming, the extent and clarity of the documentation should be carefully scrutinized before purchasing. Stay away from programs in which the documentation seems to assume prior knowledge about jargon you are not familiar with.

The displaying of graphics material on the screen can use one of two methods. Most computers use a technique known as "bit mapping" which breaks the screen up into a series of small dots, or "pixels," which can be controlled to generate the graphics. On the other hand, a few computers control these dots in small chunks or blocks; these screens are said to be "memory mapped." To assess the resolution of a graphics package, the total number of pixels the screen is broken down into are used as a measurement. A rating of 160 × 100 (horizontal dots × vertical dots) is considered low resolution and is usually satisfactory for the generation of bar graphs. Medium resolution is usually considered in the range of 320 × 200 dots. This amount of resolution is adequate for pie charts and simple graphs. High-resolution graphics will approach 640 × 400 dots. This type of resolution is needed to draw complex figures and detailed charts.

Be aware that there may be discrepancies between the resolution achieved on and off screen. The resolution that can be obtained on a printer may be very different from that obtained on the television screen. Likewise, if the program supports a plotter, be sure that the resolution on the plotter is equivalent to what is being seen on the screen. Finally, the availability of color graphics should also be assessed. As with resolution, be sure to determine whether the program supports the color graphics during the hard copy output. Besides availability, points to consider should include the number of different colors and whether or not they all can be displayed on the screen concurrently.

Hardware Considerations

More than any other type of software, graphics packages may place specific requirements on the hardware needs of a system. For example, in some computers, color graphics on the screen can be supported only if an additional integrated circuit card is present in the machine and a special graphics monitor is used. In addition, color graphics will be supported only if the monitor itself is a color monitor and is not monochromatic—a point that is often overlooked. These considerations should be assessed as part of the overall cost of adding computer graphics to the system. Except for the color monitor, the other hardware needs will probably be used only by the graphics program, and, therefore, the real cost of graphics' capabilities should include these items.

Another problem is incompatibility between software and peripheral hardware devices such as printers and plotters. Especially when planning to use a plotter, it is imperative to determine which plotters are supported by the software and which ones are not. Plotters from different manufacturers may require very different commands and support programs; thus, most graphics programs support only a few plotter types.

In a graphics system, a plotter is a worthwhile investment if the program is used extensively. Although slower than a printer, the quality of the graphics on a plotter is much better because continuous lines and solid letters as well as multiple colors can be obtained. Unfortunately, plotters can be an expensive addition to a computer system. Both the initial investment and the upkeep costs are great. In addition, plotters are not as sturdy as printers and tend to require more repairs per document produced. Likewise, they also require more user attention in order to achieve adequate results and prevent breakdowns.

With the acquisition of a graphics package, it is usually a good idea to purchase a print buffer. Currently, external buffers can be obtained that can be used with both printers and plotters to prevent duplication. A print buffer can significantly speed up the execution time of a program by allowing information to be dumped and forgotten by the main computer. Thus, availability of a buffer makes the graphics package easier to use and less time-consuming.

SUMMARY

The utilization of word processors, spreadsheets, data bases, and graphics software allows physicians to manage information more completely than ever before. With proper use of the software, report generation is made much easier and less time-consuming. Extensive paperwork, which at one time piled up, can now be efficiently managed with these electronic tools. The easy access to large amounts of information offered by these tools fosters increased efficiency and economy.

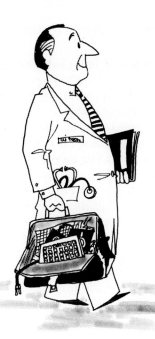

F O U R

Basic Tools

Jonathan Javitt, M.D.

If a computer is being purchased to do a specific job, such as manage an office or collect data in a hospital unit, and the software provided with the computer does that job adequately, the user of that machine needs to know very little about the material in this chapter. If, on the other hand, the computer is being approached as a tool for enabling work and generating new possibilities for working, it is worth having a context within which to view the software products that flood the market today. No book can offer up-to-the-minute reviews of specific products. Products change and advance far too rapidly. However, one's approach to them should be dictated by common sense and a realistic assessment of their capabilities, rather than by the marketing fanfare that precedes their introduction. This chapter provides an approach to evaluating software products for yourself.

THE PAPERLESS OFFICE

The introduction of microcomputers into the office and laboratory is revolutionizing the ways in which professionals approach their jobs. Although tools such as word processors, electronic spreadsheets, and telecommunications software allow more thorough and efficient handling of information, they are simply electronic tools that duplicate the same functions (and add many more) of devices that are already a staple in the professional environment. This effective duplication has sparked an ongoing debate in the computer industry. Should software lead to more productive methods of information management, or should it simply reproduce the more traditional and perhaps inefficient methods that exist today? The decision has not been easy. As a solution, the software industry has invested a large amount of time, research, and development toward the replacement of traditional office practices with electronic equipment while maintaining a minority of products that are on the cutting edge and can be said to be truly innovative.

Professionals need not feel threatened by the infiltration of computers into the office environment. Electronic tools like the word processor and spreadsheet do not change the tasks that are normally performed; however, they do make them easier. For example, the word processor has ideal features that make it a good replacement for the typewriter. Although a word processer does not greatly decrease the time for the initial typing of a manuscript or letter, it can significantly increase the speed of error correction and editing. Editing a manuscript on paper is a slow and inefficient process that can stifle creativity. Word processors, however, allow an individual to be more liberal and meticulous when making changes and rearrangements. Typically, computer generation of documents retains all the features of a typewriter and adds useful services such as computer editing, automatic duplication, and efficient storage.

A desk calculator is a common fixture in every office today. However, just 15 years ago they were an uncommon sight. Just as the calculator replaced the adding machine, the electronic spreadsheet may soon replace the desk calculator in many of its roles in the professional environment. The spreadsheet is more than just a calculator. It is a calculator, ledger pad, and data processor in one complete package. As a calculating device, it acts as a hybrid between a calculator and a word processor. It not only makes instantaneous calculations but is capable of storing and transferring the results to other devices such as data bases and word processors where the information can be utilized. In this manner, the spreadsheet is a more efficient replacement for a calculator because processed data and information need not be manually transferred to reports, thus incurring duplicated and wasted effort.

Unlike other electronic replacements for current office tools, the spreadsheet is capable of replacing several devices. It acts as an intelligent ledger pad by offering the speed and accuracy of a calculator, retaining the organizational features of a ledger pad, and performing the ancillary tasks of a secretarial assistant. Spreadsheets can keep running totals as data is being added into the spreadsheet, and they can perform recalculation of numerous variables with many different data sets at the touch of a few buttons. Ultimately, this type of capability means that medical professionals will be able to make better decisions because data can be more meticulously examined.

An unfortunate misconception about electronic spreadsheets is that they are simply tools for financial assessment or management. This reputation was derived largely because economists and financiers recognized the usefulness of this tool long before other professionals, and thus, for quite some time (and even partially today), advertising and software features were directed toward the finance market. Obviously, the spreadsheet is not just a financial tool. It can increase efficiency in both laboratory and clinical data processing as well as in the office. Like the word processor, the spreadsheet is a generic tool that can be customized to fit any application.

The way in which data is presented can be as important as the development of the data in the first place. Translating data into graphs, charts, and other representations makes the trend or thrust of the data immediately clear. Many currently available spreadsheets also have the capability to prepare data for presentation. Most of these software packages have at least limited graphic capabilities that allow the generation of pie charts, bar graphs, and the like. This ability eliminates the time, expense, and occasional hassles that can be incurred when dealing with a professional illustrator. Likewise, it allows manuscripts to be prepared with the graphics and associated figures instantly inserted.

Although word processors and spreadsheets provide a means for efficient processing of textual and numerical information, neither type of software package provides an efficient means of storing and retrieving different types of information that share a common association or linkage. For example, all patients' files may contain laboratory values, previous correspondence, and progress notes. In most offices, the organization of this information is performed by using manila folders and a filing cabinet. Although this system allows for easy accessibility through organization, it prevents a quick review of information common to all patients' files, such as addresses, telephone numbers, billing information, and vital statistics. An electronic data base management system is designed to organize these types of information in a manner that allows them to be both easily accessible and swiftly manipulated at the same time.

The management of the large amounts of information generated in the medical office is the principal reason most of the personnel are employed. In addition, at least half of a physician's own time is spent creating, evaluating, and using data for the benefit of patients. Data base management provides a means for managing and organizing files of data, a process otherwise known as file management.

Data base management systems also provide capabilities that reach far beyond those usually associated with file management systems. Although file management systems can be a useful tool, this type of software is mainly concerned with eliminating the need for the conventional filing cabinet. True data base management, however, gives the user the capability to reach into a file and pull out specific information on command. For example, a vascular surgeon might routinely store thousands of patients' medical records over the years and then need to know: "How many claudicators have I had over the age of 60 who had diabetes and an ankle-brachial index of less than 0.4?"

If the surgeon were to manually pursue the answer to that question by reviewing old records from a conventional filing system, he or she would probably spend weeks gathering that information. With a properly structured data base program, the answer to that question could be determined in a few minutes. Theoretically, data base management systems can be set up to keep track of virtually all the information in a medical office, but it may not be necessary or even feasible to do so. The value of a data base management system to a medical practice is limited only by the way in which the system is planned and designed. Setting up a data base management system requires a review and evaluation of conventional information filing procedures. A thorough evaluation can reveal procedures that need improvement and will identify areas in which cross referencing and linkage are most important.

Data base management systems can be expanded and used efficiently to track and organize patient information in the hospital as well as in the office setting. Coupled with a local area network, a data base management system could not only provide access to all the information about a patient anywhere throughout the hospital but would also allow laboratory tests and other procedures to be immediately updated. This type of system eliminates the bothersome delays that are encountered in waiting for medical records. Through cross referencing and associations, vital statistics on patients with similar diseases are instantly available;

this is an important capability in view of the implementation of diagnosis-related groups. Moreover, information from a data base can be merged easily with a form letter from a word processing program. This might facilitate the follow-up of all patients on a particular drug therapy or even automated billing.

Computerizing hospital records can have effects on the way medical information is stored in the private practice. Currently, patient information is either duplicated and then stored with the private physician or it is not accessible for several days or weeks while the physician awaits arrival through the mail. The duplication of hospital records allows ready access; however, such practices take up a large amount of storage space. Through the use of telecommunications software with a data base management system, the physician can have the best of both worlds. Telecommunications allows information to be instantaneously accessible without requiring storage space. If necessary, this information can be sent to a printer, where a hard copy can be obtained. Thus, hospital records can be treated as an external data base much like those that are accessed during a library search. Ultimately, this type of procedure reduces expenses by minimizing personnel and making more efficient use of one's time.

Telecommunications and public data base access can add important capabilities to the medical armamentarium. Public data bases are now being used for many enterprises besides simply organizing and indexing journal entries. Data bases are being used to monitor organ availability for transplantation as well as to track disease epidemics. For the physician and hospital alike, the acquisition of this type of information is limited by the availability of the proper telecommunications hardware and software. At the very minimum, a modem and a communications program will be necessary in order to access public data bases from a private microcomputer. Modems and communications programs vary widely in their ability to make your link to the outside easy to implement and convenient to use. Although the acquisition of this equipment will not be discussed in great detail in this chapter, a few minor points that differ from the acquisition of word processor and spreadsheet software should be considered.

INTEGRATED SOFTWARE PACKAGES

A big advancement in the personal computer industry was the introduction of integrated software packages. These packages are extensive programs that incorporate word processing, spreadsheet analysis, graphics, data base management, and telecommunications software. The programs are written so that information may be transferred from one program type to another. For example, graphics data can be integrated into a word processor file, or spreadsheet analyses can be transferred to the graphics package. Currently, the most advanced integrated packages allow the computer to run more than one program at the same time. This is performed through the use of windowing or screen splitting.

With this feature, word processing can be performed in one window, spreadsheet analysis in another, and telecommunications access to a public data base in a third. In this way, information from all three sources can be viewed at the same time. This capability can be extremely valuable in the generation of manuscripts. By allowing information from multiple programs to be viewed at once, tedious program and data file transitions are avoided. Likewise, the use of an integrated software package also prevents discrepancies in file formats when trying to transfer data, as from a spreadsheet to a word processor program.

Integrated software is not without its drawbacks. When windowing is used, for example, the screen is continually cut into smaller and smaller pieces. Although information can continue to be viewed, the amount in each window decreases as the screen is divided. This can be bothersome and annoying. In addition, if multiple programs are running in different windows at the same time, processor speed can be somewhat slowed down, and the amount of memory available to each program is divided by the number of programs running in the system. Finally, establishing windows and moving from one window to another can often be a difficult and time-consuming process that unnecessarily wastes effort.

Although the feature of integration may outweigh other considerations for some users, the individual components of integrated packages are not as powerful as the best separate word processors, spreadsheets, and data bases. There is simply not enough memory in a microcomputer to hold three or four full-featured components within one package. Thus, to construct a large data base of hundreds of patients with many pieces of information on each using an integrated package would be cumbersome at best. Similarly, attempting to write a book with an integrated package when full-featured word processors are available would be foolhardy. At the risk of being repetitious, the greatest power of integrated software is in integrating. Thus, data from a large data base may be imported into an integrated package for analysis on its spreadsheet. Similarly, text from a word processor may be converted to the format recognizable by that same integrated package. The data and text may then be readily combined, perhaps with the addition of graphics, into a finished report.

Integrated software packages have one significant drawback: they tend to be expensive. This should not be surprising, considering the number of different software packages and capabilities that are provided in the integrated package. Still, they constitute a substantial initial investment and therefore require a careful review of the physician's needs before purchasing. The expense, however, only begins with the cost of the software. All the packages available today require hard disks and maximum memory to be present in the computer in order for them to run efficiently.

INTEGRATED SOFTWARE APPROACHES TODAY

Even considering the drawbacks, integrated packages tend to be wise investments. Their ability to allow information to be manipulated in every way without interruption significantly increases the efficiency of the user, and this is the ultimate goal in electronic information management. Although this chapter is not designed to be a comparison of specific products, there are relatively few products in the integrated software arena presently, and they embody different approaches, which are worthy of mention.

In 1984, an integrated software package called Symphony (developed for the IBM PC) was released by the Lotus Development Corporation. Symphony is a fully integrated package that includes and improves upon the Lotus 1 2 3 spreadsheet, graphics, and data base capabilities while adding new word processing and data communications environments. Symphony allows the user to take advantage of windowing techniques so that more than one program may be run at once. In Symphony, the layout of the windows can be as small as one character or as large as the screen. The master environment in Symphony is a 256-character column by 8192 row spreadsheet. From this environment, the user may either use the spreadsheet or use the word processing, graphics, data base, or communications software. The program is menu-driven and allows data to be shared among the several environments in different windows.

In late 1984, another competitive integrated package for the IBM PC and its compatibilities called Framework was released by Ashton Tate. Much like Symphony, Framework contains word processing, spreadsheet, data base, graphics and communications capabilities. Likewise, Framework also allows windowing and multi-tasking. Framework is different from other programs of its type because it treats each task as a frame, much like a piece of motion picture film. Each frame is capable of being expanded to contain as much information as necessary. Each cell in the master environment is a frame. Each of these cells can contain an entire word processing file, graphics, data, formulas, and so on. With its word processing program, Framework can be particularly useful in developing an outline for a manuscript because each line in the outline can be a separate frame. Because each frame has a unique label (or address), frames can be taken apart and reassembled in any order by referring to the label. Coupled with the capability to expand upon each frame, the word processor allows entire segments of the document to be moved around or copied into other documents. With these features, the entire manuscript can be generated by simply expanding upon each line in the outline and arranging them in the appropriate order for printing.

Also, in 1984, Apple released its version of the integrated personal computer with the introduction of the Macintosh computer. The Macintosh is a portable, user-friendly, personal computer based on a new generation of current microprocessors. It evolved from Apple's first attempt at integrated computing with a machine called Lisa. The Macintosh and Lisa computers were at the forefront of windowing technology and therefore make extensive use of this tool. The most notable feature of the Macintosh orientation is its visual approach. The user has complete control of the screen by moving a pointer, called a mouse, around the screen and pointing to commands. In this way pieces of text may be moved, options may be specified, and files may be opened and closed.

Unlike many of its competitors, the Macintosh uses its operating system capabilities to integrate the many programs that run on this computer. Software developers are aware of the Macintosh's capabilities and design the programs so that they work within the integrated architecture. Although programs are purchased individually, programs can communicate information to each other because of the integrated nature of the operating system. In this way, multi-tasking is supported and programs may still be acquired individually as needs arise.

Recently, IBM PC compatibility has been offered to Macintosh owners through the acquisition of an additional piece of hardware at a moderate price. Therefore, much of the software base available to IBM PC owners may now be used on the Macintosh.

AN APPROACH TO SOFTWARE EVALUATION

Although there are fewer options today if you want an integrated software package, the options in stand-alone word processors, spreadsheets, and data bases are legion. The remainder of this chapter offers an approach to these products that will help you to be far less susceptible to advertising hype and far more critical as a consumer. In evaluating the major, nationally advertised packages, "good" and "bad" are not very useful terms. Large amounts of development money have been spent, generally on competent programming teams. The important issue to address is the design philosophy behind the product and specifically whether that philosophy is suited to your needs. There are three ways of answering that question, all of which may be pursued simultaneously. The first is by following the guidelines below. The second is by reading the latest reviews in the press, but with a modicum of skepticism. The third is by directly contacting those who are using the product. If all three are followed with reasonable diligence, you are unlikely to make an unwise purchase.

WORD PROCESSING—WHAT TO LOOK FOR

Word processing makes writing significantly easier and more efficient because the program frees writers to set down their thoughts as they come to mind, knowing that they can make changes quickly and intelligibly. Many professionals believe that word processing has made their writing better because they are able to revise and polish their work at will, spared from the burden of retyping successive drafts. This results in clearer and more cost-effective printed communication.

Word processing is likely to be one of the most vital capabilities the microcomputer offers. For most professionals, the word processing program will be the central focus and all other programs, such as spreadsheets and graphics packages, will need to communicate their results with this program. As the crux, the word processing program ties together all other applications software by ultimately merging their information into the reports generated in this program. Thus, an important consideration in choosing a word processing program is its ability to function as part of an integrated package or its ability to accept common data file structures that the other applications programs can generate.

As stated before, word processing does not realistically reduce the amount of time it takes to type in an original draft. After all, the typing of information at the initial stage is no different from using a typewriter. However, because the text is held temporarily in computer memory, the document can undergo significant editing. On-screen editing is fast and neat. It economizes the editing process by eliminating the duplication of effort that is associated with making changes on paper, cutting and pasting, and then transferring them to the typewriter.

Generation of Routine Letters and Reports

An important attribute of word processing programs for medical professionals is their ability to generate personalized form letters. Mail-merging programs (as they are called) are capable of taking data files with name and address information and then inserting that information into the appropriate spots of a form letter. With this capability, information from the history and physical examination can be easily organized and recorded on a standard form, routine follow-up notices can be sent to patients, and even prescription notes can be created. In fact, any document or letter that is regularly utilized in the medical practice can be efficiently duplicated and personalized. By reducing the amount of duplication and effort involved in these processes, fewer secretarial personnel are needed in the organization of the medical practice while the quality of health care provided to patients is maintained. Thus, the computer pays for itself by both economizing the physician's time and reducing the number of support personnel.

Speed and Efficiency

Word processing software offers features that also make it useful for the generation of routine correspondence in which duplication of effort is not an important issue. Through storage on electronic media (particularly floppy and hard disks), word processing software offers a compact and economical way to store information. With current technology, a floppy disk stores over 300,000 text characters. On the other hand, a typical 8½ × 11 inch sheet of paper can store only approximately 5000 characters at its maximum, which is rarely, if ever, reached. After considering the difference in volume between a floppy disk and a sheet of paper, one finds that disk storage requires 30 times less space than its corresponding nonelectronic media. This estimate probably represents a minimum. With the evolution of more efficient disk drives and the need to store columnar, numerical data, the increase in efficiency with electronic storage media probably approaches 1000-fold.

A search of a typical 300,000-character floppy disk, which stores approximately 200 single-page letters, takes less than 3 seconds from the issuance of the command until the file has been recalled. Even a well-organized conventional filing system would probably take several minutes to retrieve the same information. Once again, the electronic capabilities offered through the word processing software represent tremendous increases in economy and efficiency. Clearly, these capabilities can offer a significant increase in performance power for the medical professional in the management of text.

Editing Enhancements

Different word processing programs running on the same type of computer have different capabilities. The programs differ not only in the number of features but also in the speed at which functions are carried out, even when being performed on the same computer. In many packages, at least two thirds of the commands are intended for use in editing or in formatting a document. This is typical of most word processing software. Considering this, it is not surprising that these programs are capable of reducing the amount of time it takes to edit a document. With a few key strokes, typical programs allow paragraphs to be moved and sentences to be rearranged. Cursor functions include moving or deleting to the right or left by one character, one word, and one sentence. In the vertical direction, the cursor may be moved up or down by one line, one screen, and even one page. Even if just these few simple commands were offered (and there are many more), words could be swiftly added or deleted and spelling errors could be easily changed. The most powerful packages allow for the generation of "macros." This allows the user to specify a particular sequence of commands under one label, thus greatly reducing the number of key strokes for frequently performed tasks.

Currently, most programs offer many additional features that allow unusual formatting and highlighting to be easily performed. With just a few key strokes, boldface type, underlining, subscripts, superscripts, and even customized symbols can be inserted into the text. Unlike using a typewriter, centering a line is very simple. By changing margins and spacing, blocks of text can be separated from the main document. In addition, certain programs offer convenient features that allow headings or running feet (special bottom lines) to be automatically inserted as well as convenient placement of footnotes and pagination.

Spelling, Punctuation, and Style

In conjunction with word processing software, additional programs can be purchased, such as those which check grammar, punctuation, or spelling. These programs can all but eliminate the proofreading process. In particular, spelling programs can give information about the number of words in the manuscript and the number of different types of words and may even correct misspellings. To perform these processes, spelling programs maintain a set of dictionaries that are user-created and stored on disk. Usually, the user adds and deletes words from the dictionary after the document has been searched for misspellings. Any word in the document that is not in the dictionary can either be corrected, if it is misspelled, or used to update the dictionary. These programs can proofread a document with greater rapidity and accuracy than any individual. The punctuation and style checkers work by comparing the document in question to a list of the most common grammatic and syntactic errors. The software then shows the user the sentence in question, along with the supposed error, and leaves the user the option of rewriting it.

Major Considerations in Purchasing Word Processors

In selecting a word processing system, you should make certain that the "bells and whistles" of features do not cloud your judgment so that you overlook basic considerations. Like high fidelity stereo equipment, hardware and software are often bought and sold on the basis of how pretty it sounds, how many colors it offers, or the friendliness of the salesperson. Although each of these points affects system performance to some degree, they are usually the least important system characteristics. Although the salesperson's friendliness may reflect upon a firm's willingness to back their products' warranties, honesty and candidness will be more useful in helping to choose the right system. Unfortunately, the computer industry is flooded with sales personnel who know little more than the names of their company's products. It is unreasonable to expect a salesperson to push someone else's product, especially because it is most likely that his or her company has a competent product in a particular category. This should not be surprising, for example, to anyone who has dealt with a drug company representative. Each of the major drug houses has an approved antibiotic for almost any indication; if you look to the detail sales repesentative for antibiotic advice, you will generally buy that company's product. The only way to choose the product intelligently is to research the literature with your own criteria in mind and use the drug company representative to answer specific questions. Testing a salesperson's basic knowledge about software in general, however, may determine which one can provide an objective viewpoint. Generally, such a salesperson will be invaluable in helping to distinguish between those programs and products that look good and those that are good.

An often-used criterion when purchasing software is its ease of use. This criterion is hard to define and is highly subjective. It is not wise to assess software based on its ease of use at first exposure. Such a judgment does not take into consideration the opinions of other individuals who may be using the system or the increases in efficiency that may be obtained with more complex software once it is learned. It is surprising how fast uninitiated individuals can learn to use a computer. User-friendly program features that at first seem helpful and necessary may ultimately become tedious. Then the program that was once easy to use becomes inefficient and burdensome when compared to other products. The important point is not to underestimate the speed with which the user will become experienced and will be able to appreciate the power of more complete and perhaps complex software.

Industry analysts project that approximately 60 per cent of all personal computers being sold are for word processing applications. In light of this and the fact that word processing programs serve as the integration point for information from most other types of software, the word processing program is likely to be the most utilized type of software by the physician. One of the most important considerations when purchasing this type of software is the extent and quality of the program documentation. Before buying any program, the instructional materials provided with the software should be reviewed. The consumer should be able to easily follow the guide without seeking further clarification. If the documentation materials seem more like a glossary than a tutorial, they may not provide enough information to the inexperienced user. In addition to instructional materials, summary cards that list commands in a glossary-like fashion should also be included in the documentation but should not be a basis for them. The summary cards will soon be very useful as users become experienced with the system and do not want to search the manuals for a simple command.

To assess the documentation or any aspect of a word processing program, take any rough draft to the supplier and ask to see the commands that will edit the document into the finished product. Compare commands of different programs in order to determine if the documentation is straightforward and adequately describes the use of each command. In addition, this type of analysis will allow one to determine which commands are less awkward and confusing.

The use of documentation and its associated materials is not the only method by which an uninitiated user may learn to use software. Before the introduction of the microcomputer in information management, individuals could go to data processing schools to learn how to use large mainframe systems. Now that this technology has been usurped by the microcomputer industry, many of these schools have switched their curriculums and now teach the use of the most widely accepted word and data processing programs. In addition, many software developers in association with marketing agencies are offering in-house training, for a fee, in large installations. This offers a convenient method to quickly expose hospital personnel to a particular system. In smaller settings, such as a medical practice, secretarial personnel often can be sent to regionalized training centers for intensive training with particular software packages. The availability of training programs or in-house teaching can make a big difference in a user's proficiency with a particular software package. Thus, the availability of such programs should be an important factor in choosing a software package.

Other considerations besides a program's documentation should be considered when assessing software support (where questions should be directed). For example, some software is supported by the original vendor, and others by the distributor or retailer. Unless the software package is very popular or extensively used, software support by the original developer is usually preferable to that which is supported by the retailer. The original developer will usually have both hardware and software engineers to troubleshoot when you have a problem. On the other hand, the retailer can rely only upon personal experience with the program or must contact the original developer when difficult problems arise, thus encountering a delay.

Fortunately, most large-scale software developers now provide telephone assistance to users who have problems. A few manufacturers even offer a toll-free telephone number; others, such as Hewlett-Packard, offer 24-hour service. However, this service is not always free. For example, Hewlett-Packard, which at one time offered free assistance, now charges a substantial fee for each problem they solve. Software manufacturers and computer developers have been forced because the use of such help-lines has increased drastically and partly because this service can be profitable.

It is important to determine not only the type and amount of software support but also the level (engineer, experienced user, inexperienced user) of support that is available. Although software engineers can be very knowledgeable about troubleshooting when an unusual problem results, they are generally unwilling to answer basic, fundamental questions about the use of their product. For this reason, telephone software support is usually provided by experienced users that are trained by the software vendor. Nonetheless, the availability of an engineer should be noted when assessing support in case such assistance is needed.

Another important feature of word processing software is the availability of program updates. Most current software developers are offering annual or biannual program updates for a fraction of the original program cost. Because it is difficult to prevent software from being copied and distributed among several different users (which is an infringement of copyright law unless otherwise stated), software vendors are issuing identification numbers to buyers so that only the original purchasers will receive updates or support. This service is being offered as a means of curtailing software piracy. In addition, updating prevents potential consumers from waiting until more advanced programs are developed, thus removing the fear of missing out on significant developments.

When considering a particular software package, the availability of software updates should be weighed against the expense and frequency of their release. Updates should be promised at least yearly and should cost no more than 10 to 15 per cent of the original purchase price of the package. In addition, be aware of how many updates you are entitled to receive and whether or not there is a time limit on receiving such updates. Finally, remember that updates may provide significant developments that can increase system performance, especially in word processing, in which the program acts as the focal point of the information management system.

Aside from the extent of documentation and support, different word processing programs can differ significantly in their speed of application. One aspect of performance speed is the keyboard response. Some programs utilize keyboard buffers, and others do not. Keyboard buffers allow a user to continue keying in information (to a certain extent) even when the computer is busy performing another operation such as moving a paragraph or deleting a sentence. Although this ability prevents the user from waiting for the system, it can also cause redundancy because missed words or characters will have to be retyped. Typically, most keyboard buffers accept between 1 and 80 characters. When that limit is exceeded, the additional information is either forgotten or written over the information that already exists in the buffer (a phenomenon known as keyboard rollover). This scenario exists any time the computer cannot catch up to the typist. If it continually goes unnoticed, such an error can create havoc with a document. Likewise, when the computer is so busy that it can only keep up with the typist after the buffer is partially full, there may be a continual lag between what is typed and what appears on the screen.

Software performance should also be assessed with respect to text manipulation. Functions that are significantly affected by system response time include inserting and reformatting as well as saving and retrieving text. Speed of operation can be influenced by hardware as well as software. Obviously, microprocessor speed can affect any computer function. However, the speed of saving and retrieving text is affected by the operating system involved and the amount of software manipulation the text must undergo before being displayed or stored. Although still dependent on hardware to some extent (particularly the microprocessor), inserting and reformatting text is largely dependent on software. Ask the salesperson to demonstrate these features. Be wary of any software package that requires more than a few seconds to insert a paragraph or change the margins and reformat a section of text.

Software performance can be dependent upon hardware in many ways. Computers with the same microprocessors running at different speeds can have significantly different system response times when running the same software with the same information input. In addition, hardware extras such as coprocessors, print buffers, and intelligent peripherals can make software performance seem better than it is. Therefore, it is imperative to compare software packages on the same machine or same type of machine when trying to choose between different programs.

System speed can also be affected by other features. For example, is the word processor disk- or memory-based? Memory-based systems can store and retrieve text 20 to 30 times faster than a corresponding disk-based system. In addition, disk-based systems are much slower at searching documents and take more of a risk when moving sections of text within a document. If possible, ask the salesperson to show you how the system performs with a large document. Differences in performance between programs may be noticeable only when working with large documents. This is particularly true when comparing disk- versus memory-based systems. Under these conditions a disk-based system will bog down fast.

It is essential to assess software speed by testing all the previously mentioned components of program performance. Usually, no single program is outstanding in every one of the features. Trade-offs are made in each area of the software to achieve the balance that is most satisfactory. The physician must assess which trade-offs are most important and then find the software package that most closely fits these needs.

System capacity is an additional component of word processing software to be assessed. Like execution speed, system capacity is also somewhat determined by hardware capabilities. However, the magnitude of random access memory will affect only the total amount of information stored and not the characteristics of the way in which it is stored. Certain memory-based systems place limits on the size of the document or the total number of lines or characters in any one file. When searching for the "right" word processing software, estimate the maximum number of pages that the program will be asked to manipulate. An adequate software package should be able to handle at least twice as much information as your maximum estimate. This prevents underestimation of future growth and needs. Likewise, the consumer should also determine whether the software will be expected to generate manuscripts, simple correspondence, or both before attempting to select a program.

Although disk-based systems may be slower than memory-based systems, they are usually capable of handling much larger documents with only the floppy or hard disk as a limit. Although a given word processing package may not place a limit on document size, there may be other bothersome capacity limitations, such as limiting the number of characters per line or the number of lines per page. Most good word processing packages allow the page to be any length (thus accommodating unusual paper sizes) and allow at least 256 characters per line; some programs allow much more. Other limitations that can be annoying include limits on the distance that a block of text can be moved within a document. This limitation can significantly increase the time it takes to move a block of text long distances within a manuscript because moving the block would require hopping (moving the block of text its maximum distance several times in order to place it in the appropriate location).

System capacity adds another trade-off that must be considered when software engineers design programs. Although memory-based systems are fast, they present limitations on the amount of information the system can hold, and this is often a significant drawback. Initially, with first- and second-generation microcomputers, programmers made a more extensive trade-off on system speed in order to achieve high-capacity storage that included large documents. With the evolution of large, inexpensive random access memories and 16-bit microprocessors, fewer trade-offs on speed are being made, and software is becoming more memory-based. Still, many currently available programs have one or more of the preceding limitations owing to program idiosyncrasies or attempts to increase system speed.

A small but significant factor in a software purchase is the price. Prices range from $30 for individual basic word processing package to thousands of dollars for an integrated system. The cost depends on several factors. Increasing the number of professionals who share a particular software package (in a multiple practice, for example) can significantly reduce the cost per person. In addition, the amount of use a given program receives is also important. One is more likely to make a significant investment in a word processing package that integrates information from many programs as opposed to a graphics package that has limited capabilities. Naturally, differences in speed of operation and system capacity as well as the number of features will also greatly alter the purchase price. Because software is competitively priced with regard to its features, the appropriate package can be found only by establishing one's needs and assessing the trade-offs.

The Two Types of Word Processing Packages Currently Available

There are two types of word processing packages currently available. One is a screen formatting or "type-as-you-go" program. With screen formatting programs, the printed material on the monitor is exactly as it will be seen on a hard copy printout. This is the most popular type of word processor because it is easy to learn, operate, and understand. Some offer menus that list the functions that may be activated at any point in the program. Thus, the user is not expected to memorize every function. Experienced users have the option of limiting the amount of help in order to increase program speed and allow more information to be presented on the screen at one time. Screen formatting programs are most useful when generating short letters, memoranda, and straightforward manuscripts. Footnotes and switching formats (changing margins often or line spacing) are not as easily accommodated, although still possible. Also, the format of the typing environment, such as preset tabs, margins, and line spacing, may not be preserved from day to day and must be reset each time the machine is turned on.

Screen formatting programs may be slower than other types of software. Because the program has to both store and format the information at the same time, keyboard rollover can sometimes be a problem, and the user may occasionally have to stop and wait for the computer to finish a task. At other times, screen formatting programs can actually save time. Programs of this type can usually print a previously established file and allow a new file to be typed in at the same time because the file being printed requires little processing time, since it has already been formatted before storage on disk.

A criticism of screen formatting packages used to be that information that had been accidentally erased could not be immediately recalled. However, many of the newer packages include the capability to undo the last several commands. Because it can prevent a major user-related accident, this program feature should be considered as important as the ability to insert or delete words when assessing the capabilities of various software packages.

The other type of word processing package available is known as a printer formatting program. In these programs, the final format is created during the printing of the document. This is popular among technical writers because it easily accommodates footnotes and awkward formatting. Besides making footnotes easier, printer formatting programs are also much easier to use for such things as curricula vitae and bibliographies. However, this type of word processing program is more difficult to learn than screen formatting packages and can be awkward because the user cannot see the final format until it is printed. In addition, the intermediate interpretive step can cause problems if formatting problems are encountered. This is often frustrating and wastes time.

Keyboard rollover is rarely a problem with printer formatting packages because the computer can pay full attention to the typist. It is not trying to interpret commands, manipulate text, and receive text at the same time. Unfortunately, a previously stored file cannot usually be printed at the same time that a new file is being keyed in because the file to be printed requires computer interpretation. On the positive side, this type of word processing program usually tends to have fewer and more generalized commands. Thus, there is less information for the user to memorize, making the program easier to operate.

An unfortunate problem with both screen and printer formatting word processing programs is the loss of information that occurs with a system crash. Certain programs, particularly disk-based ones, tend to lose less information than others. Many programs have automatic disk storage of the current file being edited. With this type of program, those parts of the file that are on disk when the system crashes (perhaps due to a power loss) will not be lost. Stay away from programs that automatically update disk contents without being told to do so; they may cause unwanted loss of information. In contrast, program features such as automatically backing up files with the most recent, previously edited version can prevent a minor glitch or user error from wasting one's time and effort.

In deciding whether to purchase a screen or printer formatting program, the physician must assess the extent and type of tasks that the program will be asked to perform. For example, a screen formatting package would be a necessity if it was going to be used to design templates (standard forms) into which information could be inserted, as in the process of recording a history and physical examination. Generally, it is also more convenient to use a screen formatting package in the generation of simple letters and correspondence because the information can be viewed on screen as it will be printed. On the other hand, it may be more convenient to use a printer formatting package if the program was being used to write and update manuscripts, texts, and curricula vitae (as in an academic setting). Many physicians will have a need for both types of software packages. A medical practice with both types of software needs would probably do best to purchase an individual printer formatting program as well as an integrated package that contains screen formatting software. In this way, all needs are satisfied. However, remember that files generated on one type of word processor are generally not accepted by the other type.

Comparing Features and Performance

There are several word processing features that have been developed over the last 10 years and are now considered essential in all word processing software. A program should be suspect, though not necessarily fatally flawed, if it is deficient in or lacks availability of one or more of the following.

The rearrangement of sentences and paragraphs is a common need when editing a document. Programs refer to this cutting and pasting process as "block movement," in which the sentence or paragraph is the block of text. To perform this function, most programs place an identification marker at the beginning and end of the block. By moving the cursor to the appropriate location and then typing the proper command sequence, the block of text can be moved, copied, deleted, or even moved to a separate file on disk. Several problems can occur with this process, depending upon the program. An unfortunate drawback of certain software is the inability to break up lines when moving a block. With this limitation, the identification markers can demarcate only whole lines of text and therefore extraneous fragments at the beginning and end of the block must be trimmed and corrected after the process is completed. Limitations on the extent of block movement within a document are also annoying because they necessitate hopping, as mentioned previously. In addition, the paragraph in which the block was inserted may need to be reformed (that is, words are moved around; this is done with a separate command) because the insertion process can disrupt margins. This latter problem occurs only with screen formatting programs. Finally, an assessment of the block movement function can derive a great deal of information about the software because it can test the program's speed of operation as well as the awkwardness of its commands.

Simple editing functions that all programs should support are insertions, deletions, and overtyping. These functions are slightly more difficult in screen formatting than in printer formatting programs. Text editing in the middle of a formed paragraph with screen formatting software also requires the additional step of reforming the paragraph. Overtyping simply allows you to type over the screen printed text, so program speed cannot be accurately assessed with this function. Insertions, however, are a useful means for assessing software speed because the program has to move a segment of text following the insertion in order to make room for it. Different programs move that block of text with different techniques; therefore, response time varies. Any program will seem to have a good response time if only a few sentences follow the insertion point. Differences between systems can be adequately appreciated only if several paragraphs or pages of text follow the insertion point; this is the way in which it will be used in normal practice.

The command sequences for insertions, deletions, and overtyping should be simple and straightforward. These will be the most frequently used editing functions, and their ease of use is a most important consideration in the choice of software. The number of necessary keystrokes required to perform a function should be carefully scrutinized. For example, some programs use no more than two keystrokes to delete a word, paragraph, or sentence. On the other hand, other programs may not offer intermediate deletions like word deletion; thus, to delete an average six-character word requires six keystrokes of the character delete key. A similar problem will occur with the sentence delete command if a paragraph delete function is not offered. Typically, the number of keystrokes per function performed provides a good measure of software performance.

An editing option that can be of great value in the generation of technical manuscripts and texts is the search and replace function. This command allows the user to tell the computer to look through a document for a particular name, word, or phrase and to change it as you specify. This function is particularly useful to scientists and physicians because it prevents the writer from having to type out long, often-used phrases. For example, the abbreviations DOE or COPD are often used in writing a medical history and physical examination. With only a few keystrokes, the physician who uses these abbreviations could have the phrases "dyspnea on exertion" and "chronic obstructive pulmonary disease" automatically inserted throughout the document wherever the abbreviations appear. In essence, a physician could create a whole series of abbreviations that could be used to make the writing of such information almost no work at all. The search and replace function can also be used to update old documents or to change names and addresses within documents. Not only does this make updating faster, but it also makes it more accurate because the computer is highly unlikely to miss the phrases it is replacing.

Editing a document requires functions that allow the user to scroll through the text without necessarily making changes. Screen scrolling and cursor movement are necessary and useful functions that allow a document to be quickly examined and proofread. Many programs provide varying scroll rates to allow a user to read a document as it rolls by at the selected speed. The ability to make the cursor jump to desired locations within a document is another necessary feature of word processing software. Some programs allow markers to be placed throughout a document to identify locations that can be moved to. Also, an important feature of most programs is the ability to jump to the beginning or end of the document with a single command. Many word processing programs significantly slow down when asked to jump to the end or the beginning of a long file. This is particularly true of disk-based systems. However, certain software packages use programming tricks to avoid long delays in jumping from one segment to another; therefore, some programs perform better than others.

Differences in performance speed can also be detected through the speed of cursor movement. Often, the speed of movement will vary, depending upon the direction of movement (right, left, up, down). In addition, cursor movement may also be considerably slowed when the program is in the insert mode. Because the speed of cursor movement and the type and availability of scrolling are good indicators of software performance, they should be prime considerations in the selection of a software package.

The availability of unusual formatting capabilities such as subscripts, superscripts, underlining, and boldface type can make the difference between a dull monograph and a well-understood paper. However, these features can be utilized only if the printer is capable of taking advantage of them. Many office consultants and industry experts suggest that software should be the first aspect of a computer system that is selected so that hardware requirements can be matched to the software capabilities. Although not as important as other functions, the number of keystrokes required to perform each formatting option should be assessed along with their absence or availability.

Currently, all word processing software offers the capability to print justified text. Text that has been right justified has a smooth edge on both the right and left margins. This option allows a document to look more like a professionally typeset manuscript. Justification adds formality to a document and may make it easier to read. All word processing programs provide justified text only as an option because justified text is inappropriate in many settings. For example, unjustified text appears more natural in letters and other correspondence. In addition to justification, many programs also allow text to be aligned on the right. Right alignment keeps the right edge of the text flush and allows the left edge to be ragged. This can be useful in writing letters because addresses and signatures can be held flush with the right margin.

Screen formatting word processors have several indigenous characteristics that should be assessed; among them are word wrapping, soft-hyphens, on-screen page breaks, and a screen-oriented display. Word wrapping allows the user to type a continuous ribbon of text with no need to pay attention to margins, carriage returns, or line feeds. With this function, the program automatically moves any partially completed word at the end of a line to the next line as the user keeps typing. As an adjunct feature, many programs will ask the user whether or not a particularly long word should be hyphenated when it does not fit within the margins at the end of a sentence. This is helpful because it avoids large gaps in justified text or long spaces at the ends of lines. These hyphens are called "soft-hyphens" because they may be removed by the software if the paragraph is reformed and the whole word should fit on a line.

On-screen page breaks can be helpful to the writer because they indicate how information will be separated on the printout. An often frustrating process with printer formatting programs is the inability to determine where information will be separated. More often than not, an initial draft is printed to determine how to restructure the text so that certain information appears on the same page as it is needed; then the final draft is printed. Page breaks in screen formatting programs allow instantaneous modification of the text so that less time and paper are needed. In addition, since the editing process often involves inserting sections of text, page breaks allow the user to determine how the insertion has affected all the pages of information following it.

Even screen-oriented programs frequently do not display print enhancements such as underlining, boldfacing, and italics on the monitor. When they do, it is often at the expense of speed and performance. In this regard, their output is no better than that from a printer formatting package. Also, many current programs do not allow different type fonts to be displayed on the screen. Often, programs that do take advantage of these unusual formatting capabilities require additional hardware. Although screen-oriented display of these special features may be useful, such capabilities are generally considered luxuries and do not yet play a significant role in selection of software.

Large-scale text manipulation in the form of generating personalized letters from a form letter and a data file is an important feature of word processors. The generic letter, or boilerplate, as it is called, specifies the type and location of information that is to be retrieved from the data file. A separate program or subroutine merges the boilerplate with the file that contains the variable information. The personalized letters are created during the printout, are never stored, and therefore do not occupy disk storage space. The file merging program usually comes as an additional program, and usually an additional fee must be paid. Its utility cannot be overstated; it is usually worth the investment.

Important file-related features of word processing programs include the availability of automatic file backup and concurrent printing and editing. Automatic file backup is a useful feature because it prevents the user from wasting time manually creating backup copies. In addition, it prevents loss of information due to either bad storage media or an electronic glitch. Generally, if the computer system crashes when you are trying to write or read from a disk file, information can be permanently lost. In the case of a large document which was being stored after being edited, this would be a disaster. With the backup copy, at least those parts that were present prior to editing can be retrieved. The only drawback to a backup system is that it realistically halves the amount of information that can be stored on a disk.

Concurrent with the evolution and demonstrated need of multi-tasking, software that could print a file and edit a separate file at the same time was introduced to the market. The usefulness of these programs may rely on the amount of hardware support that they receive. Programs that can rely upon a print buffer to receive a large amount of information at one time are much more efficient than those that must continually feed information to the printer. Without a print buffer, there may be a significant incidence of keyboard rollover accompanied by a lag between what is keyed in and what is seen on the screen. Also, programs may not function well because a particular processor speed is too slow to handle the multi-tasking. Again, selection of the appropriate hardware is necessary in order to receive the maximum from the program and the system.

Programs that check grammar, punctuation, and spelling greatly decrease the amount of time it takes to proofread a document and increase the accuracy of the process. Although each program can easily cost as much as 50 per cent or more of the word processing program cost, they can pay for themselves (in the amount of time they save) faster than any other individual part of the system.

Unfortunately, no single, currently available program contains every positive feature of each of the previously listed attributes. Indeed, such a feat would be impossible because trade-offs are made to achieve superiority in certain areas. The "right" program will be found only with a thorough review of the user's needs and preferences. Watch for good documentation and avoid programs that seem too simple. As experience is gained, simple programs become tedious and cumbersome. Be wary of programs that can be operated only with menus that are an integral part of the command system. In these programs, one has to wait for the machine to offer a menu and ask for a selection. In this situation, too much help is as bad as too little. The same corollary holds true for computer software in general; the key is to find the right middle ground.

ELECTRONIC SPREADSHEETS

Important Considerations

As with all software, program documentation is an important consideration when selecting a spreadsheet program; each of the points mentioned in the assessment of word processing documentation hold true for spreadsheets as well. Unlike a word processing program, which may be used with some degree of proficiency without reading the manual or having any degree of experience, spreadsheet usage is not all straight-forward and requires good documentation. Well-written manuals and tutorials are needed in order to acquaint the user with simple commands and spreadsheet basics. Most popular programs are menu-oriented to a limited extent. Unfortunately, the abbreviations and phrases in the menu are not always self-explanatory, and complete descriptions of these functions can be provided only in the documentation. Obviously, pro-grams that are command-driven are at the mercy of their documentation to an even greater extent. Good spreadsheet documentation should include a summary card, a tutorial, and a reference guide.

Additional hardware compatibility problems can arise other than conflicts between the software and the microprocessor or manufacturer type. A commonly overlooked problem is the amount of memory a program requires in order to be used effectively. Lotus 1–2–3 requires 256,000 units of memory in order to provide a useful worksheet. The program itself uses almost 70,000 units of memory to store its instruc-tions. At the other end of the spectrum, VisiCalc works comfortably within computers with 64,000 units of memory or less. Obviously, there are considerable differences in program capabilities between the two programs.

Additional hardware incompatibilities may arise in areas besides memory size. In programs such as Lotus 1–2–3, which offers an extensive graphics package, it is important to determine whether or not a special monitor (for color, high resolution) and integrated circuitry will be necessary to display the information. Also, spreadsheets that offer tele-communications may require a modem and other associated hardware in order to be utilized to their fullest potential.

Choosing the proper spreadsheet requires a careful analysis of the type and magnitude of the tasks that it will be performing. These estimates are important because they will narrow the list of potentially usable spreadsheets based upon the maximum number of data cells needed.

An additional dimension to be considered in choosing an electronic spreadsheet is the cost:benefit ratio. Perhaps 16,000 cells will present enough data storage and work space for a physician working with a small amount of data and a limited number of calculations. If this is the case, it is unlikely that a large investment in an expensive spreadsheet will be beneficial. However, it is surprising how fast cells can be filled in a worksheet when working with even a moderately sized set of data. Not only does each piece of data occupy one cell, but each intermediate sum and calculated value as well as formulas, labels, and final results also occupy a cell. Moreover, larger data sets are more difficult to manipulate, and a user may benefit from the additional functions offered by more expensive spreadsheet software. These additional functions and increased worksheet size need to be weighed against the additional expense of the software.

Spreadsheets — What They Do

The physician needs to have a thorough grasp of the abilities and inabilities of spreadsheet software before selecting a program. A spreadsheet is not an adequate substitute for a desk calculator. Although it could perform the same functions and more, the spreadsheet would be more time-consuming and cumbersome to use than a calculator for simple calculations. However, spreadsheets are quite useful in situations that require iterative calculations. Because spreadsheets use numbers in much the same way that word processors use text, spreadsheets have been informally termed "numeric word processors," a term that reflects the way in which spreadsheets work as well as the end result of their activity. Spreadsheets conveniently allow data sets to be edited and updated with a minimum of effort by simply moving the cursor around the worksheet. In addition, they are capable of performing instant recalculations of all the formulas in the spreadsheet after editing or when switching between different sets of data. In this way, different scenarios and settings can be tested without manually recalculating every formula in the spreadsheet. Instant recalculation of all formulas in the spreadsheet prevents small changes in the data set (forgotten data that is subsequently found and added to the sheet) from becoming a large headache.

Spreadsheets are also likely to be more accurate than other manual means of data processing. Before the final calculations, all the data can be checked for accuracy and stored on disk. If questions should arise in the future about the quality of the data or calculations, the worksheet can be recalled for review. This ability to recall results and intermediate calculations can be invaluable. In addition, calculation of values from a verified data set prevents arithmetical errors or errors due to typing in a wrong number on a calculator.

Spreadsheets — The Basics

An electronic spreadsheet is a two-dimensional matrix of cells that make up a grid of rows and columns. In many ways, the spreadsheet resembles a ledger pad. In most programs, the columns of the spreadsheet are labeled with a letter of the alphabet; after "z," columns are labeled "aa," "ab," "ac," and so on. Likewise, each row is given a number starting with "1." The letters and numbers appears on the screen across the top of the rows and down the left side of the columns. With this system, each cell in the matrix has a unique address. By referring to a cell's address in a formula, the contents of that cell are accessed and may be used in a calculation. Every cell in the worksheet may contain only one item of information. The information may be a value—either a number or a formula telling how to calculate a number. It may also be a piece of text—a sequence of characters used to label a formula, highlight certain pieces of information, or describe the data.

The ability to recalculate an entire worksheet when even a single number is changed is what gives spreadsheets their power and value as forecasting and "what if" tools. However, the spreadsheet is not limited to just being used as a forecasting tool. Because data sets can be stored and retrieved independently of the formulas and format of the spreadsheet, it is also a powerful data processing tool. For physicians, such capabilities might be useful in the assessment of pulmonary or cardiovascular status, in retrospective analyses, and in the determination of descriptive statistics about a private patient population.

In many ways, electronic spreadsheets act as programming languages. The user gives the spreadsheet a set of instructions and the spreadsheet executes them. Unlike a programming language, spreadsheets are meant to be used interactively so that information can be derived from the instructions instantaneously. Unlike a programming language, most of the instructions are easy to understand and use. For example, instructions like "max" followed by a list of cell addresses will return the maximum value of the contents of those cells. Likewise, the command "average" followed by a range of cell addresses will return the average value. When a command is inserted into a cell, the result of that command, and not the command itself, is keyed into that cell. When the cursor moves to that cell and highlights the result, the command that obtained that result is usually displayed at the top of the screen. Thus, when viewing a worksheet, the user sees only a worksheet of data and results; none of the formulas is displayed unless a cursor highlights a formula-containing cell.

Simpler functions such as addition and subtraction; logical boolean operators such as "and," "or," and "not"; and conditional "if . . . then" statements are universally supported commands in all spreadsheet programs. By using these commands appropriately, a physician can customize a spreadsheet to any application. Although the process is compared to programming, the limited instruction set and logical commands allow spreadsheets to be used by even the most naive computer novices. More importantly, because all programs allow a worksheet to be stored on disk and recalled at a later date, an application never needs to be programmed twice. The worksheet may be reused as needed, allowing each set of data with results to be stored separately.

Besides an extensive set of calculation functions, most spreadsheets also support a set of instructions that allow the user to design the hard copy output. With these features, only the information that is most important to a presentation or report need be printed. In addition, output formatting commands may be used to direct results to the appropriate word processing software in a multi-tasking environment. The ability to tailor the output of a spreadsheet program is essential, and those programs with limited or minimal capabilities for manipulation of the output should be approached with caution.

A spreadsheet template is a worksheet environment that has been developed for a particular purpose and is usually purchased independently of the program. A series of related templates for a spreadsheet program is known as a model. For example, a model might be used to determine the amount of income tax returns or to evaluate a stock portfolio. When many professionals share a common problem that can be solved with a spreadsheet, a template is usually standardized and made available for purchase. A packaged template saves the user from working out formulas and structuring them into a workable spreadsheet. The nominal price of a template is overwhelmingly balanced by the time and effort that it saves.

Attributes of Most Spreadsheets

The following characteristics outline several important attributes of electronic spreadsheets which should be assessed when choosing between programs. Software packages that do not support some of the following considerations should be carefully scrutinized.

Macros and Programming. Because all spreadsheet programs require a series of commands to carry out the various functions, any command that reduces the number of keystrokes necessary to manipulate the data could be very useful. Commands that perform these functions are referred to as "macros." A macro is a single command that executes a set of instructions that have been previously stored by the user. A macro could be used to cut down on the amount of keyboarding required to fill a worksheet with data. For example, a macro may include a set of instructions to retrieve data from a file, place it appropriately in the worksheet, and then initiate worksheet recalculation. By using only a few keystrokes to activate the macro, the user may have saved several minutes of manual labor.

As macros have become more powerful, spreadsheets have actually evolved their own programming languages. These languages consist of strings of macros that may direct large and repetitive tasks. The difference between this type of programming and that in a standard computer language is that in this case the spreadsheet itself is handling the basic mathematical calculations, whereas in the traditional languages hundreds of lines of code would be needed to specify those calculations. For instance, with a spreadsheet macro language the user who wants to use the sum of a column of figures in a formula needs only to call upon the cell on the spreadsheet containing that sum. In traditional programming the user would have to define variables and instruct the computer to add them together to perform the same operation.

Floating Point Arithmetic. Another desirable spreadsheet feature is the ability to round off data values in a spreadsheet to a specified number of decimal places. Most programs will allow rounded numbers to be displayed but will retain the unrounded numbers in memory and use them in all subsequent calculations. This is a critical point to assess in a spreadsheet program. If the software retains only the rounded numbers, inaccuracies may appear in the result owing to the loss in precision. On the other hand, data tables and results may be difficult to read if a program does not offer a rounding feature or if the feature is not used because of its effects on accuracy. In assessing this function, it is also necessary to determine whether numbers sent to the printer or disk for storage are also rounded. Storage of rounded numbers will cause inaccuracies when working with the data set in the future, even though the current results may be valid.

Statistical Operations. The recent availability of built-in statistical functions in some spreadsheets has significantly enhanced their utility to the basic and clinical researcher. The statistical features offered are not extensive; however, they usually include mean, standard deviation, standard error, and confidence intervals. Statistical functions, which are a part of the spreadsheet instruction set, prevent mistakes (and wasted effort) when programming these features into a worksheet. Naturally, the presence of these features is not as important to the private physician as it is to those in academic medicine.

When setting up a worksheet for a particular application, the contents of cells are continually being revised and additional cells are being added. An important utility that makes this process much simpler is the ability to readily take the contents of some cell(s) and move it to some cell(s) in a different location of the worksheet. This feature prevents user error that may occur in the process of manually copying a cell's contents. This may be particularly important in the design of a large template in which manual movement of cells could be very time-consuming. Thus, this feature's availability and relative ease of use should be a prime concern of the buyer.

Error Checking and Speed. All spreadsheets provide some form of error detection. However, the extent of detection varies significantly from program to program. At the very minimum, the software should be able to determine and then notify the user when a cell is missing a numeric entry or if text is where a number is expected to be. Unfortunately, many programs can detect these errors but cannot notify the user. Therefore, inaccurate results are recorded, and the user is unaware of the problem. Occasionally, a keyboarding error can call for calculations that are mathematically impossible, such as dividing by zero. A good program should be able to not only detect an impossible calculation but also notify the user of its occurrence and identify the cell in which it has occurred. Quite often, software performance can be easily assessed by testing the amount of error detection a program offers. As a general rule, a hallmark of well-written programs is high-quality error detection. In contrast, poorly written programs usually do not detect errors well; thus, an assessment of the extent of error detection is one clue to the quality of the spreadsheet program.

Multidirectional scrolling is an important capability that is not supported by all spreadsheet software. Because only 20 rows by 8 to 10 columns can be displayed on the screen at any one time, the ability to scroll the worksheet in four directions allows all sections of the worksheet to be viewed quickly on the monitor. Poorly written programs may allow screen jumping only when trying to move in certain directions. This prevents areas of border-zone information from being viewed together.

The speed of the software as the cursor scrolls across a filled worksheet is another indicator of program performance. In this situation the program must completely rearrange a full screen of information (perhaps several thousand characters), and, thus, the speed of the scrolling software can be used to differentiate between software packages. Unfortunately, the demonstration models salespeople use to sell their products may not always utilize the worksheet as extensively as it ultimately will be used. To circumvent this problem, ask for a complicated template such as "accounts receivable" to be demonstrated and use a large data set. In this way, the system performance can be objectively assessed with regard to its calculation as well as editing speed (scrolling).

Output capability is a standard feature of all spreadsheets. However, like many other things, the quality of the output software may vary considerably. Some programs allow complete customization of the printout, yet others use a standard format every time. With a personalized output, spreadsheet results can be directly incorporated into a report without the further manipulation that would be required with a standardized output. Output capabilities should also be available for the transfer of data to disk and for linkage with other programs. This allows important results to be shared between programs and within an integrated package.

DATA BASES

Local Versus Public Data Bases

The recent introduction of high-quality microcomputer data base software—or local data bases—has brought many useful capabilities to the microcomputer that were once offered only on mainframes. Currently, mainframe data base systems that can be reached through the telephone lines—or public data bases—are used almost exclusively in applications that require a large memory capacity, such as searching for journal articles. Although mainframe data base systems exist on time-sharing computers, many features make them unusable for private data manipulation. For example, public data bases usually limit their users to "read only" access of information. Thus, users cannot add information to an established data base that subsequently may be needed by them. Also, public data bases have a fixed data structure that allows a search to proceed in only certain directions. Such data bases do not allow the user to create additional associations between categories when needed. Likewise, the limited command set offered to users does not permit establishment of data files for manipulation of private information. Therefore, most public data bases are used for a single purpose (bibliographic indexing, monitoring disease). This is unlike the typical environment of time-sharing systems in which each user is performing widely varying tasks. The "read only" nature, rigid structure, and specific focus makes public data bases most useful as electronic libraries.

Private data base management is offered on time-sharing computers separately from public data bases. However, such services are usually reserved for large corporations. No physician or group of physicians could afford to maintain a large data base in a mainframe facility owing to the prohibitive cost. For the doctor, such capabilities can be economically performed on a microcomputer. Aside from the initial programs cost, data base management on a microcomputer incurs its only cost in the acquisition of storage media, such as disks, and in using electricity, which is minimal. Local data base software can be customized to any application and expanded at will. Local data base systems may be used to maintain patient records, manage research data, or track appointments, staff assignments, and patient follow-ups.

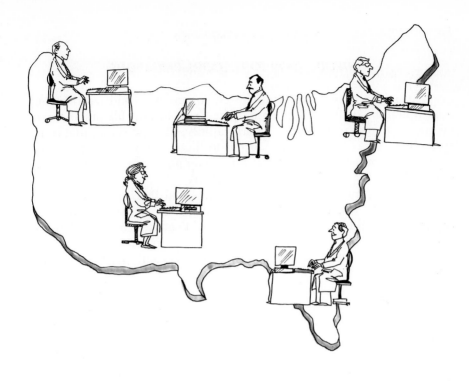

F I V E

Use of the Electronic Network

Charles E. Stewart, M.D.

INTRODUCTION TO TELECOMMUNICATIONS

Physicians have already purchased computers to aid with the business functions of the office, employing them to bill, fill out insurance claims, and produce "form" letters rapidly. The power available to a computer user is in direct proportion to the amount of data the user is able to manipulate and collect with that computer. That power does not end with writing checks and collecting bills.

Imagine a medical library in your hospital that holds over 10,000 volumes of the latest works on medical research, statistics, and current drug therapy, all within 1 to 3 months of publication in a medical journal. Now imagine that all these publications are linked together so that looking up data on a subject in one will also pull all volumes with related data off the shelf and open them to the proper page. Further imagine that you can search these volumes for any word, phrase, or topic that you desire, and that you are not limited to just index entries. Now imagine that you can enter this library, at your convenience, at home or at the office.

That library is available now, using any standard personal microcomputer and a telephone interface. Physicians can dial into huge, up-to-date medical data bases so quickly and efficiently that this concept threatens to make medical textbooks and journals obsolete. In recent years, private companies have begun providing information networks or data banks specifically for physicians with individual data bases covering everything from pharmacy to dentistry. It is no great exaggeration to predict that the traditional journals and printed medical references may someday be replaced by a microcomputer with telephone access devices.

There is a lot of technical jargon involved in telecommunications that makes for intimidating reading. This chapter proposes to answer three basic questions:
- What sort of hardware and software will be required to use these new developments?
- What kind of information is available to me right now?
- What does the future hold?

The technical information in this chapter is meant to allow choices of operational details rather than a complete explanation of how and why the systems work. If a more detailed explanation is required, please check one of the books listed at the end of the chapter.

To access any of the data bases noted in this chapter, you do not need to invest in a computer. Purchase of a modem and a simple display terminal will allow access with reduced capabilities. The computer with appropriate software allows saving the data and reusing it without retyping it. It also will allow quicker and more convenient access to the data.

FUNDAMENTALS NEEDED FOR EFFECTIVE COMMUNICATION

Let's begin with a short definition of telecomputing as the transfer of information between two or more computers using the telephone network as the medium of communication instead of direct cable communication. This transfer of information will require a microcomputer capable of data transmission through a "serial" pathway to the telephone. What this means is that the 8-bit code defining a character will be sent one bit a time to the receiving computer, followed by the next character's code. This stream of bits does not spill forth haphazardly. Both ends of the system must agree on how each of the characters will be coded, how fast they will be sent, and how the characters will be separated.

In the most commonly used system of serial data transmission, the computer adds a "start" bit to mark the start of a character and a "stop" bit to mark the end of a character. The receiving computer does not therefore need to have you type at a steady rate, but can tell where the beginning and the end of a character are by the start and stop bits. This method of separating characters is referred to as *asynchronous communications* because the transmitting computer does not have to be synchronized with the receiving computer to separate each character.

In *synchronous transmissions* characters are not sent one at a time, but rather, they are sent as a large block of characters. This means that each character does not need a start and stop bit. The computer knows that another character will follow immediately after the current one with no gap between until the end of a block is reached. This makes for more efficient use of the communications line but also requires more sophisticated hardware and software. Synchronous computer communications are not required for communication with any of the services described in this chapter.

Most systems for the physician are set up to allow asynchronous data transfer. The asynchronous hardware and software are cheaper and more widely available than with the synchronous protocols and hardware.

Obviously, the two computers must agree on how fast each character will be transmitted. There are two standard ways of specifying the transmission speed of data: baud rate and bits per second. Baud is a measure of how many signal transitions are transmitted per second, and bits per second (bps) is a measure of how many units of information are transmitted. Technically, the two terms aren't the same, but at the lower speeds usable on telephone lines, they can be interchanged. Table 5–1 notes common baud rates.

Modems

Moving from the computer to the telephone system requires a change from the transistor direct current logic of the computer to an alternating

Table 5–1. Common Baud Rates

Low speed
   100 baud (10 characters per second)
   300 baud (30 characters per second)
   600 baud (60 characters per second)
Medium speed
   1200 baud (120 characters per second)
   2400 baud (240 characters per second)
High speed (usually computer to computer)
   4800 baud (480 characters per second)
   9600 baud (960 characters per second)

tone frequency acceptable to the telephone system and back to the computer's direct current at the far end. This modulation of the outgoing pulses and demodulation of the incoming pulses is accomplished by a small device called a *modem*. Modems were invented to translate digital square waves into a form compatible with telephone equipment. There are multiple specifications for the frequencies to be used for receiver and transmitter based upon speed of transmission, country, the transmitting computer, and the receiving computer.

The rate-limiting step of the telecommunications process is the telephone system. The frequency range of the phone has been designed to allow maximal intelligible speech transmission in the frequencies of 300 to 3300 cycles per second. The telephone network therefore provides only 3100 hertz of bandwidth. This small bandwidth limits the rate of information that can be transmitted. The modulated signal needs a bandwidth or range of frequencies that is greater than the rate of change of the carrier (the baud rate). A 300-baud modem needs at least 300 hertz of bandwidth, a 1200-baud modem needs 1200 hertz of bandwidth, and a 9600-baud modem needs at least 9600 hertz. To impose binary data on the audio carrier at the higher rates, a more complex modulation scheme is needed than that used for changing frequencies. This more complex modulation scheme means more complex electronics, higher costs, and more possible errors. Unfortunately, these schemes are also based on a reliable bandwidth of 3100 hertz. Real phones have noise, echos, and poor connections. Reliable transmission is limited to 1200 baud on most telephones, with noisy lines limiting some users to 300 baud because of frequent errors at higher rates. Special "conditioned" lines are required for transmission of data at higher speeds. These conditioned lines are too expensive for small computer users. Although higher speeds are available, they are not yet practical. Low- to medium-speed 300 to 1200-baud modems are the most popular choices (Table 5–2).

An important point to note is that the originating modem will transmit on the frequencies that the answering modem expects to receive on. The same relationship holds true for the originating modem's receiv-

Table 5–2.

Bell 103 low-speed protocol
Originate modem (sending)
binary 1 = 1270 cycles per second (hertz)
binary 0 = 1070 hertz
Answer modem (transmitting)
binary 1 = 2225 hertz
binary 0 = 2025 hertz
CCIT low-speed protocol

ing and the answering modem's transmission frequencies. The proper name for this kind of modulation is frequency shift keying, or FSK.

Low-Speed Modems (Under 1200 Baud). For many purposes, 300-baud modems offer the best bargain value. They are relatively inexpensive ($100 to $200) and work with almost all telephone systems and computers. Some subscription services charge less for 300-baud service. Unfortunately, 300-baud modems are frustratingly slow if you are looking at the data as it is transferred or if you transfer large files often.

Medium-Speed (1200 to 4800 Baud) and High-Speed (>4800 Baud) Modems. The 1200-baud modems are about four times as fast but cost two to three times as much as 300-baud modems ($200 to $300). A 1200-baud modem should be considered if you are going to transmit or receive data frequently or use very large files. As mentioned before, on some telephone lines, even 1200-baud rates are too error-prone for effective use. Now 2400-baud modems are becoming available, but most information utilities are not yet equipped to transmit or receive at this rarified rate; and the modems cost at least twice as much as the 1200-baud modems. Modems over 2400 baud are specialized devices that no hobbyist or small business user is likely to need or afford. Although for a mainframe computer, high-speed modems start at 9600 baud, a high-speed modem for the microcomputer user is generally considered to be anything over 1200 baud.

Protocols commonly used for medium-speed communications are the Bell 212A and Racal-Vadic 3400 standards. Both of these standards use a four-phase modulation but at different carrier frequencies. Both ends of the communications link have to be using the same standard at the same speed. Many of the higher quality medium-speed modems will automatically recognize the frequency and change between protocols rapidly and can also operate at the Bell 103 standard for 300 baud.

Modems for microcomputers may be either "stand-alone" (a small box that sits beside the computer) or internal (a circuit card that is inserted in your computer). There are advantages to both types: Internal cards do not take up valuable desk space, and they use the computer's power supply. External modems may be used with several computers and may be kept when updating to a new computer. External modems are also available with cups for the earpiece of a telephone so that they may be used with multiple-line telephones or phones without modular plugs (acoustic modems). For most people, the difference between an internal and external modem is solely a matter of personal preference. The internal modem makes for a neater computer installation but occupies a slot in the computer that might be needed for other purposes. When the modem is purchased, ensure that the dealer provides the appropriate cables and connectors for your modem and your computer(s).

Programs

After the modem, the computer and the cables are purchased, installed, and attached, the parts will function as a "dumb" terminal. The machinery will work only in a crude fashion to transmit and receive data without appropriate software to connect the parts in a logical fashion. To give the computer intelligence, the parts must all be made to work harmoniously together. With effective communications software, you can automatically dial, receive messages, log into an information service, proceed to the data base of your choice, make a preplanned search, and save all the data retrieved on a disk. All these functions and more are available with modern communications software at the press of only a few keys on the computer keyboard. The cost of the programs ranges from free to hundreds of dollars, but cost is not a good indication of the power of the software. Because programs are revised with new features and new, more powerful programs are frequently introduced for the most popular computers, it would be appropriate to consult with the local "computer gurus" or dealers to find the ones most useful to you that are available for your computer. Some of the best communications programs are available as programs from public domain or free software included with the modem.

Table 5–3 lists programs that have been found to provide superior value and are available for free or at very low cost.

The Data Forwarding Services

If you are living in New York and a data base service is in California, 20 minutes of long-distance communication at daytime prime telephone rates may be quite expensive, regardless of whether you or your computer uses the phone. Fortunately for us, services exist to allow inexpensive forwarding of computer communications between distant cities. Like Sprint and MCI, the data forwarding services have filled a need for long-distance high-speed communications. The prototype for these services

Table 5–3. Commonly Available Communications Software

Ward Christenson's MODEM7
Available for most CP/M systems
Free (see your local computer club)

PC Talk III
Available for IBM PCs and most compatible machines
Free (contribution of $35 requested) (superb value)

KERMIT
Available for many computers
Free (See your university computer center)

Crosstalk
Available for the IBM PC
Included with some modems for free

Smartcom II
Available with all DC-Hayes modems

---

was ARPANET, a network developed to handle communications for the Department of Defense research projects in universities in many cities. Three major data forwarding networks in the United States provide service to the data base services of most interest to physicians. These networks are Tymnet, Telenet, and Uninet. In Canada, Datapac provides a similar service.

Typically these services have established high-speed digital communications networks throughout the world. You can call a computer in Pittsburgh that is constantly linked with computers in San Francisco, Paris, Sydney, New York, and even Cleveland. The charges are quite reasonable, about $4 to $6 per hour.

The networks allow a local or short-distance call into a city "node" via a low- or medium-speed modem. The node computer collects messages for a distant computer and sends it by dedicated phone lines or satellite broadcast to the distant computer at very high speed. Your message might be interspersed with several other messages to achieve the lowest cost rate. As best you can tell, however, you are directly connected to the distant computer.

Now that you have purchased a modem, have connected it to your computer or terminal, have acquired an appropriate software package to make the magic happen, and have the number of your local data transfer network, whom do you call?

THE DATA BASE SERVICES

Medical Data Base Services

There are three basic types of data bases available today: medical literature data bases, collector data bases, and full text data bases. The first type, literature data bases, allows users to search for information from government publications, theses, research papers, journal articles, conference proceedings, monographs, bibliographies, and technical reports. The two most popular medical data bases for the practicing physician are the National Library of Medicine's MEDLINE and the competing Excerpta Medica, produced by a Netherlands-based company (the Medical Database Publishing Division of Elsevier Science Publishers). Printed versions of both of these services are found in most medical libraries. The printed references will contain about 60 per cent of the sources that are available on the computer version. Other medical literature data bases available include conference paper indexes, Epilepsyline, Drug Info/Alcohol Use/Abuse, Health Planning and Administration, Pharmaceutical Literature, Bioethicsline. Depending upon which data base is used, the physician can review on a computer screen abstracts or bibliographic data on any desired subject.

The second type, collector data bases, stores statistics, indicators, and demographics. It has not only search but also comparison features. Using such systems, for example, the physician can request information on adverse reactions to a specific drug or summon up a wide spectrum of case histories to compare symptoms in cases with similar presentations. An example of this type of data base is AMA/Mednet's Disease Information or Drug Information Services. Again, these data bases are available in printed form, but the computer services are updated more frequently and contain more citations than the printed matter. For example, newer diseases such as AIDS and toxic shock syndrome are included in the disease data base but are not available in the printed equivalents.

The third and newest electronic data base is the full text data base. Currently available only through BRS, The Critical Care Medicine Library is a series of reference books on critical care medicine that have been adapted for computer searching. Entire texts are placed on-line. This prototype service allows searching of all on-line texts for the desired subjects and retrieval of either the full text of the paragraphs containing the subject or the bibliographic citation of the works. If this concept becomes as popular as BRS hopes, entire libraries of texts and journals will become available.

The dramatic advantages offered by any electronic data base as compared to the labor-intensive searches of the traditional library are as follows:

1. The speed at which the information can be sought, found, and delivered.

2. The efficiency produced by having data on topics from a cross section of diverse sources, sometimes spanning several decades.

3. The currency of information. Updating the computer version may take only a few minutes, and all who access the computer will have the

current version, yet the publishing process for a book or journal can span a year or more for updates.

In addition to these many advantages, there is the more mundane advantage of being able to do it all from your home or office without going to a central library.

A few words of warning are appropriate, however. These data bases are entered by human beings and are therefore subject to human errors. This means that some data will be entered incorrectly and be improperly indexed. Occasionally, dosages will be in error, and calculations may sometimes be incorrect, just as in printed material. Of course, the errors can be corrected much more easily when found. Searching commands are still unsophisticated and can be frustrating. Such frustration can cost you money as you try to find an article you know is in a journal that is indexed by one of the data bases.

We now are ready to discuss the specific data base services that are available, what they offer, strengths and weaknesses, and their prices.

Dialog and Dialog's Knowledge Index. Dialog is the oldest and largest of the on-line information data base services. A subsidiary of Lockheed Corporation, this collection of over 200 data bases developed from an in-house information retrieval service started in 1963. In 1969, this service was expanded when Lockheed received a NASA contract to organize a half million documents from the space program into a coherent data base. Subsequent government contracts added more information to the system, and a specialized command language was created for searching through this electronic library. The language, Dialog, became the name of the commercial service offered to the public by Lockheed in 1972. Dialog now has indexed some 60,000 journals in addition to dissertations, research and conference reports, patents, government publications, and corporate financial reports. This information adds up to over 70 billion characters of data, which is available to the public for searching. Within Dialog there is a medicine and biosciences group. This group consists of eight data bases for biology, eight data bases for medicine, three collections of pharmacy data, and a zoologic data base (Table 5–4).

In most cases you have the ability to order a copy of an article after you find it. This copying service from Dialog is called DialOrder. It records the request for a copy of an article in a file and transmits this file to a service that will copy and send the article to the user. If translation is required, this can also be arranged at the same time. This service is not cheap! A 10-page article will cost about $8, but it may be the only source of documents from obscure publications or events.

If the number of citations found are more than you would like to print on-line to your home computer, the citations may be printed by Dialog's ultrafast printers and sent to your home for review. This option

Table 5–4. The Dialog Database Family

Biosis Previews (3 files)
CA Search (5 files)
Chemsearch (7 files)
Excerpta Medica (3 files)
Health Planning and Administration
International Pharmaceutical Abstracts
Life Sciences Collection
MEDLINE (3 files)
Mental Health Abstracts
Pharmaceutical News Index
Scisearch (3 files)
Telegen
Zoological Record
Medical Files in Knowledge Index

will often be cheaper for a large citation list than paying for the computer time to download them from Dialog.

Rates: Dialog does not charge a start-up fee, but, at the time of writing this chapter, recommends both their training seminars at $130 and their manuals at $20. The day and a half training seminar is worthwhile, has free search time both at the seminar and afterward at home, and includes a comprehensive training manual. Fees for the Dialog data bases range from $15 per hour to over $100 per hour, with an average fee of about $1 per minute. Medline costs $35 per hour to use from Dialog.

A less expensive service is offered by Dialog to users of microcomputers and is called Knowledge Index. It costs $35 for start-up fees (manuals included) and a flat $24 per hour for every data base available. Knowledge Index is limited in the number of data bases available, and has hours limited to the "after peak" evening hours. Knowledge Index has eight data bases that are designed specifically for the medical profession. The reprint ordering and off-line citation printing services are not available for Knowledge Index. Keep in mind that Dialog is much more expensive, more difficult to use, and uses a completely different set of commands from those of Knowledge Index, but Knowledge Index has a small number of available data bases and shorter working hours.

For an accomplished searcher on Dialog, searches are quick and specific. Commands may be abbreviated, concatenated, and easily reviewed. The search is from the full text of the article's bibliographic citation and abstract. This full text citation search allows articles that have a new disease or symptom not yet indexed to be retrieved easily by selecting articles that merely mention the disease, drug, or search word in the abstract. This "false positive" may result in citations not desired by the searcher, but it also results in a more complete search of the subject. Typical times for an experienced medical searcher to find a specific subject are about 5 to 10 minutes per search at a cost of roughly $10 to $15 to retrieve both bibliographic citations and abstracts. Contrast this with driving to the medical library and spending an hour going through the *Index Medicus* for the last 6 years for citations alone and finally starting to look up the articles that are available in the stacks of the library.

Another word of warning: Do not try to use the service on a weekday afternoon. Hundreds of searchers across the nation will be using the system at that same time, and the search times are prolonged by the multitudes of users. Unfortunately, the clock and the rate meter are continuing to run, and the wait for your slice of the computer can be expensive. If you plan your search beforehand and pick the proper time to access Dialog, even the most expensive data base becomes relatively inexpensive to search. (See equipment section also.)

BRS, BRS/Search, BRS/Colleague Medical, BRS/After Dark. BRS is also a full service, multispecialty data base supplier, just like Dialog. If Dialog is the Hertz of data base services, then BRS is the Avis. Dialog caters to the professional searcher and assumes that you know what you are doing before you log on and start to search. BRS caters to the professional who is using the computer as a tool, but is not necessarily a computer "hacker" or a library or information sciences major interested in remembering every command and nuance of the search strategy.

BRS was inaugurated in 1977 with 10 data bases. The BRS product line now consists of over 80 data bases and caters to three recognized levels of searchers. Institutions and information professionals may choose BRS/Search, which has a relatively complex search language and services available. BRS/Search is comparable in services, price, complexity, and rapidity to Dialog. Generalists may choose BRS/After Dark, which caters to relatively naïve users with limited frills and extensive menu-driven searching at a very low price. Intermediate users can select BRS/Colleague which has ability to order off-line printing of the search and the ability to access the nonmedical data bases at extra cost.

BRS seems to have focused on the medical community as their primary marketing target. Because of this focus, and with the innovations that BRS has started in pricing structure and full text search services, BRS is more useful to most physicians. If a physician wishes to subscribe to only one data base service, then BRS/Colleague should be that service.

BRS started the low cost searching revolution with BRS/After Dark. After Dark uses the BRS computers after work hours. The company can charge a lesser fee because the equipment and service costs are already established to serve the peak time daily users. The extra customers during the low use periods provide essentially "free" income from equipment that has already been committed for peak use times.

To simplify searching for relatively inexperienced users, BRS/After Dark makes extensive use of menus and text displays. The new user will find the command structure simple and easy to remember. Searching capability is excellent, but off-line printing, document retrieval, and complex commands are not used. Sophisticated searchers may stack commands by separating anticipated responses with semicolons. This stacking is somewhat cumbersome, but it does speed the process.

BRS/Colleague caters to the professional who wants to do his or her own searching without intermediaries and without memorizing a complex command language. BRS/Colleague is menu-driven with menus similar to After Dark and is midway in price, complexity, and utility between the Search and After Dark services from BRS. On-line training and tutorials are provided with 1 hour of free searching. Free telephone support is given to those who need further help at all times that the computers are operational. Even with slow menus, the average search among current users takes 10 to 15 minutes for an average cost of $4 to $8.

BRS/Colleague recently inaugurated a new service jointly with W. B. Saunders, medical publishers, providing the full text of 30 textbooks "on-line" as an initial offering. This service has been rapidly expanded to include the full text of a number of medical journals "on-line." These journals include the *New England Journal of Medicine, The Annals of Internal Medicine, Lancet, The British Medical Journal, Drug Information Full-Text,* and *The Medical Letter.* Needless to say, graphics, ECG's and radiographs are not yet available. Currently, the user does not have the option of selecting a single text or browsing through a single journal easily.

The search strategy for full text involves a subtle logic change from that for bibliographic citations. If you search for a myocardial infarction in bibliographic citations, you use the boolean operators "and" and "or." The "and" means to include all articles that have both myocardial and infarction in the article. If this operator is applied to full text, any paragraph with both of these words in it is selected, even though the words are not related in the paragraph. Many physicians who have mastered the techniques of bibliographic searching will be frustrated at the inappropriately high number of articles retrieved that are not related to the question when the same techniques are used with full text.

Only a limited number of data bases are available under the low-cost terms of the subscription, but these include the common medical data bases such as Medline and Health Planning and Administration data bases. Another feature not found in any other service is PRE-MED, BRS's own bibliographic listing of 109 core journals within 10 days of publication. If the subscriber wishes, he or she may access the other 80 or so data bases offered by BRS, but at a substantially higher cost and greater inconvenience. The other data bases will require use of the search language used by the main BRS/Search service.

Rates: BRS/After Dark charges are currently the lowest in the business, with $50 start-up and manual fees and only $6 per hour per data base. The user is also charged for telecommunications and royalties on all data bases, so most use averages about $10 to $15 per hour. BRS/Colleague start-up fees are $50, with monthly minimums of $15 per month. Rates for the medical data bases are $20 to $32, depending upon the access times requested. An additional hourly charge and citation display charge are levied when using "non-core" nonmedical data bases. Off-line prints are 25 cents per page of citations.

Minet and GTE Telenet Medical Information Network. GTE Telenet, in conjunction with the American Medical Association, also offers an on-line data base for the medical profession called Minet. With the vast experience of GTE Telenet in computers and the experience of the AMA in medicine, you would expect a rich, full-function data base combining the strengths of both organizations. Unfortunately, the hybrid appears to be weaker than either of its parents.

Instead of using MEDLINE and the National Library of Medicine as information sources for the data base, Minet has chosen a subset of the Excerpta Medica called EMPIRES (Excerpta Medica Physicians Information Retrieval and Education Service). The EMPIRES service supplies only selected publications from 1981 to the present date. Other organizations such as Dialog provide the full Excerpta Medica, containing all the "back files." The MEDLINE service covers more journals and spans a greater period. MEDLINE is available on all major services.

A subscriber to Minet can access the Harvard Medical School Laboratory of Computer Science's Continuing Medical Education Programs for category I CME credits. There are 20 or so simulations that provide individualized, self-paced learning based upon computerized patient simulations. Computerized simulation cases allow the user to explore different approaches to diagnosis and treatment, including "what if" decisions, without causing harm to a patient. (This may be the most useful service on Minet that is not available on other data base services at this time.)

The AMA also has presented on-line versions of the *Physician's Current Procedural Terminology, AMA Drug Evaluations,* and *Current Medical Information and Terminology.* These sources are updated on a yearly or twice yearly basis.

The drug data base allows you to request information about medications using the generic name, trade name, use, adverse reactions, toxicity, or interactions. The drug information handouts that the AMA has prepared for patients taking some of the indexed drugs are also available in this service. Several drug companies are now providing a companion service to the AMA drug evaluations called PHYCOM, which is an electronic version of the familiar *Physician's Desk Reference.* This portion of the service is available on a free subscription to physicians requesting it. Recently, the AMA has purchased the rights to the *Medical*

Letter and added full text searching of this drug information journal to the Minet services. The collected drug information services are valuable but are also found for lesser cost on other services in similar form.

The current medical information data base DISEASE allows you to obtain a short summary of the causes, symptoms, physical examination, laboratory data, and course of over 3500 diseases. The information is cursory but serves as a quick review.

Several other services are available but seem less useful. These include a listing of current socioeconomic literature and MED/MAIL. MED/MAIL is a subset of GTE's TELEMAIL that will not support hard copy transmission or transmission to nonsubscribers. MED/MAIL messages may also be sent with the free PHYCOM subscription. The PHYCOM subscription will charge for user-to-user mail but allows free user-to-drug company mail.

Users of the AMA service complain of high costs and relatively unproductive searches. The AMA is currently charging $100 per year annual membership fee and monthly minimum charges of $45 for each registered user. This means that the user is paying a minimum charge of $640 per year. For the physician who wishes to subscribe to only one service, Minet should not be that service. For the occasional user, either BRS/Colleague or Dialog Knowledge Index will provide more in-depth coverage of the literature data bases at far lower rates. For free, the PHYCOM subscription cannot be matched, but it offers very limited services.

Other Services Available

Physicians may use other information and communication networks that are not medical data base services. These other networks provide airline schedules, investor services, news, and communications services. They do not cater to literature searches, data base searches, or research. The three most used commercial networks are Dow Jones, The Source, and Compuserve. Typically, these organizations will charge a start-up fee and may charge a small monthly maintenance fee. They will often have larger fees for the daytime hours of use. Frequently, they will charge more for 1200-baud use. See the end of this chapter for details on how to contact them.

Although it is clear that the non–data base networks are not designed for reporting medical problems, the first medication recall to be triggered by intercomputer medical consultation occurred on Compuserve. The withdrawal of Zomax (McNeil, Zomepirac) from the commercial market was speeded by multiple reports of allergic reactions noted on the MEDSIG (medical special interest group) bulletin board on Compuserve. Indeed, because of MEDSIG's quick reaction, the FDA has announced that they will allow physicians to send them adverse drug reaction reports (ADR) via Compuserve or the AMA/GTE computer network. Physicians involved in the MEDSIG are convinced that it is a unique way to flag pharmaceuticals with side effects before the drugs cause too much damage. They note that telecomputing allows physicians to share favorable experiences and techniques that have not yet been published in the formal literature. The MEDSIG members feel that this method is far superior to the usual government agency surveillance methods.

Numerous privately based smaller networks are found in schools, universities, and private homes in the form of computerized bulletin board services (CBBS). These CBBS are set up by an individual or small organization to provide local dissemination of computer and civic information, free communication at all hours, and recreational use. The organizations and individuals providing such services literally change on a daily basis.

THE FUTURE

Where do we go from here? AT&T is installing new networking computers in the University of Pittsburgh, their "campus of the future." The new computers will allow communication via "light pipes" at unprecedented speeds between mainframe computer and end user. IBM, Apple, and others have chosen other campuses for innovative technology. The National Library of Medicine is funding innovative projects in medical library networks to link student, faculty, and librarian together. Organizations are experimenting with transmission of pictorial data via the telephone lines to microcomputers. Other organizations are working to link small microcomputers together in inexpensive networks in offices and clinics.

Researchers are trying to model information retrieval systems that are responsive to the individual researcher and to learn from individual idiosyncrasies in typing and syntax. These systems will automatically correct the "hte" that is typed for "the" and will continue with the search. Better searching strategy programs will soon be able to understand a search for "fortune telling" when you ask for "telling fortunes" and to anticipate alternative choices and searches for the physician to consider when looking for data. These systems act as a trained member of the team, anticipating the flow of events, rather than as a passive source of data.

The capacity for meeting the information needs of the health professions has been radically affected by this rapidly evolving electronic information technology. The new technology of the computer may also mean a shift from paper to electronic publishing and the evolution of medical education tailored to the health care practitioner.

Medical Letter, Lancet, British Medical Journal and *The Annals of Internal Medicine* are currently offering "on-line" versions of those journals. It is easy to visualize the specialty journals rapidly following suit in electronic publishing. These electronic journals are easier to update and may prove to decrease both the costs and the time between acceptance of an article and its publication. As more rapid data communication becomes available, these electronic journals may offer pictures, electrocardiograms, and radiographs by telephone. It is easy to see that for expensive, small, specialty journals, electronic media may be the quickest, cheapest, and most widespread form of publication available.

Medical education may also undergo radical changes in two fields because of this new technology. With the development of large bases of medical knowledge, coupled with rapid computer-driven access of this data and the addition of "artificial intelligence," expert medical advice by computer may become available. The information processes involved during diagnosis can be managed by computer. Symptoms are charted, signs and physical examinations are recorded, and laboratory procedures are requested via computer. Computer programs capable of accepting these kinds of data and producing a list of diseases from which a differential diagnosis might be chosen can be expected to become available in the near future. When such a diagnostic program is being used, it can assume that the physician wants to choose a course of therapy. Here the information system can include factors concerning treatments suitable for each of the diseases on the list, and information on the pros and cons of particular therapeutic choices. The physician can modify the list with data on the family history, occupation, epidemiology, and social situation of the patient. Then new therapeutic possibilities are presented to the physician. These systems are covered in greater detail in other chapters in this book, and they will most likely be implemented as dial-up services from the physician's office.

Given an adequate form of information service installed in a hospital, the physician could call from home to get pertinent data from the patient's medical records. More sophisticated networks would allow graphic representations of data trends of critically ill patients with computer monitoring, and reception of digitized electrocardiogram and radiographic data at home on video terminals.

Lest we think that all the technology has only good effects, we should look at some grave concerns about the burgeoning data and information services. These concerns center around access, privacy, and accuracy. If only those students and practitioners who have access to computers or terminals are able to use this technology, what happens to those folks who do not have these devices? If the standard of care requires that you submit a difficult diagnosis to an "expert" system for aid and possible resolution, what happens to the qualified physician who does not, and makes an honest error? If the affluent medical student is able to tap into an expert learning system and practices daily with it, how will some poorer peer compete? There is a real concern that if the rich can afford these tools, and the poor cannot, there will be a widening of the inequality.

If all medical records are computerized so that physicians, researchers, and of course, administrators have access to them, who will protect the patient's privacy? Who will prevent unauthorized release or, worse, unauthorized changes to medical records? Security of data has even been breached by computer users in classified defense projects and electronic banking transfers. What measures will be taken to prevent such breaches in medical data?

If the literature is updated on a monthly or daily basis, what can prevent a third party from dissemination of deliberate falsifications? The publishers of books are well aware of third party interests, and they obtain scrupulous reviews. It is difficult to add data to a printed document after it is published. Adding data to a computerized data base would be very easy for an accomplished programmer or systems analyst. Will unscrupulous drug companies be willing and able to pay to "filter" all bad references and to add favorable reviews of their product? Will government bodies be able to suppress data in the "national interest"? Could all reports of "Agent Purple" cancer–associated deaths be "filtered" before release of an updated data base? What measures will be taken to ensure continuing accuracy in electronic publishing?

Despite these grave concerns, the probability exists that the easy access to information given by the medical networks will provide a great overall benefit to practitioners and patients alike. Certainly, it is much easier for the physician to acquire information about a topic than in the past, and this is a direct product of the computer age. This information access represents power to patient and physician alike.

APPENDIX OF SOURCES DISCUSSED

Data base services
   BRS
   1200 Route 7
   Latham, NY 12110
   800-833-4707

   Dialog
   3460 Hillview Avenue
   Palo Alto, CA 94304
   800-982-5838

AMA/Mednet
1500 Walnut Street
7th Floor
Philadelphia, PA 19102
215-875-4650

PHYCOM
Fisher-Stevens, Inc.
Campus Road
Totowa, NJ 07512
201-790-0700

Dow Jones News/Retrieval
P.O. Box 300
Princeton, NJ 08540
800-257-5114

ORBIT
SDC Information Services
2500 Colorado Avenue
Santa Monica, CA 90406
213-820-4111 x6194

GTE TELENET Communications Corporation
8229 Boone Boulevard
Vienna, VA 22180
703-442-1000

Uninet, Inc
1125 Grand Avenue
Kansas City, MO 64106
816-474-0856

Nexis
Mead Data Central
9333 Springboro Pike
Miamisburg, OH 45342
513-865-6800

MCI Mail
2000 M Street NW
Third Floor
Washington, DC 20036
800-MCI-2255

Compuserve Information Service
5000 Arlington Centre Boulevard
Columbus, OH 43220
614-457-8650

Suggested equipment specifications for data access
Transmission mode: Asynchronous TTY
Code: American Standard for Computer Information Interchange (ASCII)
Speed:
    300 or 1200 baud modem—1200 preferred
    110 to 300 bps, compatible with Bell 103
    1200 bps, compatible with Bell 212A or VADIC 3400
Data Terminal Settings:
    Parity: No parity
    Transmission mode: Full duplex
    Block mode off

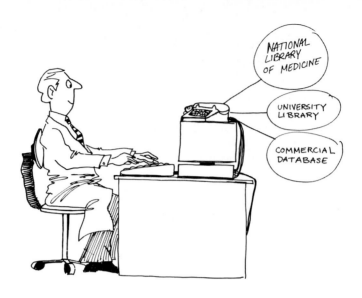

S I X

The Computer As a
Personal Bibliographic
Retrieval Tool

Ernest Beutler, M.D.

Keeping abreast of the biomedical literature is one of the most important and yet one of the most vexing requirements in any field of research. It is necessary not only to know current happenings in one's field of interest but also to have ready access to the foundation of knowledge as represented in the scientific literature.

Access to this information is required not only to properly plan and execute experiments but, quite importantly, in presenting the results of one's studies. Every scientific discovery is based upon previous discoveries, and it is the obligation of the publishing scientist to provide the background that puts his or her work into an accurate perspective. This task has never been easy, but with the proliferation of scientific journals and accumulation of scientific knowledge at ever-increasing rates, the retrieval of scientific information has reached a point at which its scope staggers the imagination. Fortunately, the development and availability of computers has, in recent years, paralleled the growth of the scientific data base and offers some possible solutions to the dilemma faced by the working and publishing scientist.

Accessing the scientific literature must be approached from two points of view. The first of these is access to the world's entire literature on all subjects. This important topic is covered in Chapter 5 by Dr. Charles Stewart. The second consideration is the storage and retrieval of references from a small subset created for the benefit of a single investigator or for a small group of investigators working together.

THE PERSONAL DATA BASE

The use of a personal data base may be divided into three major operations or functions. First of all, it is necessary to store the references. Second, the stored references must be retrievable. Finally, if the references have been electronically encoded, it is desirable to be able to use them directly in the preparation of a document such as a journal article, book, or grant application.

The first two of these functions can be performed without the use of a computer. A variety of noncomputerized techniques have been utilized by investigators for many years. At one extreme is the stacking of journals around an office. Frantic shuffling through piles of papers for a specific reference is a usual component of this search algorithm. At the other noncomputerized extreme is the use of punched cards to record references to be retrieved. In between these extremes of chaos and order, many other strategies have been used. These include the use of ordinary file cards and, very commonly, the filing of reprints in folders. It is somewhat surprising to me how often the latter, very inefficient technique is employed by investigators.

The principal difficulty with noncomputerized methods for reference storage is that retrieval under multiple subject headings becomes very cumbersome and that authors other than the first are difficult to find. Various methods of cross-indexing can be used but at the expense of considerable overhead to the system. Even the use of data retrieval systems with punch cards places severe constraints upon the number of topics that can be coded and the extent to which cross-indexing is possible.

The availability of computers has almost entirely removed these constraints. Clearly, computerized systems are the best way to maintain literature files, and with the advent of remarkably inexpensive microcomputers, this method of literature storage and retrieval is within the reach of even quite junior investigators whose financial resources are very limited.

THE IDEAL BIBLIOGRAPHIC SYSTEM

Compatibility

Transportability among computers is highly desirable. It should be possible to obtain versions of the program to run on all computers—micros, minis, and mainframes. The data bases that are created should, of course, be freely transportable among different computer types. Thus, it would be ideal for a junior investigator to be able to begin building a personal data base on a $200 Commodore home computer and then upgrade successively through a variety of microcomputers, finally putting the data base on the institution's mainframe computer.

Data Input

The ideal system should be able to add references either through keyboard entry or electronically from other data bases. There should be no limitation upon the number of authors, the number of key words attached to the reference, the length of the title, the length of the journal designation, or the length of notes appended to the reference. The ideal program should have the capability of "downloading" references from any data base, distinguishing authors from titles and page numbers from year of publication. In so doing, it should ignore the useless and redundant information usually offered by national data bases, such as issue number and month and day of publication. The user should be alerted when a new author, new journal, or new key word is entered. This minimizes the entry of inappropriately abbreviated journals, misspelled authors' names, and misspelled or redundant key words. The user should be alerted when entering a reference that has been entered before. The ability to enter references by transferring from one data base to another is very desirable. It should be possible to do this either by entry number or by retrieval of a data set.

Retrieval should be extremely rapid, regardless of how large the personal data base is. For practical purposes, this means that retrieval must be based on index tables rather than on sequential searches. It should be possible to retrieve on multiple parameters using [and], [not], or [or] as logical connectors. Author or editor names should be accessible regardless of whether the initials are known, and retrieval by virtue of the appearance of any word in title or notes should be possible. It is desirable for the program to be able to remember previously retrieved data sets so that subsets may be retrieved without taking the time to retrieve the basic set each time.

Good editing capabilities are essential. One of the major advantages of a computerized bibliographic data base is that the accuracy of the references may be continually upgraded, as correctly entered references remain accurate while references with errors are corrected as the errors are detected. The ideal editing module should make it possible to correct an entry with a minimum of effort. If an error exists in a title or in notes, re-entry of the entire item should not be required. Word processing functions should be incorporated into the program so that words can be inserted or deleted with ease. Global changes (the capability of changing a key word or a journal name wherever it appears in the data base) should be possible.

The program should contain functions that facilitate evaluating, maintaining, and improving the data base. The generation of alphabetized lists of authors, editors, key words, and journals allows the user to scan these parameters, easily detecting duplications and misspellings. If the program does not have the capability of detecting duplicate entries at the time of entry, it should be able to identify duplicates in the data base.

Aiding the author in preparing a completed manuscript that is ready for submission to the publisher is a valuable feature of the ideal bibliographic system. It should be possible for the system to create a list of references in the exact format specified by the publisher. Because the number of formats is nearly as large as the number of journals, this requires enormous flexibility. Items which must be considered include, but are not limited to, the number of authors cited, punctuation after initials, punctuation after authors' last names, whether initials precede or follow the surnames, whether authors' names are capitalized entirely or initially, whether periods appear after journal abbreviations, whether page numbers are inclusive, the punctuation after reference numbers, and many more. The program should also have the capability of modifying the text itself so that the references cited in the bibliography are correctly identified. The program should be capable of numbering articles in the sequence in which they appear in the text or alphabetically by authors' names and should even be able to insert the authors' names into the text, as required by some journals. Reformatting the new manuscript and list of references to take into account changes in spacing that occur when one number is substituted for another or authors' names are inserted into the text is desirable but can usually be accomplished by using the word processing program in which the manuscript was originally created.

EXISTING BIBLIOGRAPHIC SYSTEMS

In about 1972, the author of this chapter, feeling ever more acutely the need to efficiently manage a personal data base, developed a bibliographic retrieval system for the PDP-11/40 computer. Use of this system for a period of about 10 years provided background with which to develop an entirely new microcomputer-based system, incorporating the desirable features of the original system and adding features that had not been present but whose need had been felt. The new set of programs, first made commercially available in 1984, was designated Reference Manager. In this chapter this program will be discussed in detail. In part, greater emphasis is given to Reference Manager because of the author's greater familiarity with the program. It is probably not unreasonable, however, to consider it the program against which others must be judged.

To the extent that the information is available to us, let us see how existing, microcomputer-based programs measure up to the ideal standard:

Reference Manager (Research Information Systems, 2707 Costabella Drive, La Jolla, CA 92037) is distributed in a compiled form of CBASIC. Versions are available that can be executed on any microcomputer using PC-DOS, MS-DOS, CP/M, or CP/M 86. Other operating systems including UNIX, those of Apple computers, and those of mini- and mainframe computers are not supported. Apple computers with a CP/M card or minicomputers with suitable emulators may be used. Version 2.3 of the program requires only approximately 48K of transient program area and therefore will execute in an 8-bit, 64K microcomputer. Later versions of the program containing certain enhancements require larger internal memory and are available only in the MS/PC-DOS version.

This program is able to incorporate references into its data base either through keyboard entry or by "downloading" from national data bases. There are some constraints with respect to the number of authors permitted and the number of key words, but these are very liberal. A total of 26 authors, 27 different key words, and 22 editors are accommodated per reference. There is no limit to the length of titles, the length of notes appended, or the length of names and editors or authors or of key words. Reference Manager can download MEDLINE, as obtained directly from the National Library of Medicine, and MESH, MS78, MS74, MS70, and BIOSIS Reviews files from BRS Colleague. In the case of

BIOSIS Reviews, an algorithm in the program changes the upper-case format in which the references are transmitted to an upper- and lower-case format. This, of course, needs to be edited to change terms like "Atp" to "ATP." The program lacks the capability to download files obtained through other services such as Dialog, Knowledge Index, or ISI. However, disk files created from other data bases may be reformatted in a word processor to simulate one of the data bases that are supported and may then be entered. Reference Manager also has the capability of transferring references from one Reference Manager data base to another.

Once data have been entered, either by downloading from a compatible data base or through the keyboard, they may be edited by the user prior to being written on the disk. The user is warned by the program when an author, editor, key word, or journal are used for the first time. This feature is very helpful in avoiding degradation of the data base by the gradual accumulation of misspelled names and redundant key words. For example, if the journal abbreviation "New Engl. J. Med." were entered when the correct abbreviation is "N. Engl. J. Med.," a flashing star would appear next to the entry to warn the user that something might be amiss. When entry is completed, the user has the option of obtaining a printout of the newly entered references, and here the new names are marked with asterisks, a useful feature for those fortunate enough to have someone else enter their references for them.

Retrieval is very rapid because names of authors, editors, key words, and journal names are all indexed. Up to nine or even more search parameters may be used in a search, and these may be connected by [and], [or], or [not]. Searching by defining words or characters in the text of notes and titles is also possible; however, because this search is not an indexed one but rather is sequential, it is not as rapid as searching for indexed parameters. It is quite rapid once an indexed parameter has narrowed the field of search to a few dozen references.

Entries may be edited, either individually or globally. Except for global editing of titles, global editing can be carried out only during execution of the data restructuring utility. It has the capability of changing the name of a key word, author, editor, or journal name whenever it appears in the data base.

Reference Manager offers a variety of utilities that aid the user in reviewing and maintaining the data base. For example, it provides the user with data base statistics. It is able to check the data base for duplicate entries using an algorithm that detects most near-duplicates as well so that minor typographic errors in titles, for example, do not permit duplicates to continue to reside in the data base. A data base compression and restructuring module squeezes out of the data base dead space that has accumulated during editing and corrects pointer errors that may have occurred as a result of computer malfunction. The program will generate alphabetized lists of authors, editors, key words, and journals. It is possible to record the date a reprint has been requested and then to have the program report which reprint requests are pending from a specified time period.

A major feature of Reference Manager is its ability not only to create bibliographies but to process text files of manuscripts so as to include citations to the bibliography in the text. Because the program operates directly on the text file in the computer, this function is largely (but not entirely) independent of the word processing system that has been used to create the manuscript file. The program parses the text file and interprets numbers following "(" or some other user-defined token, such as "{", as a reference number unless it has been marked as a nonreference by the user. A duplicate file is created in which the reference number is substituted for the computer number. The names of the authors and year of publication may be substituted if the user so specifies. The format in which the bibliography is created is specified by the user and can be made to conform to almost any journal. There are exceptions, however. *Science*, for example, lumps several citations under one footnote, and Reference Manager is unable to cope with this aberration.

BiblioTek (Scientific Software Products, Inc., 5726 Professional Circle, Suite 105, Indianapolis IN 46241) is a personal bibliography management system written in BASIC exclusively for the Apple II microcomputer. The capabilities of the program are limited by the hardware that supports it. The program has been designed to take maximum advantage of the limited disk storage space that is available. Thus, the key words that are employed are user-defined in advance, and instead of actual entry of a key word, a number from a preconstructed list of key words is used. Entry of new data is possible only from the keyboard; downloading from national data bases is not supported. The number of authors is limited to 10, with up to 25 characters per last name, and to three initials. The length of the title is limited to 224 characters. The name of the journal, book, or conference is limited to 120 characters, and numbers representing eight key words may be entered per reference. Up to 200 characters of comments may be entered. Entries may be edited using various control codes.

Searching is sequential, not indexed, and [and], [or], and [not] logic may be used. Lists of references can be prepared and sorted by author names, by dates, or manually. The format in which a bibliography is printed may be defined in some detail by using "tokens" to represent the various parts of the reference. No direct interaction with a manuscript is possible. Because it is written in uncompiled BASIC, the program is quite slow in execution and is best suited for limited bibliographies.

Bookends and Bookends Extended (Sensible Software Inc., 6619 Perham Drive, West Bloomfield, MI 48033) is another Apple II program, but it is written in machine language. All Apple II–compatible computers are able to implement Bookends, but Bookends Extended requires the full 128K and 80-column display of the Apple IIc and the IIe. An IBM PC version of Bookends Extended is under development but is not yet available.

References may be entered into Bookends either from the keyboard or downloaded directly from files created from MEDLINE, BRS, and selected data bases from Lockheed Dialogue. Each reference is allocated 760 bytes, and these may be distributed in any way between authors, editors, journal designation, title, or notes. The user is not warned of the addition of a new author, journal, or key word, nor does the program check for duplicates. Global changes are not possible. References created from one Bookends data base may be transferred to another, and data bases may be merged. Retrieval is possible by multiple parameters using [and] and [or] but not [not] logic. Subsets of previously retrieved data can be recalled. Searches are sequential but because they are carried out in random access memory (RAM) they are extremely rapid once the entire data base has been loaded. Although it is possible to search from disk to disk, loading of sequential blocks of data greatly slows such searches. Word processing functions are built into the program. The program formats references in unlimited types of formats. It cannot, however, interact with a manuscript to insert citation numbers or authors' names into the text.

REF 11 (DG Systems, 32 Prospect Avenue, Hartford, CT 06106) appears to be available for a greater number of different computers than any of the other bibliographic systems. It is not only distributed for microcomputers running MS/PS-DOS and those using CP/M 80, but also the Digital Equipment minicomputer series using operating systems such as RT 11, RSX 11, and VAX/VMS. CP/M 86 and Apple computers are not supported, however. References may be entered from the keyboard or from a text file. In the latter case, however, the references must be assembled by the user into the form expected by the optional utility program that downloads them into the REF 11 data base. The number of authors is limited to eight. In areas of science in which as many as 15 or 20 authors are not unusual, as in cancer chemotherapy, this could prove to be a serious handicap. Four editors may be entered, and the length of editors' and authors' names is limited to 26 bytes. The name of the journal or other source may occupy up to 134 bytes, and a title may use 268 bytes. There are 240 bytes allocated for notes that may be appended to the reference.

The program does not warn the user when new authors, journals, or key words are entered, nor does it check for duplicates. Thus, automatic protection against pollution of the data base is not provided. References created in one REF 11 data base can be transferred to another REF 11 data base.

Retrieval by multiple parameters is possible, but [not] logic is not supported. Subsets of previously retrieved data can be recalled. A major disadvantage of this program is the fact that searches are sequential. Thus, finding an author from a data base of 660 references on an RX-02 floppy disk consumes 86 seconds, a task that would consume less than 1 second with a program using indexed author files. Because the length of time required to find a reference bears a linear relationship to the number of references searched sequentially, the delay in finding a reference in a large data base would be truly intolerable. Some word processing functions are intrinsic to the program. Global changes are not possible. The program is able to generate alphabetized lists of authors, but not of editors, key words, or journals. The program has a capability of formatting journal citations and can interact with a manuscript by inserting citation numbers. It can store an unusually large number of references on a single IBM PC floppy disk. This is undoubtedly due, in part, to clever programming but also to restrictions in the length of titles and number of authors.

BiblioFile (Martz Software, Inc., 48 Hunters Hill Circle, Amherst, MA 01002) is available for CP/M 80 and MS-DOS computers but not for Apple or CP/M 86. References are not entered directly into the program, but rather, a text file is created with a word processing program and this file is read into the program. Downloading references from national data bases is possible only after editing to fit BiblioFile's input format. The number of authors or editors is limited only by the number that can fit into a 500-character field. This is an ample allotment and should suffice for virtually all purposes. The length of the journal and title fields are also a generous 500 characters each, but notes are also limited to 500 characters, a length insufficient for a complete abstract of many papers.

The program does not warn the user when new authors, journals, or key words are entered and does not check for duplicates. However, global changes are possible. References can be transferred automatically from one BiblioFile data base to another. Searching is sequential and is, therefore, relatively slow. Subsets of previously retrieved data can be recalled, and retrieval is possible using all the boolean connectors [and], [not], and [or]. Alphabetized lists of parameters are not produced by BiblioFile, but alphabetization can be achieved by using the BiblioFile programs in conjunction with a program such as "Super Spellguard." BiblioFile does format references in a large number of different formats. It interacts with manuscripts inserting sequential citation or alphabetic citation numbers but not authors' names.

SciMate (Institute for Scientific Information, 3501 Market Street, Philadelphia, PA 19104) is a comprehensive bibliographic retrieval and storage system available for IBM PC XT/AT computers and CPM 80 computers with 8 inch disk drives. A separate set of programs, designated the SciMate Universal Online Searcher, is used to download references from national data bases. SciMate attempts to combine the characteristics of a general data base management system with those of a system for the storage of bibliographic references. In doing so, a system that is more flexible than other bibliographic storage systems has been created. At the same time, the system is more difficult to use because the user is required to define his or her own fields, creating a series of "templates." A different template is required for each "host" computer. The system does not incorporate automatic warning for entry of new authors, journals or key words, nor does it check for duplicates. Transfer from one data base to another is supported.

Retrieval can be indexed and [and], [not], and [or] connectors may be used. Limited word processing capabilities are incorporated into the program, but global changes cannot be made. Generation of alphabetized lists of parameters is not possible; however, printed output of selected subsets of a data base is possible. The fields of a record to be printed may be specified, but the content of an individual field (such as authors) may not be manipulated.

In the form available at the present writing, interaction with manuscripts is not supported, nor can the references be reformatted to fit the specifications of journals. A third set of programs, the SciMate Editor, is being prepared for early release and, according to the publishers, will support these functions.

SUMMARY AND CONCLUSION

It is apparent that none of the programs available for use in constructing bibliographies meets the ideal standard in every respect. Given the constraints of current computer technology, it is unlikely that any of them could ever do so. The diversity of operating systems and the heterogeneity in the manner in which national data bases are presented preclude the development of an ideal program.

All the programs reviewed here represent major advances over card shuffling. All require some effort to learn to use them. The choice of the correct one is of critical importance to the investigator. Considerable portability of references within each program exists, but transport of references between programs cannot be readily achieved. Thus, commitment to one or another program represents an investment that the serious investigator should not make without careful consideration.

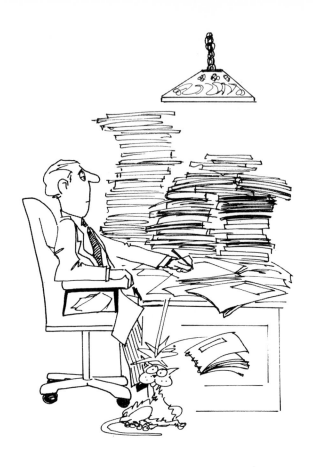

SEVEN

How to Computerize a Medical Office

Jonathan Javitt, M.D.

Physicians are rapidly reaching the day when it will no longer be feasible to maintain an uncomputerized office. By the end of the decade, all records, accounting, inventory, and payroll functions will be electronic. Ten years may be a long time off, yet there are numerous reasons to computerize an office today and numerous tasks that today's microcomputers are ready to take on.

The most commonly available computer application in a medical office is patient accounting, billing, and insurance for generation. There are numerous programs on the market that fulfill these basic functions and add features such as electronic scheduling, electronic submission of insurance claims, and generation of patient recall notices. At the time of this writing, there are no microcomputer management packages that provide an intelligent and comprehensive approach to clinical record keeping. Of course, this remark may be obsolete by the time this is published. The problem has generally been the lack of uniformity from office to office and specialty to specialty in terms of determining what information must be stored for a given patient. Thus, any software packages that have come out so far that purport to store comprehensive clinical information have been disappointing. A few packages do include the ability to store patient medications, allergies, diagnoses, and active problems, along with free form progress notes. These features are quite useful but are clearly only a supplement to a paper chart on each patient.

As medical practice costs rise and the supply of physicians increases, practices will need to pay increasing attention to productivity and to marketing functions. Most good office management packages make it easy to generate productivity reports by practitioner, by procedure, even by piece of equipment. It becomes an easy matter to determine whether the practice is running a particular piece of diagnostic equipment at a profit or a loss and to make management decisions on that basis. Similarly, the time expended in various procedures and treatments can be correlated with the billing for those procedures in determining what services to offer and at what price.

One of the most difficult aspects of practice management is patient follow-up and recall. Although good patient care dictates tracking down individuals for needed appointments and tests, the realities of manual record keeping systems and chronically overworked office staffs make this nearly impossible. Computerized record keeping makes it a simple matter to mail one or more reminder letters to patients and to track those who don't respond. Similarly, as the supply of physicians increases, practices will have to pay more attention to building and maintaining a stable patient population. The facility of a computer for generating patient newsletters, health alerts, and similar communications can make an enormous difference in the degree to which patients perceive being taken care of on an ongoing basis.

We are living in the midst of a communications revolution in which instant access to information is as close as the telephone. A computer is an instant link with a world of information stretching from the hospital records of one's patients to the extensive data base of the National Library of Medicine. Up-to-the-second conferences on a variety of topics are available to anyone with a computer and a telephone. Within the next few years, electronic mail will be the simplest way for physicians to share information about patients. Mailing charts, consultation letters and test results will soon be as passé as bloodletting. Right now, extensive data bases of information are available to any physician with the ability to access them.

HOW TO COMPUTERIZE SUCCESSFULLY

The selection of a computer system for a medical office need not be a painful, protracted, or even inordinately expensive process. If the process is approached logically and systematically, it may even turn out to be somewhat enjoyable and informative. If at all possible, find a consultant who is experienced in medical office systems. The cost of mistakes in system selection is far more expensive than any consultant's fee! By consultant, I mean someone who is familiar with the products on the market in the medical management area and with the computer systems needed to run those products. I do not mean a programmer who offers to write a system for running your office. With the latter, you will pay thousands of dollars needlessly and will most likely wind up with a suboptimal system for all your efforts. If you have a problem with it, you had better be able to find the original programmer because no one else will be able to help you!

The process of office computerization breaks down into five steps:
- Needs assessment
- Writing system specifications
- Vendor selection
- Delegation of tasks within the office for computer operations
- Arrangements for system support.

Although these items may seem obvious at first, each one is crucial, and bypassing any of them is an invitation to disaster. If at all possible, do not change their order. It is especially important to avoid allowing the vendor to be the determining force in system selection. The vendor's priorities are clearly different from yours.

THE NEEDS ASSESSMENT PROCESS

It is crucial to involve all office staff in this process from the outset. A computer system is only as capable as those who use it. If the staff is unenthusiastic about the system from the outset, the chances of success are minimal. All too often, the office staff first encounters a computer system when it is delivered to the office in boxes. The other side of this caveat is equally important. Often the office staff knows far more about office work flow than the physicians in the practice. They will be able to spot inadequacies in the system while they can still be corrected with an eraser and notepaper. "If only I'd known . . ." is an expensive utterance when it comes to computerizing a medical office.

The essential question to ask at the outset is, "What jobs do we expect the computer to do for us today?" It is essential to be specific and to be absolutely certain that the system is capable of those tasks. This specification should include exactly which pieces of information the system will be expected to store on any given patient, which report functions the software must be able to write, and so on. The second question is how expandable the system will be for future needs.

Right from the outset, it is essential to determine who is going to be using the system and how the flow of information in and out of the computer will be managed. It is totally impractical to have people sharing terminals on any regular basis. In the end, the cost is far greater than the $1000 to $2000 for the extra work station. A related question that will have implications later on in the system selection process is how many users will be on the system at once. The answer to this question will determine the computing power needed in the hardware.

The last of the four initial questions is that of budget. A well-designed office computer system can not only save staff time and administrative costs while improving cash flow, it can actually lead to increased revenue through more efficient management of relationships with the practice's patient pool. The only intelligent approach to budgeting for this project is to sit down with the practice's financial advisors and determine the monthly cost of the system (whether leased or financed) versus the projected return on the system. In all likelihood, the calculations will justify a system large enough to handle the office's needs. Once these questions are answered, the place to start designing the actual system is with its software.

MEDICAL MANAGEMENT SOFTWARE

The major decision point in software selection for the medical office is the level of information to be stored on the proposed system. The current state of the medical management software market is that there are several packages that can do highly competent accounting and production management. The ability of those packages to store clinical information on patients in a useful fashion is extremely primitive at this time. Although the concept of a paperless office with all patient data stored electronically is highly attractive, it is not practical on microcomputer systems in 1985. At present, that level of data management is available only in the minicomputer environment.

The reason for this situation is twofold. The major factor is that software development is driven by market demand. At present, relatively few medical offices have sophisticated microcomputers. Management information is relatively standard from one medical practice to the next. Thus, the same software package can accommodate surgeons and psychiatrists. Only the diagnosis and treatment codes must be changed when the package is installed in order to render it appropriate. The nature and structure of clinical information vary enormously from one medical specialty to the next. It is simply not possible to design a clinical data base that is generic enough to be useful to a large segment of the market and yet is specific enough to be useful for anyone.

There are packages that accommodate specific items of clinical information. In this way a practice may designate 10 or 20 items that must be known on each patient and configure data fields to store those items. Similarly, it is possible to store lists of diagnoses, medications, and allergies on each patient. Some packages allow for visit notes to be entered as free text in addition to the structured data. In the long run, what is needed is a relational data base that is able to track clinical parameters over time and to correlate them with other parameters. This level of sophistication has not been developed under current microcomputer operating systems and is currently available only under UNIX and MUMPS (see Chap. 13). As a larger base of computer users develops within the medical world and more powerful operating systems become available on microcomputers, there is no doubt that specialty-specific clinical data bases will be developed to run on microcomputers. There is, however, an enormous amount a microcomputer can do today in any practice. Any of the good management packages is able to maintain a general ledger for each patient. It is important to make sure that the package also keeps a complete audit trail for each account. By storing the insurance carriers for each patient, one or more carriers can be automatically billed for each account payable. A major way in which the computer system will rapidly earn its keep is in its ability to track and age accounts receivable. By billing with the computer on a staggered basis rather than monthly, it is possible for a practice to maintain a much smoother cash flow than by hand. The availability of this ledger information makes it simple to develop management reports to determine the economics of the practice's fee structure, particular pieces of equipment, or procedures. Look for a software package that not only offers these reports, but makes it possible to devise your own reports as you go along.

A well-designed software package can be an enormous asset in enhancing communication with patients. By combining scheduling functions with automatic patient recall, it is possible to automatically send reminder notices to patients before any scheduled visit, test, or procedure. This makes it far easier to periodically recall patients with chronic conditions such as hypertension or diabetes, for the appropriate clinical tests. This type of followup is nearly impossible using manual methods. The mailmerge functions of these packages make it simple to generate a patient newsletter to report new services offered, important medical news, and similar information.

The preceding functions are dependent upon a word processor. Make sure that the package you consider either contains a good one or interfaces easily to a standard word processor. There are several packages on the market that make it enormously difficult to change a form letter or recall notice.

A major factor to consider in any of the software packages is the human engineering involved. Unfortunately, many packages on the market are adaptations of hospital mainframe computer packages. They mostly run in batch mode, which means they are designed to perform a type of function, such as entering new accounts, posting charges, or writing bills. This is enormously difficult to use if you want to enter one patient's account, post a charge, and generate a demand bill. Make sure that you select a package that is primarily record oriented in this fashion so that you are not constantly switching from one module to another simply to perform the above-mentioned operation.

At the same time, batch mode is excellent for certain operations. It is enormously useful to be able to post the hospital charges for an entire hospitalization in one operation or to post the charges for one day's rounds with a single command. Similarly, it is important to be able to print all outstanding insurance forms at once. Look for a package that can operate in this type of batch mode as a secondary option.

In evaluating software, pay little or no attention to the publicity material and advertising for the product. The only valid data is provided by current users. Many software packages have attractive demonstration programs that dealers are only too happy to show. These programs accommodate a small number of patients, run fast, and never lose data. The story may be quite different when the software is loaded with information on 2000 to 5000 patients. Any reputable company should be willing to provide any physician with the names of colleagues who are successfully using the software. If they are not willing to do this, look elsewhere.

Always determine ahead of time who is going to service the software and to what extent. It is unrealistic to expect a dealer to know as much about a package as the company that developed it. Similarly, a dealer who sells only a few copies of a product cannot afford the time to learn it inside and out. Unless the product is directly and completely supported by the publisher, it is a risky investment. This risk is compounded by the tendency of dealers to reorganize, restructure, and go out of business.

If the company that wrote the software is not supporting you directly, you are in serious trouble. At the same time, the dealer should know the software well enough to install it competently and train your staff. Always ask the dealer to supply you with the names of people who have bought this particular product and make sure you call those people.

It is unreasonable to expect full software support for free; no company can afford it. A company that guarantees to keep your software running, even if they have to put a support person on an airplane to do it, is entitled to charge a monthly fee for this. Any company that provides this level of service without charge is trying to finance the support out of future sales and is most likely headed for serious financial trouble. More often, however, the company simply does not provide the support staffing that is promised. Full software support and revision are worth the price. Too many have learned that lesson the hard way.

Medical management packages are time-consuming to install, and installation times vary greatly from one package to another. In the initial phase, the personal data on each physician in the practice must be entered as well as the particulars of each insurance carrier with whom the practice deals. A complete list of diagnoses and procedures used in the practice must then be entered along with the appropriate procedure charges and ICD diagnostic codes. The most painless way to do this part of the installation is to maintain a list of all diagnoses and procedures encountered during the month prior to installation. A major time saver is a package that learns previously unknown diagnoses and procedures as it encounters them instead of forcing the user to leave the current module and enter new codes.

A major amount of installation time can be consumed in designing billing forms and insurance forms. Look for a package that comes preconfigured with all forms needed in your state. Even better, some packages even include the paper on which those forms must be printed. This can easily save 20 hours of installation time in a busy practice.

One misleading feature of several packages is that of electronic claims submission. At the time of this writing, there is no standard protocol provided by the insurance carriers. If the package makes provision for this feature, do not expect to use it in the immediate future. Look rather for a package that is strong in its other features and backed by a stable company. As electronic claim submission becomes a reality, any strong publisher will rapidly update the package to include this feature. In other words, when shopping for software, do not be influenced by "bells and whistles" you cannot use today. If the product is stable, those features will be added as they become practical.

SYSTEM HARDWARE SELECTION

Only after the software has been chosen is it reasonable to consider system hardware, for the first question will be what operating system the software functions under best. In a single-station, single-user system running under CP/M or MS-DOS, hardware selection is straightforward. Most likely, however, a competent office system will have several work stations and the issues then become much more complicated. The problem centers around the lack of standardization in multi-user or networking operating systems. The software designers are rapidly struggling to keep their products compatible with these operating systems as they evolve.

It is essential, early on, to determine the quantity of information to be stored. This is based on the number of patients and the amount of information stored for each one. An office that fills up its mass storage in 2 years and is then faced with a major financial expenditure for more disk space has clearly made some mistakes at this stage of the selection process. The only intelligent solution is to determine the actual number of bytes needed per record stored and to multiply that by the projected number of patients over the next 5 years.

The companion question to how much mass storage is needed is how it will be backed up. The cost to a medical office of an unprotected hard disk crash is incalculable. Although hard disks can be backed up onto floppy disks, discipline on the part of the office staff is required. Murphy's law guarantees that the day back-up is not performed is the day the disks will crash. The only safety lies in iron clad rules about daily back-up, preferably with a tape streamer. Similarly, make sure to invest in a backup power supply in case the failure is on the part of the local electric company. The investment in security is well worth it in this environment.

In evaluating hardware systems, be somewhat conservative. The tested product is generally a safer bet than the newly released product with the same feature added. There is no shortage of maturing products that will provide all the power any office needs. Only by a year or two of experience in field situations can a manufacturer work out the final "bugs" that develop under the pressure of daily use.

In buying a microcomputer, do not be concerned about whether it will ever break. I promise that sooner or later it will. The essential question is how fast will it be fixed and by whom. Repair turnaround must be promised to you in terms of working hours, not days. An obvious point is not to consider operating without a service contract with a firm willing to make this commitment.

In avoiding work jams, clients all too often equip themselves with adequate numbers of terminals and adequate storage, only to fall short in the simplest and cheapest area—the printer. Dot matrix printers are getting less expensive and more reliable by the day. A medical practice needs to print on several types of paper. There are insurance forms to be filled out, demand statements to be printed, and letters to be printed on letterhead or bond paper. The sensible approach is to purchase several printers so that the office staff is not continually installing and aligning different types of forms in one overworked printer. The minimal equipment cost is rapidly offset by the savings in terms of staff time.

SELECTING A DEALER

Careful selection of a dealer is an essential aspect of the overall system acquisition. Although most dealers are honest and have good intentions, there are vast discrepancies in their ability to follow through on promises that are made regarding installation, training, and support. Because of the enormously high cost of inventory in computer dealerships, cash flow problems can often be a fatal blow, and the rate of dealership failures is high. Look carefully at the business record of the dealer with whom you undertake the project. Ask for bank references and for the names of satisfied customers. By all means, call the manufacturer's sales division and tell them you are considering buying their product through a specific dealer. Often, you will get a clearer impression of the dealer's reputation and stability.

Any promises regarding training and support must be part of the initial sales contract. Training and installation time to be provided must be specified in terms of both hours and who the personnel will be. If the dealer promises that this will be sufficient training time for the office staff to competently operate the system, this also should be in the sales contract. If service is provided through the dealership, find out whether the technicians involved are employed full time or whether this service is being subcontracted. It is essential to set up service in a way that ensures that all components will be serviced under the same contract. You do not want to find yourself in the position of having the computer serviced by one party and the printer by another. They will quickly start to argue about whose equipment is causing any problem, leaving you in the middle.

OFFICE TASK ASSIGNMENT

The last aspect of office computerization is the actual process of integrating the machinery into the office. All too often, office personnel come in one morning to be confronted with a stack of ominous-looking boxes that they are told to learn how to use. Effectively integrating a computer system will take some time, and provisions should be made for staff overtime and a reduced work load to allow for this.

There must be one person in the office who takes overall responsibility for system installation, training, and maintenance. This must be someone who is enthusiastic about the project in the first place and is likely to remain on the staff for some time. If installation is planned in advance, it will be a much smoother process. As indicated above, a month before the system arrives, all diagnostic and procedure codes should be recorded at the time of patient visits. All insurance company information should be collected, along with relevant physician identification numbers. Although it is tempting to try to enter all patients in the practice into the computer, in general, this is not a good time investment. Instead, the best approach is to enter all patients with open accounts during the initial installation. Other patients can be entered as they appear for appointments and thus generate accounts receivable. In this way, staff time and storage space are allocated primarily to those patients with active accounts in the practice.

Although there are some caveats expressed in this article, the process of office computerization is enormously worthwhile and likely to be highly successful. If the preceding guidelines are followed, the chance of untoward surprises is minimized and the most likely question to arise will be, "Why did we wait so long to do this?"

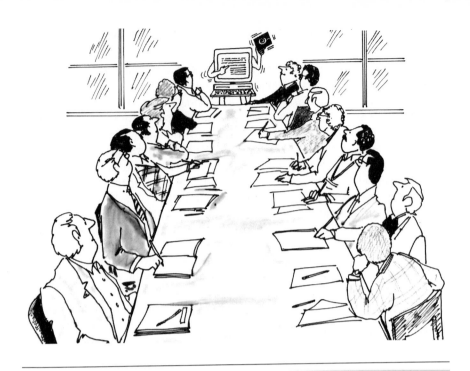

E I G H T

The Integration
of the Computer
Into Medical Education

J. Jon Veloski

Robert S. Blacklow, M.D.

How can an understanding of computers help the medical student in the pursuit of competence? When should individuals acquire computer-related skills? Before entering medical school, as medical students, or as residents? How might computers and related technology best be applied to make medical education more efficient and effective for both students and faculty? The revolution in computer technology in the 1980s and the growing number of relatively inexpensive personal computers bring with them many new opportunities for the use of computers in education. Although this trend has aroused new curiosity about computers in medical education, there is a body of literature on this subject that has been growing steadily ever since computers first became widely available in the 1960s.[11, 12, 15, 20, 75, 89, 95, 99] In this chapter we will review what has been learned from some of the early deliberations over, and experiments with, computers in medical education. New approaches to making the best use of the vast computing capability now available will also be examined.

Before addressing these questions, it is important to remind the reader that the terms "medical education" and "computers" can be used quite loosely. Medical education does not consist simply of 4 years of medical school. In its broadest sense, medical education refers to a sequence of learning experiences that begins with a selection of courses in a baccalaureate program. After earning a bachelor's degree, a student pursues an undergraduate medical education in a medical college. Completion of the required medical school courses is then followed by graduate training in a residency program, and even further training is required for subspecialization. Then there is the continuing education required throughout every professional's career. The distinctions between phases of medical education are even less clear in medical colleges that offer combined B.A./M.D. programs in which the premedical and medical phases of education are fused into a 6-year program.

The role of computers in medical education may be quite different in the early years of medical school when contrasted with their uses in later clinical, graduate, and postgraduate training. Even within a medical college, classrooms and lecture halls must be distinguished from laboratories and hospital sites when considering the use of computers for education. Each environment offers unique opportunities and challenges. When these variables are taken into consideration, it is insufficient to ask whether computers can be used to improve medical education. One must investigate, at each point in the curriculum, how they can be used to augment or replace specific lectures, laboratories, clinical experiences, small group discussions, or independent study activities. Although undergraduate medical education leading to the M.D. degree will be emphasized in this chapter, the differences between the levels of undergraduate and graduate medical education will be highlighted where appropriate.

The term "computer" needs to be examined. A decade ago a computer referred to a large and expensive machine located in a controlled environment. In present usage, "computer" usually refers to a general-purpose digital computer such as the desktop personal machine that can be used to execute a wide variety of programs stored on magnetic media such as disks. We will assume this to be the meaning in general. However, there is increasing realization that special-purpose computers (microprocessors) are found almost everywhere in instruments such as clocks, thermometers, cameras, diagnostic equipment, office machines, and complex laboratory devices. When an obstetrician uses a fetal monitor, is this physician using a computer? Many of the most capable clinical instruments would be useless without their computing components. Furthermore, because spectacular developments in all aspects of electronics are blurring the distinctions among computers, audiovisual materials, and communications technology, it must be recognized that it is becoming less meaningful to discuss the use of computers in education without considering the impending merger of computers, video technology, and communications systems.[2, 3, 29] One should be aware of the changing definitions of computers when evaluating any new developments concerning their use in medical education.

In analyzing and defining the role of computers in any type of education, it has been customary to differentiate the routine uses of the machines from their creative uses. The routine use of computers in education enables students working *with* computers and other instructional technology such as video disks to study a variety of topics in an educational program without the need to understand how a computer actually works. Creative uses, on the other hand, refer to the curricula and resources that can be provided for students to learn *about* computers as potentially powerful tools for collecting, storing, managing, and analyzing many types of data. This dichotomy has been proposed because it seems inappropriate to assume that, while using computers to review independent study lessons, to take self-assessment tests, or to solve simulated patient management problems, students will acquire the skills needed to use computers as general-purpose tools throughout their professional careers. The latter has been sometimes referred to as computer literacy or computer familiarity. Conversely, an academic policy that requires every student to buy and learn to use a certain type of computer for word processing, spreadsheets, data bases, and other types of programming will not necessarily assure that the computers will be used effectively for learning. Competent instructional materials must be developed for or recommended to students by the faculty. It can be argued that separating routine and creative uses is arbitrary and unnecessary, for students who are able to learn to use computers as tools for managing information may discover many new ways to use them in medical school, residency, or later. At the present time, many of the issues concerning the role of computers in medical education nevertheless can be clarified more easily if these two uses are addressed separately.

LEARNING WITH COMPUTERS IN MEDICAL SCHOOL

Throughout the 1970s, there were pockets of intense enthusiasm for the use of computers, with advocates promising that portions of medical education could be made more effective and efficient through automation.[10, 86] In many cases these investigators were able to demonstrate empirically the expected benefits. Representative evidence can be found in the literature of many disciplines and areas of specialization such as anatomy,[44, 92] anesthesiology,[46] biochemistry,[83] biostatistics,[32] cardiology,[40] emergency medicine,[41] family practice,[23] general practice,[64] hematology,[30] immunology,[4] internal medicine,[14] microbiology,[27] neurology,[13] pathology,[34] pediatrics,[76] pharmacology,[45, 53] physiology,[8, 48, 51, 61, 90, 91] psychiatry,[96] rheumatology,[22] and surgery.[36]

Several features of this early work are noteworthy. Most report the intense efforts of a small group of faculty members over a short period of time rather than the results of projects involving an entire department or medical school. Cooperative arrangements among institutions were not conspicuous. Computer programs were developed using the computer hardware and software that was available locally in each medical school, and as a result, there was great variation in the technical characteristics of these programs. Mainframe and minicomputers were used; general-purpose microcomputers were not available. The results of the projects were often evaluated by measuring the satisfaction of faculty and students, and in some cases by the results of students' performances on written examinations. There was little attention given to the long-term effects of the projects and their impact on students' careers.

During the 1980s the level of interest in computers in medical education has increased. The continuation of earlier work on computerizing medical education as well as examples of new investigations can be found in anesthesiology,[30, 39, 60, 68, 80] cardiology,[1] clinical chemistry,[71] emergency medicine,[24] family practice,[17, 73, 74] medical decision theory,[81] nephrology,[19] pediatrics,[52, 77] pharmacology,[67] physiology,[69] and radiology.[38, 42]

One of the earliest, most comprehensive, and most carefully observed experiments in the computerization of an entire component of medical education was conducted at the Ohio State University College of Medicine.[28, 94] Beginning in 1966, members of the faculty prepared computer-based instructional packages for portions of the basic science curriculum using a mainframe computer with simple typewriter terminals. Instead of attending lectures some medical students studied the basic sciences independently using both the computer system and faculty advisors to help guide their learning. A significant component of the system included self-assessment tests that provided information about students' strengths and weaknesses to both students and faculty members. With external financial support the system was implemented at Ohio State, and a few other medical colleges were able to use these and other programs by means of a national communications network that was being developed by the Lister Hill Center for Biomedical Communications and the National Library of Medicine.[68, 97, 98] A narrower, but no less intense, project was developed at the Kansas State Medical College in the Department of Pharmacology.[67] Another ambitious project at the University of Illinois used a mainframe computer and the PLATO system,[65, 82] and Harvard Medical School began to offer continuing medical education credits to physicians who used computer-simulated patient management problems through a nationwide communications network. Several excellent summaries on the use of computers in medical education have been published during the 1970s and 1980s.[27, 29, 57, 84, 85, 86]

When the efforts to automate medical education over the past 15 years are reviewed, it is apparent that "computer-assisted instruction" cannot be meaningfully discussed or evaluated as a single entity. To many readers the phrase computer-assisted instruction has connotations of a teaching machine that alternates between displaying information and asking questions of the student. The richest opportunities for the use of computers in medical education can best be discussed by separating them into the following broad categories of instruction: fundamental biologic processes, simulated patient management problems, student testing (either for formal evaluation or for self-assessment), and interactive teaching dialogues. This differentiation does not assume that these four broad types of computer-based instruction cannot be combined. However, because many successful efforts have emphasized at least one of these techniques of designing instructional programs, we will use these as a framework to describe the opportunities to introduce computers and to analyze future trends.

Models of Biologic Processes

The complexity of the biologic processes studied in the basic medical sciences has attracted the interest of computer enthusiasts in a number of disciplines.[72] Recognizing the potential to put to use the inexpensive interactive computational power that is available in desktop personal computers, these educators have proposed that life-like computer models of parts of the human body, such as the cardiovascular system, can provide students with a valuable opportunity to learn about the dynamic behavior of complex systems. By varying and observing important parameters in the models, students are able to conduct experiments to test their own understanding of the biologic processes.[67] At the cellular and molecular level, models of pharmacological phenomena may enable medical students to examine the effects of different drug doses.[7] When contrasted with the use of laboratory animals as teaching models for organ systems, the advantages of computer models are significant. Not only might the long-term economic cost of computer models be lower, but the concerns of antivivisectionists may be reduced. Other advantages include the opportunity for greater student involvement when each student uses a separate computer rather than groups of students sharing a limited number of laboratory animals. Students are able to generate hypotheses and test their predictive power by manipulating variables in the computer model. Rather than memorizing selected relationships among variables, students can discover them by experimentation. By controlling the speed of processes, computer models allow students to conduct a number of lengthy experiments in a shorter period of time, or to extend the elapsed time of a very brief experiment so that they can better understand the processes being illustrated. Experiments can be stopped to study intermediate results and restarted at the student's direction. They can even be reversed. Experiments that might expose students to dangerous organisms, chemicals, or radiation can be carried out safely through modeling. Finally, students may be given the opportunity to learn by varying parameters at levels which would injure live animals.

Uses for models of biologic processes have been found not only in the basic medical sciences but also in those clinical specialties and subspecialties concerned with the precise regulation of these processes in individual patients. Examples include maintaining electrolyte balance, determining insulin dosage in diabetics, and regulating pulmonary function. Although often thought of as tools for independent study, such biologic models could also be used by faculty members to enhance the presentation of an existing lecture, laboratory, or conference. The motivation of students might be heightened if, after a computer model were demonstrated and interpreted by an expert lecturer, each student could use his or her own computer to explore further the behavior of the biologic process being studied by using "trial and error." During the demanding schedules of clinical clerkships and residencies, accessibility to such models would be an asset for students and residents who need to reinforce or update what they learned in the basic science years of their medical education. Some limitations in present continuing medical education programs might be overcome if simulation models were made available to practitioners.[54] Accurate, affordable, and easy-to-use models of the most important biologic processes can be used for teaching at all levels of medical education.

With the many advantages of these models of biologic processes, why then have they not gained widespread acceptance in medical education? One reason is that their validity has been challenged. The reduction of a complex biologic system to a series of differential equations stored in a computer often yields a model that is somewhat less than perfect, although proponents argue that the loss in accuracy is insignificant compared to the advantages. Another reason may be attitudinal. Some faculty members may feel that experience in a wet laboratory is an indispensable part of medical education, and they fear that computers may infringe upon laboratory time, which is already felt to be inadequate. Proponents of computer models respond by asserting that using these models may be better than no laboratory at all in situations in which laboratory time has already been cut back.[55] It is possible that a lack of familiarity with computer technology may discourage some faculty members from delegating teaching responsibilities to computers. Yet in other fields, such as engineering, in which faculty members were among the first to use computers in research and practice decades ago, there is still, unfortunately, a dearth of educational software.[26] Although less important at this time, a major reason for the limited use of computer models in the past was the scarcity and high cost of computer hardware. While this is now less of a constraint, the most complete models still require monitors capable of displaying high-resolution color graphics supported by more powerful microprocessors than are found in many affordable personal computers. A fifth factor may relate to the increasing role of standardized tests in medical education, since the methods used to evaluate medical students greatly influence their approach to learning.[70] If the written multiple-choice examinations used for promotion, certification, and licensure in medicine tend to measure the students' knowledge and ability to deal with static representations of biologic processes, there may be less reward for the kind of knowledge gained from studying dynamic computer models. More will be said about the present and future role of computers and student testing in a later section.

Simulated Patient Management Problems

Inspired perhaps by the proven capability of flight simulators for training in aviation, many teachers in medicine have long been intrigued by the possibility of producing powerful patient simulators that could be queried, diagnosed, and treated by medical students, residents, or practicing physicians. Even before computers were widely available, a few people were experimenting with manual patient simulators based on stacks of cards[21] or latent images that could be exposed with a special pen.[58, 59] One of the first attempts to automate patient management problems was reported by investigators at the University of Illinois.[37] Now the increasing availability and falling prices of computers have been accompanied by a crescendo of interest in these simulations.

In the traditional patient management problem a student first reads a description of a hypothetical patient's presenting complaint. By requesting further information about the patient's medical history or physical findings, or by ordering diagnostic tests, the problem solver attempts to formulate a diagnosis. After a diagnosis is made, many of the patient simulations also require that the problem solver proceed to evaluate alternative plans for management of the patient. Early simulations were labeled as either "linear" or "branching" simulations. Linear problems guided the student through a fixed sequence of data collection, diagnosis, and finally, treatment of the patient. A student could often rule out certain diagnoses by skimming ahead to see which treatment options would be offered. Although cumbersome in paper form, early branching simulations were able to present students with treatment options only after a diagnosis had been made. Deeper levels of branching attempted to simulate the consequences of management decisions.

Although a few computer systems developed in the 1970s made attempts to use typewritten natural language as input, most presented menus or lists of codes for history, physical examination, and laboratory tests that were used by the student to make selections. In the 1980s advocates have begun to envision high-fidelity computer-based simulators that would accept spoken words from students, produce their own voice output with synthesizers, and display images from video disks. Imagine a modestly priced personal computer with a color video disc player connected to a monitor and voice input/output device that, when queried about the patient's chief complaint, would display a video image of a 45-year-old man talking about his abdominal pain and pointing to the location! Using such a system, a medical student could ask further questions, examine the results of laboratory studies, select appropriate treatments, and observe the results. The months or years normally spent by the physician managing a complex patient problem could be reduced to a few hours for the benefit of the student.[1, 9]

Simulated patient management problems have met with controversy, especially when used to evaluate students or physicians. Compromises in their design, often imposed by limitations in the available technology or budget, led to questions about their validity.[33] Unfortunately, early patient simulations prevented students from exercising essential clinical skills, and some implementations actually may have encouraged the development of inappropriate clinical skills. It was not unusual for programs to let students make clinical decisions in ways that real doctors would never consider, leading one writer to question the quality of a particular program by speculating that "its mathematical and theoretical constructions emanate from the armchair rather than the bedside."[79] Skipping past the computer's options for the history and physical information, a student could go directly to the list of diagnostic laboratory tests and quickly gather information crucial to making the proper diagnosis. Without a penalty for the economic costs and time wasted by ordering excessive tests, the student would solve the problem quickly with a complete profile of laboratory values without an incentive to search for diagnostic clues in the history and physical examination.

These limitations have been overcome in the new simulations in which the costs of each question asked by the student are accumulated in terms of time, dollars, and patient discomfort. No longer can one order an SMA-12 or perform a bone marrow biopsy on the simulated patient without the penalties of dollars consumed and some estimate of the pain and discomfort inflicted.

The use of multiple choice options in early simulations provided cues not found in the real world, thus upsetting their validity. Fast desktop computers with large storage capacities now enable free-response input to be used instead of checklists of patient data and laboratory tests. Even in the most elegant and complex simulations today, the structure of available options and key words can still play tricks with the judgment of an experienced clinician who needs only a few subtle diagnostic clues to assemble a meaningful differential diagnosis.[25] Nevertheless, work by investigators in recent years shows that when these difficulties are encountered, they can be overcome with diligence.[1]

It is easy to imagine how high-quality simulations of patients could be used to augment or substitute portions of the clinical experiences in medical school or in certain residencies. Although many proponents of patient management problems promise that students will learn problem-solving skills, it has also been shown that factual knowledge can be increased when simulations are used for teaching.[63] Elegant and valid computer models of patients would allow students to learn by trial and error without endangering patients or consuming health care resources.[7] Patient management problems could be used to motivate medical students in the early years of their education at a time when they are eager to attack clinical problems but are not yet able to assume responsibility for real patients. Changes in the health care delivery system that are placing more pressure on hospitals might make some institutions limit their support for educational programs, and thus reduce the opportunities for students to take histories and perform physical examinations on adequate numbers of patients. Simulations can be used by teachers and students to study the diagnostic process to better understand the relative value of information obtained from laboratory tests.[87] Having a set of "standard" computer simulations available could help to assure that all students would be exposed to a proper assortment of patient problems. Thorough and creative simulations could be used to teach students valuable lessons by incorporating random errors in reporting laboratory results. Simulations could be designed to remind students of the challenge that is encountered when a patient's complaints and symptoms are exaggerated, or when a patient's noncompliance with the prescribed treatment is not reported to the physician. The occasional inclusion of spurious results in simulations would have the secondary benefit of reminding students that the crisp, clean output from any computer does not guarantee that it is accurate. Like their close counterparts—models of fundamental biologic processes—a carefully developed patient management problem could be used at many different levels of medical education. Practicing physicians might find it productive to continue their education with carefully chosen patient simulations that fit the profile of their professional practice or specific areas they wish to strengthen.[54]

Student Testing

Nowhere in the past 20 years have computers had greater impact on medical education than in the area of tests for medical students and residents. Introduced with promises of psychometric precision at a reasonable cost, the machine scoring of multiple-choice examinations has largely eliminated the use of oral and written essay examinations by most medical certifying and licensing boards. Dominating the technology of testing in undergraduate medical education is the National Board of Medical Examiners, which administers a series of three certifying examinations, a popular route to licensure for many medical students in nearly every state in the United States. In over 70 per cent of U.S. medical schools, students must take these examinations.[70] Parts of these examinations are also used for internal decision making about the promotion of students in over half of the medical colleges, and these nationally standardized tests are among the criteria used by some residency programs for reviewing applicants. Recognizing the legal and professional uses, many medical students view these or similar tests—such as the Federation Licensing Examination (FLEX)—as principal hurdles to overcome in their careers. According to a recent report, "The methods used to evaluate medical students' achievement greatly influence their approach to learning."[70] The decision of some medical colleges to use only pass/fail grading has led the directors of some residency programs to become more dependent on National Board scores to screen applicants for residencies. Passing the nationally standardized examinations is essential, and achieving the highest possible score can also open additional career opportunities as the number of residency positions dwindle. Although there is continuing controversy about how much these multiple-choice examinations really do affect the curricula of medical colleges and the study habits of students, there seems to be little doubt that they exert at least some influence.

Since 1968 the National Board has encouraged research on and development of new applications for computers in evaluating the competence of physicians. In 1985 the Board approved a recommendation of one of its committees to begin to implement computer-based testing. Current plans call for the first computer-based test to be used for the Part III examination in 1988. The Board's computer-based examination builds on the concept of the traditional patient management problem, using an interactive computer to provide an unstructured computer program to represent the interaction of a physician with a patient and the health care system. The physician (examinee) performs a diagnostic evaluation of a simulated patient and proceeds to institute management of the problem that has been identified. Unlike paper-and-pencil techniques of simulation, the physiologic parameters of the simulated patient may change in response to the physician's intervention, or in a direction that is consistent with the natural course of the disease. The Board is also planning to administer the conventional multiple-choice questions of Part III by computer.[88]

It seems unlikely that changes in the format of the National Board examinations will go unnoticed by students, residents, and medical educators. Because the Part III examination is taken by residents at the end of their first year of postgraduate training, the initial use of computer-based testing by the Board would be expected to have little impact on undergraduate medical education. In order to make this change, the Board plans to establish a nationwide network of computer testing centers where examinations will be administered. After automating the Part III examination, the Board anticipates extending these techniques to other tests. When this happens, it seems reasonable to expect that many medical schools and students will become interested in examinations administered by computer. Even if a medical school decides not to offer computerized tests, some students may use them as self-assessment instruments to prepare for comprehensive examinations in the same way that they use commercial review courses at the present time.

Interactive Teaching Dialogues

The development of this classic form of computer-assisted instruction can be traced to the idea of teaching machines introduced in the 1950s and modified to take advantage of general-purpose computer technology in the 1960s.[35] Based on theories of behavioral psychology, especially on the work of B. F. Skinner, educators reasoned that students could be taught best by administering instruction in small increments with frequent interplay between teacher (or machine) and student. With proper programming these Socratic dialogues would direct the machine to ask questions of a student, accept the student's response, and then decide the proper time to administer more difficult material or whether remediation was needed. When combined with pre-testing and post-testing of students' knowledge, it suggested that education could be automated.

One of the important theoretical foundations of instructional dialogues is that important information is to be found in students' wrong answers to questions. An experienced teacher who has a solid grasp of students' most common misconceptions in his or her discipline can develop a competent computer program that will deliver sophisticated, personalized, tutorial assistance to many students. It is assumed that such programs can guide students' learning by helping them interpret their strengths and weaknesses. These programs are expensive to develop, requiring 20 hours or more of faculty time to develop just 1 hour of computer-based instruction. More time is needed for pilot testing, evaluation, and revision. Of course, if such a program can be used productively by hundreds of students, the average cost per student may be small. Some faculty members, especially those in the rapidly changing biomedical sciences, have been concerned with the cost of keeping these programs up to date. Nevertheless the computer hardware and software needed to generate computerized instruction are available today for computers in every price range. It would seem that teaching dialogues would have greatest utility in the early years of medical education when lectures and other formal classroom teaching have been predominant. The dynamic nature of clinical clerkships and residencies and their decentralization seem to be factors that would inhibit the introduction of computerized instruction. On the other hand, computerized instruction could help to assure uniformity in educational experiences when students' clinical experiences are divided among a number of diverse affiliated hospitals.

An editorial in *The Lancet* expressed unbounded hopes for the use of programmed instruction and computers in teaching. By taking advantage of the optic nerve's million nerve fibers rather than the 25,000 fibers of the auditory nerve, it was reasoned that the visual potential of computers coupled with graphics and video technology could make learning much more efficient.[3, 18] Unfortunately, this traditional form of computer teaching has been criticized for producing programs, sometimes referred to as "electronic page turners," that offer few advantages over books when the true capabilities of the computer were not put to use.[6, 79]

Applications of Available Programs

Commonly, the introduction of computers into medical education has been accompanied by changes in the very structure of the educational programs. Proposals for innovation in medical education have often emphasized the potential role of computers.[16, 29, 43] Programs at Ohio State and Kansas State were designed as independent study programs using computers as convenient learning tools. Where computers are being used most successfully, it is not unusual to find educators grappling with the subtle distinction between learning and teaching. The actual link between the two may be limited when one finds that learning is a function largely of what an individual student already knows at the beginning of instruction as well as what is of greatest interest to the individual student. There is extensive empirical evidence produced by hundreds of studies in a multitude of disciplines that students can learn independently by a technique known as the Keller Plan. When this individually paced, mastery-oriented approach to teaching was used, it showed that students' content learning equaled or exceeded performance in traditional lecture sessions.[47] These findings have major implications in that they support arguments for the effectiveness of computerized teaching dialogues when used as a substitute for some lectures and classes.

A number of questions about the four major opportunities to use computers in medical education need to be examined in the next decade. Will published computer programs be subjected to the same degree of peer review as textbooks and other publications? If not, acceptance of computer programs may be halted by some of the same resistance that developed against audiovisual materials of marginal quality produced during the 1970s. Will computer-assisted learning tend to integrate or fragment knowledge? Just as pressures to publish the results of research have sometimes led some academicians to publish studies of limited importance, reward mechanisms for the development of computer programs may encourage faculty members to produce too many materials too quickly.[6]

Many traditional publishers of textbooks are eager to establish new territory in electronic publishing. In an era when interdisciplinary teaching is of increasing importance, might computer programs developed along traditional disciplinary lines serve to segregate rather than integrate? How will students sample a variety of perspectives on a given topic? Using the printed word, a diligent student can read carefully chosen sections on a given topic in several textbooks, or review reprints of selected journal articles. It might be impractical in the same amount of time for that student to make use of several diverse computer programs—for example, one written by a professor, one published by a nationally recognized authority in the field, and one put together by a proprietary publishing house.

Many programs have been designed with a beginning and ending without provision for browsing. Sampling different programs would be almost impossible if each program required a different brand or configuration of computer. By writing local instructional programs, overzealous and prolific faculty members might inadvertently teach students to become dependent upon a single source of information. Such dilemmas could be magnified during the transitional period when computer programs might be offered as supplements to a conventional educational system of lectures, reading, laboratories, conferences, and clerkships. If experimental computer programs in medical education are offered simply as additions to the regular class schedules, is it possible that they will be quickly judged as failures simply because time was not available to properly use them?

Faculty members must address these possibilities to assure that materials developed for students make the best possible use of all available technology. Recommendations are now being made to make medical education more effective and efficient by reducing the amount of structured classroom time in medical education in the coming years.[70] Appropriate use of computers for learning may be a viable option.

LEARNING ABOUT COMPUTERS IN MEDICAL SCHOOL

One of the earliest elective courses designed to teach medical students about the use of computers was reported from the University of California, San Diego, in 1969.[99] The broad objective of learning to identify and understand appropriate biomedical computer applications was addressed by exposing freshman students to programs dealing with fluid and electrolyte calculations, image processing, automated diagnosis, electrocardiogram processing, clinical laboratory automation, radiation treatment planning, and cardiovascular simulation. The students also learned to write computer programs in the BASIC language using terminals connected to a large time-sharing computer. With a few exceptions, special attention to computer skills has been inconspicuous in the formal curricula of most medical colleges.[29, 49] There seems to be little evidence that medical schools and physicians have given the same universal respect to computers as has been given to basic medical tools such as microscopes, stethoscopes, otoscopes, and ophthalmoscopes. Computers have not yet been embraced by all clinicians as indispensable instruments for collecting, storing, retrieving, and analyzing data.

Some of the explanations for this general lack of regard for computers may be the following:

When the first computers became available, their capabilities and the skills needed to operate them were far from being universally defined and were not generically equivalent in various settings. That is, one who learned to use an automated medical records system, diagnostic aid, or bibliographic search program in the hospital of a particular academic medical center could not be certain to find the same computer system in another setting. Some acquired skills might have been transferable, but the computer hardware and software of different manufacturers and various medical institutions frequently adhered to slightly different conventions, thereby inhibiting standardization.

The learning curve for mastering computer skills on large computer systems was often prohibitively long, steep, and sometimes endless. Again, local customs, mysterious acronyms, abstruse written documentation, periodic updates to operating systems, and the uneven capabilities of different computers discouraged many students and physicians from trying to learn to use computers.

Even after the necessary skills were acquired, computer facilities often remained inaccessible or far too expensive. Until a few years ago, it was understood by students and faculty that using a computer often meant going to a special room, or to a special building. Even when terminals were conveniently located, one had to have a user account identifier and password so that administrators could safeguard expensive resources and maintain the security of data in large computer systems. A few devoted users of computers did buy their own terminals to use in their offices, laboratories, or homes.

Traditionally, the use of keyboards and associated activities such as typing have not enjoyed high status in the medical community. Some may have avoided the social stigma attached to operating a computer keyboard. At the same time, a flawless memory has been recognized as one of the hallmarks of a skilled clinician. The use of a machine that extends the human memory may have been viewed as some sort of an admission of inadequacy.

Despite the increased reliability and availability of large computer systems, there may have been fears about becoming dependent on a large "electronic brain." Because modern medicine has copied the design of the human body and built redundancy into many of its support systems, the notion of a single central computer where all patient data would be stored was an anathema to the instincts of prudent clinical practitioners. Questions have also been raised about confidentiality, privacy, and legal issues surrounding large computer data banks.[78]

In a recent analysis of medicine's apparent lagging behind other fields in implementing new technology, one author observed: "Physicians are willing to use any reliable and effective technology. Lack of clinical use (of computers) indicates flaws in these products."[50]

What appears to be widespread indifference to the use of computers in medicine cannot be generally attributed to all specialty areas. Certain specialties seem to have attracted individuals with interests in computers and technology, or they have fostered the development of these interests. Anesthesiology, radiation therapy, radiology, and cardiology require that most practitioners be able to use certain kinds of computers routinely as components of the specialties' rapidly changing diagnostic and therapeutic technologies.[62] Certain career paths, such as research, within almost any specialty have likewise required or fostered the development of appropriate computer skills. Few laboratories or epidemiologic research centers function today without some degree of automation.

Most of the above-mentioned obstacles to physicians' use of computers are no longer relevant. Today's computer equipment bears little resemblance to that found in use 5 to 10 years ago. Computers are now easy to use, much more accessible, and simple to learn about. What were referred to a decade ago as "canned computer programs" which enabled novices to use mainframe computers have been repackaged and labeled as "user-friendly software," advertised through magazines and television and merchandised at convenient retail outlets throughout the world. In actuality, although many of today's programs share the same goals as the computer programs of a decade ago, they are quite different, as they have been designed to make effective use of the computing capability of a desktop computer, relieved of the complications introduced by large, shared systems. A distinguishing characteristic of the present computer environment is that decisions about whether or not to use computers are no longer made solely by an organization or institution. Ten years ago the decision to use a computer required managerial planning, capital investment, substantial floor space with a controlled environment, and an assurance of future funding to support maintenance and personnel. Now a department, faculty member, or student can buy a powerful machine for a few thousand dollars and add programs and capacity in modest increments. In fact, a department can buy several machines to assure that a back-up is available if one fails. This is not to say that careful planning for the use of computers in organizations is unimportant. What is implied is that there are now few obstacles to the use of computers in medical schools. As the practical utility of computers in medical practice is demonstrated, individuals in medical schools will decide to buy them.

What do medical students need to learn about computers? In the 1980's it has been predicted that the availability of computers will influence the role played by the physician.[5, 93] As described in other chapters of this book, there are growing opportunities for physicians to use computers in a variety of areas. Computer software is now available to solve real problems for physicians in some settings. Word processing, spreadsheets, data base managers, and communications programs can be used productively. Data bases of references to journal articles can be searched electronically by telephone, and selections can be transferred to a physician's or student's computer. It seems inevitable that clinicians will soon begin to use automated medical records of some sort. Therefore, they need to have an understanding of the advantages and limitations of such changes in procedure and their effects on clinical matters. Another argument is that using computers helps one to develop clear and structured thinking, which will exert a positive effect on some clinical skills.[87] There is increasing acceptance of reliance upon treatment protocols and their broader counterparts, algorithms, for clinical decision making. An indirect argument for "computer literacy" among physicians is that they will be better prepared to interpret the findings of computer-based information systems. The radical changes that are taking place in the financing of health care since the implementation of prospective payment systems with diagnostic related groups (DRGs) have been a result of quantitative models that probably would not have been developed without computers. Finally, one can see on the horizon the uses for the newest products of computer technology—robotic devices that perform microscopic surgery.

To ask exactly which computer knowledge and skills are needed by medical students may be a moot question at this time. A more important question deals with the problem of *when* a medical student or physician should begin to learn to use computers. One approach would be to teach students about computers and their application to medicine in the early years of medical school. When this was attempted by Yoder in 1969 it was reported that the lack of clinical knowledge of entering freshman medical students limited their ability to fully understand the context of biomedical computing.[95] Of course, it could be argued that computers can serve as a vehicle to teach young students basic clinical concepts. If introduced in the early years of medical school, teaching about computers must be followed by practical use. What is learned about computing in the early years of medical school may be lost unless the acquired skills are reinforced in students' actual clinical experiences. Even if the hospital most closely tied to the medical school provides facilities for students to use computers in their clinical clerkships, it may be difficult to assure that students will exercise their skills if they leave the academic medical center for clerkships in smaller affiliated hospitals or outpatient settings that may have less of a commitment to the clinical application of computers. Decentralized clinical teaching is the rule, rather than the exception, in medical colleges at this time. Finally, early learning about computers may have been counterproductive in the days when the technical characteristics of personal computers were changing almost every year. This seems to be less of a problem now, but future trends and revolutions are uncertain. The reader should keep in mind that the foregoing discussion is irrelevant to the issue of how medical students can learn *with* computers. Experience and reason strongly suggest that computers can be introduced for selected purposes at almost any point in medical education.

Should formal attention to biomedical computing be delayed until the latter part of medical school or even residency? Such a plan would assure that students receive the most current information about computer technology in the context of their clinical experiences. Although it could be argued that all students should learn certain basic computer skills, the needs for emphasis in certain topics may vary according to career plans. A student planning to enter primary care may have different expectations of computer use than a student planning to enter a subspecialty.

A panel of medical educators did give formal recognition to some of the potential uses of computers as part of a national report on the general professional education of physicians, published in 1984 by the Association of American Medical Colleges (AAMC).[70] Among the five broad conclusions of this panel was a statement that a general professional education should prepare medical students to be able to learn independently throughout their lives. To implement this goal, the panel recommended specific changes in the style of medical students' learning, accompanied by reductions in rigidly scheduled class time and lecture hours. Recognizing the growing uses of computer systems to help physicians retrieve information from the literature and to analyze patient data, the panel's deliberations also addressed specifically the opportunities for the use of computers in medical schools. To meet the needs of students and faculty in this growing area, the panel recommended that medical schools designate academic units to provide institutional leadership in the application of information sciences and computer technology. Subsequent to the publication of this report, the AAMC did sponsor a first Symposium on Medical Informatics in March, 1985, as a first step in addressing these and similar recommendations. The representation of many medical colleges at this meeting and a commitment to convene again on this topic suggests that computers will soon become more visible in the curricula of many medical colleges.

Any of three factors may serve as the catalyst for medical schools to integrate computers into the clinical experiences of medical students. First, computers are being used as tools more frequently by clinicians in the patient care environment. With or without the initiative of deans and curriculum committees, students in their clinical rotations will come into close contact with faculty members who use computers in their professional work. This is already happening in many medical schools. Another important factor is that trends in baccalaureate education in the 1980s encouraged many college students to buy personal computers as part of institutional arrangements with computer manufacturers. Many students will enter U.S. medical colleges in the late 1980s already owning and knowing how to use a computer. The final factor relates to the demands of residency programs. If certain computer knowledge and skills are deemed important in the selection of residents, medical schools will adapt to assure that their graduates can compete for the best positions.

The availability of inexpensive computers, the curiosity of many faculty members about them, and the growing number of medical students who enter medical schools already owning computers suggest that in medical colleges and residency programs computers will be commonplace. Their presence in every institution will not necessarily ensure their effective use as learning tools in the education program unless faculty members assume an active role in producing or recommending educational computer programs, and in modifying the structure of the curriculum so that students will have time to use them. There is an opportunity for creative faculty members to develop and publish competent programs that can be used not only by medical students but also by residents and practitioners. Whether or not students are encouraged by the faculty to study by using computers in medical school, they will learn about them, becoming able to use them to the extent that the computers enable them to become more productive professionals. It is becoming easier and easier to learn to use computers. Although many students will be acquiring these basic skills before entering medical school in their baccalaureate program or earlier, others may not find a need to learn to use computers until they encounter them in their clinical experiences in medical school. What each medical student needs to know about computers will depend largely on the type of residency selected and the specific type of career planned. The most important influence determining what young physicians learn about the creative uses of computers will be the manner in which computers are actually put to use in their residency training institution where work habits are refined.

The influence of the computer on medical care, education, and research is pervasive. In order to ensure that future professionals embrace this technology, it is necessary for medical educators to introduce students and faculty to the opportunities offered by computers.

REFERENCES

1. Abdulla, A. M., Watkins, L. O., and Henke, J. S.: The use of natural language entry and laser videodisc technology in CAI. J. Med. Educ., 59:739–745, 1984.
2. Abdulla, A. M., Watkins, L. O., Henke, J. S., et al.: Classroom use of personal computers in medical education. Med. Educ., 17:229–232, 1983.
3. Abdulla, A. M., Watkins, L. O., Henke, J. S., and Frank, M. J.: Usefulness of computer-assisted instruction for medical education. Am. J. Cardiol., 54:905–907, 1984 (editorial).
4. Allwood, G. G.: Computer-assisted revision system in immunology. Med. Educ., 10:512–513, 1976.
5. Antley, M. A., and Antley, R. M.: Obsolescence: The physician or the diagnostician role. J. Med. Educ., 47:737–738, 1972.
6. Arons, A. B.: Computer-based instructional dialogues in science courses. Science, 224:1051–1056, 1984.
7. Asbury, A. J.: ABC of computing. Computers in medical education. Br. Med. J., 287:887–890, 1983.
8. Barnett, G. O.: Strategies, potentials, and problems of computerized assisted instruction. Physiologist, 16:621–625, 1973.
9. Barnett, G. O.: Computer-based simulations and clinical problem-solving. Med. Info., 9:277–279, 1984.
10. Bringham, C. R., and Kamp, M.: The current status of computer-assisted instruction in the health sciences. J. Med. Educ., 49:278–279, 1974.
11. Brown, M. C.: Electronics in medical education. J. Med. Educ., 38:270–281, 1963.
12. Budkin, A. and Warner, H. R.: Computer-assisted teaching of cardiac arrhythmias. Comput. Biomed. Res., 2:145–150, 1968.
13. Burch, J. G., Heyman, A., Hammond, W. E., and Haynes, C.: Computer-aided instruction in clinical neurology. J. Med. Educ., 53:693, 1978.
14. Burnum, J. F.: What one internist does in his practice. Implications for the internist's disputed role and education. Ann. Intern. Med., 78:437–444, 1973.

15. Caceres, C. A., and Barnes, D. R.: Training and education for acceptance of the computer sciences. Ann. N.Y. Acad. Sci., 166:1038–1044, 1969.
16. Chapman, D. M.: Making medical school fun while keeping pace with science and technology. Pharos., 47:29–34, 1984.
17. Coggan, P. G., Hoppe, M., and Hadoc, K.: Educational applications of computers in medical education. J. Fam. Pract., 19:66–71, 1984.
18. Computer-assisted learning. Lancet, 1:293–295, 1980 (editorial).
19. Davidson, W. D., and Davidson, S. M.: Teaching dialysis kinetics with a minicomputer. Am. J. Nephrol., 4:19–26, 1984.
20. de Dombal, F. T., Hartley, J. R., and Sleeman, D. H.: Teaching surgical diagnosis with the aid of a computer. Br. J. Surg., 56:754–757, 1969.
21. de Dombal, F. T., Smith, R. B., Modgill, V. K., and Leaper, D. J.: Simulation of the diagnostic process: A further comparison. Br. J. Med. Educ., 6:238–245, 1972.
22. Diamond, H. S., Weiner, M., and Plotz, C. M.: A computer assisted instructional course in diagnosis and treatment of the rheumatic diseases. Arthritis Rheum., 17:1049–55, 1974.
23. d'Ivernois, J. R., Dagenais, G. R., Christen, A., et al.: Computer assisted instruction for retraining family doctors in hypertension and hyperlipoproteinemia. Med. Educ., 13:356–358, 1979.
24. Dugdale, A. E., Chandler, D., and Best, G.: Teaching the management of medical emergencies using an interactive computer terminal. Med. Educ., 16:27–30, 1982.
25. Elstein, A.: Medical Problem Solving: An Analysis of Clinical Reasoning. Cambridge, Harvard University Press, 1978.
26. Engineering professors deplore lag in using computers in their courses. Chronicle Higher Educ., 13, July 3, 1985.
27. Essex, D. L., and Sorlie, W. E.: Effectiveness of instructional computers in teaching basic medical sciences. Med. Educ., 13:189–193, 1979.
28. Folk, R. L., Griesen, J. V., Beran, R. L., and Camiscioni, J. S. (Eds.): Individualizing the Study of Medicine: The OSU College of Medicine Independent Study Program. Westinghouse Learning Corporation, New York, 1976.
29. Friedman, C. P., and Purcell, E. F. (Eds.): The New Biology and Medical Education: Merging the Biological, Information and Cognitive Sciences. Port Washington, N.Y., Josiah Macy, Jr. Foundation, 1983.
30. Friedman, R. B., Beatty, E., Korst, D., and Friedman, P.: A diagnostic aid for medical education. J. Med. Educ., 52:935–937, 1977.
31. Gibbs, J. M., and Burke, D. P.: The computer as a teaching aid: With particular reference to anaesthesia. Anaesth. Intensive Care, 10:212–216, 1982.
32. Gjerde, C. L.: Integration of computers into a course on biostatistics. J. Med. Educ., 52:687–688, 1977.
33. Goran, M. J., Williamson, J. W., and Gonnella, J. S.: The validity of patient management problems. J. Med. Educ., 48:171–177, 1973.
34. Goroll, A. H., Barnett, G. O., Bowie, J., and Prather, P.: Teaching differential diagnosis by computer: a pathophysiological approach. J. Med. Educ., 52:153–154, 1977.
35. Green, E. J., and Weiss, R. J.: Programmed instruction: For what, for whom and how? J. Med. Educ., 38:264–269, 1963.
36. Halverson, J. D., and Ballinger, W. F.: Computer-assisted instruction in surgery. Surgery, 83:633–638, 1978.
37. Harless, W. G., Drennon, G. G., Marxner, J. J., et al.: CASE: A computer-aided simulation of the clinical encounter. J. Med. Educ., 46:443–448, 1971.
38. Harper, D., Butler, C., Hodder, R., et al.: Computer-assisted instruction and diagnosis of radiographic findings. J. Med. Syst., 8:115–120, 1984.
39. Heffernan, P. B., Gibbs, J. M., McKinnon, A. E.: Teaching the uptake and distribution of halothane. A computer simulation program. Anaesthesia, 37:9–17, 1982.
40. Hoffer, E. P., Barnett, G. O., and Farquhar, B. B.: Computer simulation model for teaching cardiopulmonary resuscitation. J. Med. Educ., 47:343–348, 1972.
41. Hoffer, E. P.: Computer-aided instruction in community hospital emergency departments: a pilot project. J. Med. Educ., 50:84–86, 1975.
42. Jacoby, C. G., Smith, W. L., and Albanese, M. A.: An evaluation of computer-assisted instruction in radiology. AJR, 143:675–677, 1984.

43. Jonas, S.: The case for change in medical education in the United States. Lancet, 2:452–454, 1984.
44. Jones, N. A., Olafson, R. P., and Sutin, J.: Evaluation of a gross anatomy program without dissection. J. Med. Educ., 53:198–205, 1978.
45. Kahn, N., and Bigger, J. T., Jr.: Instruction in pharmacokinetics: A computer-assisted demonstration system. J. Med. Educ., 49:292–295, 1974.
46. Kenny, G. N., and Davis, P. D.: The use of a micro-computer in anaesthetic teaching. Anaesthesia, 34:583–585, 1979.
47. Kulik, J. A., Kulik, C. L., and Carmichael, K.: The Keller plan in science teaching. Science, 183:379–383, 1974.
48. Lal, S., and Wood, A. W.: Computer-assisted learning in the teaching of physiology [proceedings]. J. Physiol., 270:11–12, 1977.
49. Levinson, D. L.: Information, computers and clinical practice. J.A.M.A., 249:607–609, 1983.
50. Lincoln, T. L.: Medical Information Science: A joint endeavor. J.A.M.A., 249:610–612, 1983.
51. Lipsky, J. A., et al.: A computerized instructional and self-evaluation program for learning medical physiology. Physiologist, 22:31–35, 1979.
52. Lustig, J. V., and Groothuis, J. R.: Computer applications in pediatrics. Adv. Pediatr., 31:295–323, 1984.
53. Madsen, B. W., and Bell, R. C.: The development of a computer assisted instruction and assessment system in pharmacology. Med. Educ., 11:13–20, 1977.
54. Manning, P. R.: Continuing medical education. The next step. J.A.M.A., 249:1042–1045, 1983.
55. Marchand, E. R., and Steward, J. P.: Trends in basic medical science instruction affecting role of multidiscipline laboratories. J. Med. Educ., 49:171–175, 1974.
56. Margolis, C. Z.: Uses of clinical algorithms. J.A.M.A., 249:627–632, 1983.
57. Marion, R., Niebuhr, B. R., Petrusa, E. R., and Weinholtz, D.: Computer-based instruction in basic medical science education. J. Med. Educ., 57:521–526, 1982.
58. McCarthy, W. H., and Gonnella, J. S.: The simulated patient management problem: a technique for evaluating and teaching clinical competence. Br. J. Med. Educ., 1:348–352, 1967.
59. McGuire, C. H., and Babbott, D.: Simulation technique in the measurement of problem-solving skills. J. Educ. Meas., 4:1–10, 1967.
60. McIntyre, J. W.: Computer-aided instruction as a part of an undergraduate programme in anaesthesia. Can. Anaesth. Soc. J., 27:68–73, 1980.
61. Meyer, J. H. F., and Beaton, G. R.: An evaluation of computer-assisted teaching in physiology. J. Med. Educ., 49:295–297, 1974.
62. Morgan, C.: The new literacy. Anaesth. Intensive Care, 10:188–190, 1982.
63. Murray, T. S., Cupples, R. W., Barber, J. H., et al.: Computer-assisted learning in undergraduate medical teaching. Lancet, 1:474–476, 1976.
64. Murray, T. S., Cupples, R. W., Barber, J. H., et al.: Teaching decision making to medical undergraduates by computer-assisted learning. Med. Educ., 11:262-264, 1976.
65. Nelson, C. D., Sajid, A. W., and Solomon, L. W.: Diagnose: A medical computer game utilizing deductive reasoning. J. Med. Educ., 54:55–56, 1979.
66. O'Neil, T., Sewall, J., and Marchand, R.: Time-shared computer-assisted preclinical instruction: A short trial and evaluation. J. Med. Educ., 51:765–767, 1976.
67. Pazdernik, T. L., and Walaszek, E. J.: A computer-assisted teaching system in pharmacology for health professionals. J. Med. Educ., 58:341–348, 1983.
68. Parbrook, G. D., Davis, P. D., and Parbrook, E. O.: The microcomputer in self-assessment for examination of anaesthesia. Anaesthesia, 36:1136–1137, 1981.
69. Peterson, N. S., and Campbell, K. B.: Simulated laboratory for teaching cardiac mechanics. Physiologist, 27:165–169, 1984.
70. Physicians for the Twenty-First Century: Report of the Panel on the General Professional Education of the Physician and College Preparation in Medicine [report]. Washington, D.C., Association of American Medical Colleges, 1984.
71. Raj, P. P., Kricka, L. J., and Clewett, A. J.: Microcomputer simulations as aids in medical education: Application in clinical chemistry. Med. Educ., 16:332–342, 1982.
72. Randall, J. E.: Microcomputers and Physiological Simulation. Reading, Mass., Addison-Wesley, 1980.

73. Richards, J. G. Computer-assisted instruction and the use of PILOT. J. Fam. Pract., 19:255–257, 1984.
74. Rosenblatt, R. A., and Gaponoff, M.: The microcomputer as a vehicle for continuing medical education. J. Fam. Pract., 18:629–632, 1984.
75. Ross, S. E.: Programmed instruction and medical education. J.A.M.A., 182:938–939, 1962.
76. Schneiderman, H., and Muller, R. L.: The diagnosis game. A computer-based exercise in clinical problem solving. J.A.M.A., 219:333–335, 1972.
77. Schwartz, M. W., and Hanson, C. W.: Microcomputers and computer-based instruction. J. Med. Educ., 57:303–307, 1982.
78. Schwartz, W. B.: Medicine and the computer. The promise and problems of change. N. Engl. J. Med., 283:1257–1264, 1970.
79. Simpson, M. A.: Letter: Computer assisted learning. Lancet, 1:859, 1976.
80. Skinner, J. B., Knowles, G., Armstrong, R. F., and Ingram, D.: The use of computerized learning in intensive care: An evaluation of a new teaching program. Med. Educ., 17:49–53, 1983.
81. Smyth-Staruch, K., and Littenberg, B.: Using microcomputers to teach sensitivity analysis to medical students. Med. Decision-Making, 3:9–13, 1983.
82. Sorlie, W. E., and Jones, L. A.: Description of a computer-assisted testing system in an independent study program. J. Med. Educ., 50:81–83, 1975.
83. Stevens, C. B., Enzor, M., Phillips, T., and Small, P. A.: An evaluation of self-instructional package on amino acid and protein chemistry. J. Med. Educ., 48:276–297, 1973.
84. Stolurow, L. M., Peterson, T. I., and Cunningham, A. C.: CAI in the Health Professions. Newburyport, Mass., Entelek, Inc., 1970.
85. Stolurow, K. A.: A perspective on instructional uses of computing in medicine. J. Med. Syst., 6:165–170, 1982.
86. Stolurow, K. A., and Cochran, T. M.: Instructional uses of computing in the health sciences. An annotated bibliography. J. Med. Syst., 7:61–84, 1983.
87. Taylor, T. R., Aitchison, J., and McGirr, E. M.: Doctors as decision-makers: A computer-assisted study of diagnosis as a cognitive skill. Br. Med. J., 3:35–40, 1971.
88. The National Board Examiner. Philadelphia, National Board of Medical Examiners, 1985.
89. Thies, R., Harless, W. G., Lucas, N. C., and Jacobson, E. D:. An experiment comparing computer-assisted instruction with lecture presentation in physiology. J. Med. Educ., 44:1156–1160, 1969.
90. Tidball, C. S.: II. Challenges of CAE development. I. Introductory remarks. Physiologist, 16:608–610, 1973.
91. Tidball, C. S.: III. Operating systems and computer languages for educational applications. Physiologist, 16:617–621, 1973.
92. Weber, J. C. and Hagamen, W. D.: ATS: A new system for computer-mediated tutorials in medical education. J. Med. Educ., 47:637–644, 1972.
93. Weed, L. L.: Physicians of the future. N. Eng. J. Med., 304:903–907, 1982.
94. Weinberg, A. D.: CAI at the Ohio State University College of Medicine. Comput. Biol. Med., 3:299–305, 1973.
95. Weiss, R. J., and Green, E. J.: The applicability of programmed instruction in a medical school curriculum. J. Med. Educ., 37:760–766, 1962.
96. Woods, S. M.: A computerized self-assessment examination for residents. Am. J. Psychiatry, 131:1283–1286, 1974.
97. Wooster, H. V.: The Lister Hill experimental CAI network—a progress report. Physiologist, 16:626–630, 1973.
98. Wooster, H., and Lewis, J. F.: Distribution of computer-assisted instructional materials in biomedicine through the Lister Hill Center Experimental Network. Comput. Biol. Med., 3:319–323, 1973.
99. Yoder, R. D.: A course in biomedical computing applications. J. Med. Educ., 44:1056–1062, 1969.

CLINICAL APPLICATIONS OF COMPUTERS IN MEDICAL CARE

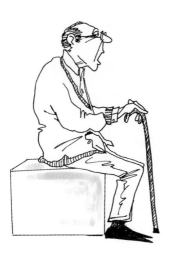
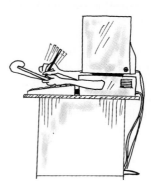

Computerized
History Taking

Edward Messina, M.D.

THE PURPOSE OF THIS CHAPTER

This textbook is dedicated to the application of computers in health care, and this specific chapter consists of the author's personal views regarding automated history taking. From the onset, it should be stated that history taking will be viewed as a diagnostic test in this chapter, rather than as a simple gathering of information. Just as an erythrocyte sedimentation rate is used to screen for abnormalities that might not have been specifically suspected, so the history, particularly the review of systems, should be viewed as a screening test as well. Indeed, a so-called "expert history," which we will later define, can serve as a means for the generalist to uncover any symptoms that might not have been suspected in terms of the chief complaint.

As the medical economic pendulum swings toward very guided work-ups, the medicolegal pendulum is swinging toward a great increase in malpractice litigation. On one hand, we physicians are being asked to run fewer tests, yet we are considered negligent if we fail to uncover underlying disease. A logical way of coping with this dreadful turn of events is to increase the amount of historical data on the patient. Physician time, however, is at a premium owing to the need for high productivity in the office to combat frozen or diminished reimbursements. One of the easiest ways to maximize productivity is have an assistant obtain a medical history or to have a patient interviewed by a computerized history-taking program in which questions are determined by physicians.

Over the years several attempts have been made by large health care organizations, such as HMOs or large clinics, to utilize pencil and paper or large mainframe computer techniques for patient history acquisition. These did not gain in popularity owing to either expense or impracticality. Fortunately we are in the midst of a literal revolution in microcomputer technology so that inexpensive units are available for most office settings.

THE MEDICAL HISTORY

Concept of the Medical History

The actual purpose of the medical history taking is the gathering of data about a patient. The questioning is sometimes guided directly by the nature of the patient's chief complaint, some of it includes necessary demographic or historical information common to all patients, and some of it is used as a screening test for underlying illness that is not related to the chief complaint. As physicians, we are trained to carefully observe the manner in which patients express themselves by observing eye contact, vocal tone, body language, movement, and so on. Our minds are constantly hypothesizing and rejecting various ideas as we converse with a patient, and sometimes our logic will branch along a given avenue of pursuit based on the patient's responses. We often modify the nature of our history to the needs of the individual patient. Our skill in history taking grows rapidly in our first years of medical school and becomes more practical and direct as we become more experienced. We all fall to the temptation of shortening the history because of time constraints and often take "short-cuts" in identifying a problem.

I can still vividly remember the first few histories I took as a second-year medical student. I would spend the entire morning interrogating the patient, break for lunch, and return that afternoon to try to formulate the information into a logical form. There was a plethora of data, and my own inexperience caused me to include a great deal of unnecessary information in my write-up. As I progressed in medical school, the actual interrogation time dropped dramatically, and as an intern in internal medicine I was able to proudly "whip through" a good history in less than an hour. When I reached my neurology residency I found that my general medical history assessment almost outweighed the part dedicated to the patient's chief neurologic complaint. As I learned more about neurology, I had a tendency to play down the "non-specialty" aspects of the patient's case and to concentrate more upon the neurologic. This was in part due to my increasing knowledge of neurology but it was also a function of external time constraints and responsibilities.

I led you through this nostalgic journey of my history-taking observations for a reason. We have a tendency to pursue areas in which we are more comfortable, and perhaps this is to the patient's detriment. A degree of sensitivity certainly should change from case to case, and our threshold for what's important should also vary. Unfortunately, time constraints might change this threshold so that we may overlook important related complaints in the face of what looks like a "more important" chief complaint such as neuropathy.

For this reason, an ideal history-taking system would approach all aspects of the patient's general care without regard for time or number of important complaints. Obviously, none of us has the luxury in our clinical practices to spend the entire day taking a history, but we can suggest that the patient invest some time in this history-taking process and that we as physicians might simply review the entire overview and then ask for specific and pertinent questions.

Source of the History

Patients are usually the best source of information regarding their own health, provided that they're not too young or demented to do so. We must look at the patient as a source of specific historical information but also as a person whose historical ability might be altered by illness. A family member's perspective is quite helpful as well, particularly if there are serious emotional issues or denial to be considered. Review of other physicians' records is also an important part of the complete medical history, as technical procedures, specific laboratory values, physical examination findings, and so on are not usually well communicated by a lay patient.

In making this information pertinent to the computerization of data, as we shall later do, we would like to simply point out that one must realize that each of the above-mentioned sources of patient history are subject to their own individual bias.

TYPES OF HISTORY

Complete History. This so-called complete history would include several parts, one in which the initial focus would be on the patient's chief complaint, if one is present, followed by a systematic review of the rest of the patient's general health.

Partial History. In the specialty setting the initial focus would again be on the chief complaint, but perhaps the systematic review of systems might be limited to those organ systems relating to a specific specialty application. For example, an ophthalmologist might not automatically inquire into the condition of one's bones and joints or history of fractures in the past, but this might be of greater interest to an orthopedic surgeon or a rheumatologist.

The partial history might be utilized as a triage tool in several settings. In one situation it might be used as a means of determining entry into a health care system such as a specialty clinic. A telephone complaint could be handled in a similiar way so that the nature of the complaint would determine whether or not the patient should come in to be seen that day or not. In a clinic setting or immediate care setting a partial history would be useful to determine whether or not a patient has an emergency problem. In the emergency room setting the degree of severity or the acuity of an illness might be initially determined by a partial brief history in order to place the patient in the proper priority category.

When the patient returns to a health care provider for a follow-up visit, an initial limited history of the patient's chief complaint is taken, and a brief review of the patient's overall health attempted, guided by known medical problems in the chart, perhaps to review medications or side effects of these medications and perhaps to go through each problem on the patient's problem list. Sometimes necessary laboratory studies, and certain protocols, would be initiated based upon this automated history. In a pediatric setting certainly one needs to systematically review the need for vaccinations or boosters.

CLINICAL USES OF THE HISTORY

In clinical settings one can use the history to explore a known complaint, as has been noted, or as a means of uncovering unstated complaints.

Exploration of Known Complaint. The problem-oriented history has been well represented in publications in recent years. For example, headache has gotten a great deal of attention by various authors who wish to shorten the amount of time necessary for an interview. Francis and associates described a system that used two types of questionnaires.[7] One was filled out by patients at the time of the headache so the information would be "fresh" in their minds, and the other was then administered in the office setting by a physician or a helper. The program they described attempts to come up with the diagnosis based on formulas, and treatment is then suggested. Stead and associates designed a computer-based self-administered interactive questionnaire for patients with functional headache.[26] The patient would respond by keyboard to questions regarding clinical systems, neurologic manifestions, prior treatment, emotional factors, and personality problems. They found that their computer diagnosis agreed with the physician in 36 of 50 patients. They wrote that the automated interview saved physician time, offered a data base for research, and provided a diagnostic aid for patients with functional headache. Freemon[8] used a computerized 30-question program to categorize headache patients into groups. He felt that computer diagnosis was feasible and appeared practical. Bana and associates utilized a comprehensive headache interview utilizing a large mainframe and telecommunications hookups.[2]

In our experience, problem-oriented histories have been extremely helpful in the clinical setting. For several years prior to the development of our original history programs for headache, backache, and other areas written questionnaires were developed and questions were tested for applicability, patient understanding, and so on. These questions, and their branching logic, were then applied to programs that are currently being used on microcomputers. Figure 9–1 illustrates sample questions from our back program, and Figure 9–2 illustrates sample questions from our headache program.

Exploring Unstated Complaints. A systematic review of systems, as has been noted, can be an extremely helpful screening test, particularly when a large population of patients is being evaluated. This is true in an HMO or large-scale health care system when a good deal of preventive action needs to be taken upon entry into the system. A program of this type was developed by A. K. Olson. He developed and tested an exhaustive review of systems inventory, which pursues all system groups and explores them in detail. Quantitation is possible owing to the branching logic, as noted in Figure 9–3. This program was tested on a cohort of patients who had virtually no previous exposure to computers. Their acceptance of the program was excellent, and the questions were easily understood because they were in lay language; a sample printout is provided in Figure 9–4. This program goes out of its way not to make a diagnosis but presents the positive and negative findings in a grouping,

Text continued on page 168

```
-------------------------
        THE BACK
     PROGRAM REPORT
-------------------------
```

PERSONAL INFORMATION:
=====================
AGE: 27
FEMALE
RIGHT HANDED
OCCUPATION: NURSE--CURRENTLY EMPLOYED
65 INCHES, 125 POUNDS
MARRIED GRADUATED FROM COLLEGE
PRESENT MEDS: TYLENOL PRN FOR H/A, ESGIC PRN FOR H/A

PAIN
====

LOCATION

RIGHT SIDE

DESCRIPTION OF PAIN

PAIN DESCRIBED AS DULL
SENSATIONS OF PRESSURE OR FATIGUE NOTED IN BACK

TIMING:
THIS IS A NEW ONSET OF PAIN
ONE DAY OF BAD PAIN PER WEEK
HAS GRADUAL ONSET

HISTORY OF BACK PAIN:
INCLUDING OCCASIONAL NAGGING PAIN

PATTERN:
PAIN IS INTERMITTENT - PATIENT HAS GOOD DAYS WITH OCCASIONAL BAD ONES

EXACERBATING FACTORS

RELATION TO POSITION:
PAIN OCCURS MOST OFTEN WHEN STANDING
PAIN GETS WORSE WHEN SITTING RATHER THAN STANDING

Figure 9–1. Sample printout from screening history of patient with back pain.

Illustration continued on opposite page

RELATION TO ACTIVITY:
THE FOLLOWING ACTIVITIES WORSEN THE PAIN: TRAUMA, WALKING, BENDING,
LIFTING, PROLONGED WALKING, WALKING UP INCLINES, WORK

RELIEF FACTORS

PRESENT STRATEGY:
POSITIONS: SQUATTING, STRETCHING, BENDING BACKWARDS
BEDREST MAKES PAIN BETTER

PHYSICAL THERAPY:
IMPROVEMENTS HAVE SHOWN FROM EXERCISES

MEDICATIONS:
TYLENOL, TYLENOL X-TRA STRENGTH, ASCRIPTIN

NUMBNESS AND PARESTHESIA
===========================
LOCATION:
IN LOWER AND UPPER EXTREMITIES INCLUDING HANDS, CHEST

PROPHYLAXIS ATTEMPTS
====================
PATIENT HAS ATTEMPTED TO LOSE WEIGHT

GENERAL MEDICAL INFORMATION
===============================
PAST HISTORY

ARTHRITIS:
PATIENT NOTICES MORNING STIFFNESS IN HANDS

PAGET'S DISEASE:
PATIENT GETS HEADACHES

SLEEP HISTORY

PATIENT USES FIRM MATTRESS
PATIENT HAS THE SAME BEDTIME EVERY NIGHT, DOES NOT TAKE SLEEPING PILLS

OCCUPATIONAL HISTORY

PATIENT'S JOB INVOLVES STRESS, LIFTING 15 POUNDS, STANDING, WALKING,
STOOPING AND BENDING
PATIENT HAS BEEN DOING THIS TYPE OF WORK FOR 1 TO 5 YEARS, ENJOYS THE
WORK, FEELS THERE IS TOO MUCH STRESS, FEELS THE BOSS EXPECTS TOO MUCH,
WORKS DAYS (DOES NOT WORK REGULAR HOURS EVERY DAY), DOES NOT CHANGE
SHIFTS FREQUENTLY

PSYCHOSOCIAL FACTORS

UNABLE TO CONTINUE WORKING DUE TO PAIN
DOES NOT CONSIDER HIM/HERSELF TO BE OVERWEIGHT

Figure 9–1. Continued

```
                ------------------------
                HEADACHE DATABASE SHEET
                ------------------------


NAME: HESTER PRYNN                                           DATE: 4/4/84
REFERRED BY DR. SARDONICUS

===============================================================================
GENERAL INFORMATION
-------------------------------------------------------------------------------
AGE: 23
RIGHT HANDED
FEMALE
OCCUPATION: MARKET ANALYST--CURRENTLY EMPLOYED
66 INCHES, 122 POUNDS
DIVORCED
GRADUATE OR PROFESSIONAL DEGREE
REASON FOR REFERRAL:      HEADACHES WHICH INTERFERE WITH LIFESTYLE
PRESENT MEDS:  ELAVIL, INDERAL
===============================================================================
CHARACTERISTICS OF THE PAIN
-------------------------------------------------------------------------------
ONE HEADACHE TYPE
HISTORY OF HEADACHES FOR MORE THAN 10 YEARS
HEADACHE OCCURS MORE THAN ONCE A MONTH
INTENSITY OF PAIN ON SCALE OF 1 TO 5 : 4
LOCATION: FOREHEAD
ONE EYE
MOST PAINFUL SIDE: RIGHT
OCULAR INVOLVEMENT WITHOUT RED EYE
PAIN NOTED AT BACK OF NECK
RADIATES FROM HEAD TO NECK
PAIN DESCRIBED AS THROBBING
USUALLY RIGHT SIDE
DURATION OF PAIN: LESS THAN A DAY
===============================================================================
PRODROME
-------------------------------------------------------------------------------
IRRITABILITY, DULL THROBBING, EMOTIONAL CHANGES
===============================================================================
AURA
-------------------------------------------------------------------------------
SCOTOMATA, ZIG-ZAGS, SPARKS
===============================================================================
HEADACHE BEHAVIOR
-------------------------------------------------------------------------------
UNABLE TO CONTINUE WITH ACTIVITIES
NAUSEA AND VOMITING
HEADACHE WORSE THAN N+V
PHOTOPHOBIA NOTED
COPING BEHAVIOR: LIES DOWN IN A DARK PLACE, A COLD CLOTH ON HEAD, RUBS TEMPLES
```

Figure 9–2. *Sample printout from screening history of patient with headache.*

Illustration continued on opposite page

```
==================================================================================
ACCOMPANIMENTS
----------------------------------------------------------------------------------
PALLOR, STIFF NECK, TENDER SCALP
MIGRATING SYMPTOMS
GRADUAL BUILDUP OF ACCOMPANIMENTS
SYMPTOMS CAN MIGRATE TO OTHER SIDE OF BODY


==================================================================================
A L L   H E A D A C H E S
==================================================================================
PRECIPITATING CAUSES
----------------------------------------------------------------------------------
THE HEADACHE CAN BE TRIGGERED OR WORSENED BY: ALCOHOLIC BEVERAGES,
CERTAIN FOODS, SMOKING A CIGARETTE, STRESS, RIDING IN A CAR OR BUS,
BRIGHT LIGHT, HUNGER, OVER SLEEPING, EATING OR DRINKING SOMETHING VERY COLD
HEADACHE OCCURS ONE HOUR AFTER A DRINK
*****PATIENT HAS PERSONAL PROBLEMS TO DISCUSS IN PRIVATE*****
==================================================================================
RELIEF FACTORS
----------------------------------------------------------------------------------
PATIENT HAS ATTEMPTED TO GET HELP FROM SPECIAL HEADACHE DIET
PRESCRIPTION MEDS TRIED IN THE PAST: WIGRAINE, CAFERGOT, MIDRIN, ELAVIL,
INDERAL, FIORINAL, CODEINE, ERGOSTAT
OVER-THE-COUNTER DRUGS: ASPIRIN, EXCEDRIN
==================================================================================
OCCUPATIONAL HISTORY
----------------------------------------------------------------------------------
ON THE JOB 1 TO 5 YEARS
PATIENT ENJOYS THEIR JOB
PERCEIVES TOO MUCH STRESS AT WORK
BOSS EXPECTS TOO MUCH
THE PATIENT WORKS THE SAME HOURS EACH DAY
DAY SHIFT
THE PATIENT'S CO-WORKERS SMOKE NEARBY
HEADACHES ARE MORE FREQUENT ON WORK DAYS
HEADACHES WORSE AFTER WORK
==================================================================================
SLEEPING PATTERNS
----------------------------------------------------------------------------------
THE PATIENT HAS THE SAME BEDTIME EVERY NIGHT
THE PATIENT HAS TROUBLE FALLING ASLEEP AT NIGHT
PATIENT AWAKENS AT NIGHT AND CANNOT GET BACK TO SLEEP
EARLY MORNING AWAKENING
PATIENT SLEEPS WITH A PARTNER
PATIENT AWAKENS BEFORE 7:00AM
TYPICAL BEDTIME = 12 MIDNIGHT
NO DAYTIME NAPS
DAYTIME DROWSINESS IS NOTED
==================================================================================
HABITS
----------------------------------------------------------------------------------
SMOKES MORE THAN A PACK A DAY
PATIENT DRINKS ALCOHOL LESS THAN ONCE PER MONTH
COFFEE DRINKER ALL WEEK LONG
3 TO 5 CUPS
==================================================================================
DIETARY FACTORS
----------------------------------------------------------------------------------
3 MEALS EVERY DAY
REGULARLY EATS THE FOLLOWING: RIPENED CHEESE (INCLUDING PIZZA), CHOCOLATE,
NUTS, PEANUT BUTTER, CHINESE FOOD, MONOSODIUM GLUTAMATE, BEAN PODS, WINE
==================================================================================
```

Figure 9–2. Continued

which makes it easy to synthesize by the physician. Likewise, a psychiatric screening program was developed by Zarumski to seek key positive findings on routine questioning and pursue them in detail as needed. Questions are asked in a nonthreatening manner, as shown in Figure 9–5, and the results are exhibited as shown in Figure 9–6, which groups them according to symptom type.

In summary, these two screening programs for psychiatric and general medical application serve the purpose of screening a population for specific illness. The benefit is that a physician is not necessary to acquire the data but certainly is essential for the interpretation of the data. It is this author's opinion that current technology is not yet able to duplicate the diagnostic acumen of a skilled clinician. Our technology is, however, able to ask very expert questions, time-consuming questions, and exhaustingly detailed questions, for example, thus benefiting the patient. An example of detailed questioning, which is usually not pursued by most of us in the clinical setting yet is welcome information, is exemplified in Figure 9–7. This demonstrates the large number of over-the-counter medications utilized by headache patients, and one is sometimes surprised by the total salicylate load consumed by these patients. This information might not be as readily apparent by simply asking a patient, "Do you take medications?" One could say that the automated history, as noted in this section, actually allows the patient to think about the illness, formulated in appropriate terminology, or even stimulate the memory regarding medication. We have all experienced a situation in which a patient will answer negatively to the question, "Do you take any medicines?" but later we may find that they take 200 to ·300 aspirin per month but didn't really consider them "medicine."

ACQUISITION OF THE CLASSICAL HISTORY

History Taking By Dialogue

By this term, we specifically mean a physician sitting down with a patient and asking a set of guided as well as very routine questions. The benefits certainly are many, and indeed, this is the classic manner in which medicine is practiced in most settings. This allows the physician to observe the patient's body language, tone of voice, breathing patterns, eye contact, and so on, and allows a certain flexibility for branching and probing questions. Unfortunately, it is a time-consuming process, and certainly one's train of thought is easily broken by the many interruptions that are part of today's practice environment. The data are either committed to memory by the physician, later to be reproduced, or notes are taken during the interview. Many patients regard the note taking as a threatening procedure, and often a patient will answer a very routine

Text continued on page 176

PERSONAL HABITS
==

DO YOU DRINK BEER?
1) YES   2) NO
 1)

HOW MANY PER DAY?
 1) ONE OR LESS
 2) TWO
 3) THREE
 4) FOUR
 5) FIVE
 6) SIX OR MORE

HOW MUCH BEER DO YOU DRINK PER WEEK?
 1) ONE OR LESS
 2) TWO
 3) THREE
 4) FOUR
 5) FIVE
 6) SIX OR MORE

PERSONAL HABITS
==

DO YOU DRINK WINE?
1) YES   2) NO
 1)

HOW MANY GLASSES PER DAY?
 1) ONE OR LESS
 2) TWO
 3) THREE
 4) FOUR
 5) FIVE
 6) SIX OR MORE

HOW MANY PER WEEK?
 1) ONE OR LESS
 2) TWO
 3) THREE
 4) FOUR
 5) FIVE
 6) SIX OR MORE

PERSONAL HABITS
==

DO YOU DRINK LIQUORS?
1) YES   2) NO
 1)

HOW MANY OUNCES PER DAY?
 1) ONE OR LESS
 2) TWO
 3) THREE
 4) FOUR
 5) FIVE
 6) SIX OR MORE

HOW MANY OUNCES PER WEEK?
 1) ONE OR LESS
 2) TWO
 3) THREE
 4) FOUR
 5) FIVE
 6) SIX OR MORE

Figure 9–3. Example of branching logic. A response of "no" to the first question in a category will cause the program to skip to the next category. A response of "yes" will cause the remaining questions to be asked.

```
------------------------
    GENERAL MEDICAL HISTORY
        DATABASE REPORT
------------------------
```

PERSONAL INFORMATION:
=====================
AGE: 27
FEMALE
RIGHT HANDED
OCCUPATION: NURSE--CURRENTLY EMPLOYED
65 INCHES, 124 POUNDS
DIVORCED
GRADUATED FROM COLLEGE
PRESENT MEDS: TYLENOL PRN FOR HEADACHE, ESGIC PRN FOR HEADACHE, TAVIST TID
FOR ALLERGIES

PAST MEDICAL HISTORY:
=====================
SURGICAL PROCEDURES: TONSILECTOMY, APPENDIX, HERNIA REPAIR OF THE ABDOMEN,
UTERUS

PATIENT HAS TAKEN OR IS CURRENTLY TAKING MEDICATIONS FOR: SKIN DISORDERS OR
ITCHING, HEADACHE, ALLERGIC RHINITIS OR HAY FEVER, INFECTION

VITAMIN SUPPLEMENTS TAKEN: NONE

ALLERGIC OR HAS INTOLERANCE TO: PENICILLIN, SEPTRA DS, PBZ, DEXATRIM, ELAVIL

PERSONAL HABITS
===============
PATIENT HAS NEVER SMOKED CIGARETTES AS A HABIT

PATIENT DRINKS THE FOLLOWING:
LIQUOR (ONE OR LESS OUNCES PER DAY - THREE OUNCES PER WEEK)
REGULAR COFFEE (TWO CUPS PER DAY)
DIET COLAS (THREE PER DAY - SIX OR MORE PER WEEK)
```

**Figure 9–4.** Sample printout from general medical history screening program.

*Illustration continued on opposite page*
```

FAMILY HISTORY
==============
HIGH BLOOD PRESSURE, HEART FAILURE, ALCOHOLISM, CANCER, EPILEPSY (SEIZURE,
FIT OR CONVULSION), MIGRAINE, ASTHMA, HAY FEVER, ULCERS, KIDNEY DISEASE,
GOITER OR THYROID DISORDER, ARTHRITIS, NERVOUS BREAKDOWN

REVIEW OF SYSTEMS INVENTORY
===========================
THE PATIENT'S AFFIRMATIVE RESPONSES TO THE REVIEW OF SYSTEMS SUGGEST
CATEGORIES OF ABNORMALITIES WITHIN SYSTEMS. THE FOLLOWING CATEGORIES ARE
MEANT TO BE GENERAL GUIDELINES FOR THE CLINICIAN AND SHOULD NOT BE CONSIDERED
ALL INCLUSIVE NOR MUTUALLY EXCLUSIVE OF OTHER DIAGNOSTIC POSSIBILITIES OR
IMPLICATIONS. THE FINAL INTERPRETATION OF THE RESPONSES MUST BE MADE BY THE
CLINICIAN IN THE CONTEXT OF THE PATIENT'S HISTORY OF THE PRESENT ILLNESS AND
THE FINDINGS ON PHYSICAL EXAMINATION.

THE FOLLOWING SUGGEST CONSTITUTIONAL COMPLAINTS:

SWEATS AT NIGHT, PAINFUL OR STIFF NECK, TIRED OR FATIGUE, INTENTIONAL WEIGHT
LOSS OF 5-10 LBS. OVER 3-6 MONTHS

THE FOLLOWING SYMPTOMS SUGGEST THE PRESENT OF AN INFECTIOUS PROCESS:

SWEATS AT NIGHT

THE FOLLOWING SUGGEST DISORDERS OF THE INTEGUMENT:

ITCHING, SCALING SKIN, REDDENING OR INFLAMMATION OF THE SKIN, DRY SKIN OR
HAIR

THE FOLLOWING SUGGEST DISORDERS OF THE EYES:

INJURY TO THE EYE

THE FOLLOWING SUGGEST DISORDERS OF THE EARS, NOSE, MOUTH, AND/OR THROAT:

CLEAR DISCHARGE FROM THE NOSE

THE FOLLOWING SUGGEST DISORDERS OF THE LUNGS AND/OR CARDIOVASCULAR SYSTEM:

COLD HANDS, COLD FEET, PAINFUL HANDS OR FEET IF EXPOSED TO COOL TEMPERATURES

THE FOLLOWING SUGGEST DISORDERS OF THE GI TRACT:

LOSS OF APPETITE, NAUSEA, BOWEL PATTERN OF ALTERNATING DIARRHEA AND
CONSTIPATION, INTENTIONAL WEIGHT LOSS OF 5-10 LBS. OVER 3-6 MONTHS

THE FOLLOWING SUGGEST DISORDERS OF THE GENITOURINARY SYSTEM:

FREQUENT URINATION, URGENCY TO URINATE, GETTING UP TO URINATE AT NIGHT

THE FOLLOWING SUGGEST DISORDERS OF THE REPRODUCTIVE SYSTEM:

PATIENT IS NO LONGER MENSTRUATING

THE FOLLOWING SUGGEST DISORDERS OF THE RHEUMATOLOGIC SYSTEM:

BACK PAIN

THE FOLLOWING SYMPTOMS SUGGEST DISORDERS OF THE IMMUNE SYSTEM:
---HAYFEVER,
SWELLING OF THE SKIN OR WELTS, FOOD ALLERGY, POLLEN ALLERGY

THE FOLLOWING SUGGEST DISORDERS OF THE METABOLIC SYSTEM:

CHANGE IN SKIN PIGMENTATION, INTOLERANCE TO HEAT OR COLD, INTENTIONAL WEIGHT
LOSS OF 5-10 LBS. OVER 3-6 MONTHS

Figure 9–4. Continued

```
                              SECTION A
============================================================================

HAVE YOU EVER BEEN HOSPITALIZED FOR A PSYCHIATRIC CONDITION?
1) YES     2) NO
 1) YES

HAVE YOU EVER BEEN TREATED WITH ELECTRO-CONVULSIVE THERAPY (ECT)?
1) YES     2) NO
 1) YES

DOES ANYONE IN YOUR FAMILY HAVE A PSYCHIATRIC DISORDER OR SEE A PSYCHIATRIST/
PSYCHOLOGIST?
1) YES     2) NO
 1) YES

HAS ANYONE IN YOUR FAMILY COMMITTED SUICIDE?
1) YES     2) NO
 1) YES

IS ANYONE IN YOUR FAMILY A HEAVY DRINKER OR DRUG USER?
1) YES     2) NO


                              SECTION A
============================================================================

HAVE YOU EVER BEEN SEEN BY A PSYCHIATRIST?
1) YES     2) NO
 1) YES

HAVE YOU EVER TAKEN ANY MEDICATIONS FOR YOUR MOOD OR NERVES?
1) YES     2) NO
 1) YES


                              SECTION A
============================================================================

HAVE YOU EVER TAKEN ANY OF THE FOLLOWING TYPES OF MEDICATIONS?
 1) YES  2) NO
----------------------------------------------------------------------------
ANTIDEPRESSANTS? (ELAVIL, TOFRANIL, PAMELOR, NORPRAMIN, DESYREL, LUDIOMIL,
NARDIL, PARNATE)
 1) YES

LITHIUM?
 1) YES

TRANQUILIZERS? (THORAZINE, HALDOL, PROLIXIN, MELLARIL, STELAZINE, TRILAFON)
 1) YES

SEDATIVES? (LIBRIUM, VALIUM, SERAX, ATIVAN, TRANXENE)
 1) YES


                              SECTION A
============================================================================

WITHIN THE PAST YEAR HAS THERE BEEN A CHANGE IN YOUR MARITAL STATUS?
1) YES     2) NO
 1) YES

WITHIN THE PAST YEAR HAS THERE BEEN A CHANGE IN YOUR JOB OR OCCUPATION?
1) YES     2) NO
 1) YES
```

Figure 9–5. Question strategy in psychiatric history-taking program.

Illustration continued on opposite page

SECTION B

==

HAVE YOU THOUGHT ABOUT HARMING YOURSELF INTENTIONALLY?
1) YES   2) NO
 1) YES

DO YOU HAVE PLANS TO HARM YOURSELF?
1) YES   2) NO
 1) YES

HAVE YOU EVER TRIED TO COMMIT SUICIDE?
1) YES   2) NO
 1) YES

HAVE YOU FELT SO BAD THAT YOU'VE HAD THOUGHTS OF HARMING OTHERS?
1) YES   2) NO
 1) YES

SECTION C

==

HAVE YOU EVER HAD A PERIOD THE OPPOSITE OF DEPRESSION IN WHICH YOUR MOOD WAS
OVERLY HAPPY OR TOO GOOD?
1) YES   2) NO
 1) YES

DURING THAT PERIOD DID YOU REQUIRE LESS SLEEP THAN USUAL?
1) YES   2) NO
 1) YES

DID YOU GO ON SPENDING SPREES (I.E. SPEND MONEY FOOLISHLY ON ITEMS YOU
DIDN'T REALLY NEED)?
1) YES   2) NO
 1) YES

DURING THAT PERIOD DID YOUR THOUGHTS COME AT A FASTER SPEED THAN USUAL?
1) YES   2) NO
 1) YES

SECTION C

==

DID YOU OR OTHERS NOTICE YOUR SPEECH TO BE FASTER THAN USUAL?
1) YES   2) NO
 1) YES

HAVE YOU EVER BEEN TOLD BY A PHYSICIAN THAT YOU ARE MANIC-DEPRESSIVE?
1) YES   2) NO
 1) YES

SECTION D

==

HAVE YOU HAD UNUSUAL EXPERIENCES - SUCH AS HEARING VOICES WHEN THERE IS NO ONE
AROUND?
1) YES   2) NO
 1) YES

HAVE YOU HAD VISIONS THAT OTHERS COULD NOT SEE?
1) YES   2) NO
 1) YES

HAVE YOU HAD THE EXPERIENCE OF BEING TOUCHED WHEN THERE IS NO ONE AROUND?
1) YES   2) NO
 1) YES

DO YOU FEEL THAT OTHERS ARE ABLE TO CONTROL YOUR ACTIONS AGAINST YOUR WILL?
1) YES   2) NO
 1) YES

DO YOU HAVE SPECIAL POWERS -SUCH AS ESP, TELEPATHY, MIND READING?
1) YES   2) NO

==

Figure 9–5. Continued

```
-----------------------
    PSYCHIATRIC ILLNESS
     SCREENING REPORT
-----------------------
```

AGE: 36
SEX: FEMALE
MARITAL STATUS: DIVORCED
RIGHT HANDED
OCCUPATION: TEACHER--CURRENTLY UNEMPLOYED
66 INCHES, 122 POUNDS
COLLEGE GRADUATE
PRESENT MEDICATIONS: BIRTH CONTROL PILL--? TYPE, ASPIRIN

I. PAST PSYCHIATRIC HISTORY:

PATIENT HAS BEEN HOSPITALIZED FOR A PSYCHIATRIC CONDITION, HAS A HISTORY OF
PSYCHIATRIC PROBLEMS, HAS BEEN SEEN BY A PSYCHIATRIST, HAS TAKEN MEDICATIONS
FOR A PSYCHIATRIC DISORDER-INCLUDING ANTIDEPRESSANTS, SEDATIVES, HAS FAMILY
HISTORY OF PSYCHIATRIC PROBLEMS

II. DEPRESSION SYMPTOMS:

PATIENT HAS BEEN FEELING DEPRESSED OR SAD, HAS HAD A RECENT MOOD PROBLEM, HAS
BEEN MORE IRRITABLE LATELY, HAS HAD CRYING SPELLS, HAS HAD A CHANGE IN SLEEPING
PATTERNS, ADMITS TO SUICIDAL IDEAS, HAS DIFFICULTY FALLING ASLEEP, STAYING
AWAKE, OR WAKING UP TOO EARLY, HAS BEEN FEELING FATIGUED, HAS LOST INTEREST IN
USUAL ACTIVITIES, HAS HAD A DECREASE IN SEXUAL INTEREST, HAS ATTEMPTED SUICIDE
IN THE PAST, HAS HAD A CHANGE IN APPETITE, HAS HAD WEIGHT CHANGE (WITHOUT
DIETING), HAS TROUBLE CONCENTRATING, HAS BEEN MORE CRITICAL OF HIM/HERSELF
LATELY, FEELS THAT LIFE IS HOPELESS, HAS THOUGHTS OF WISHING TO DIE

III. SUICIDE RISK FACTORS:

DIVORCED, HAS BEEN HOSPITALIZED FOR A PSYCHIATRIC DISORDER, HAS A FAMILY
HISTORY OF SUICIDE, HAS HAD RECENT MOOD PROBLEMS, ADMITS TO DEPRESSIVE SYMPTOMS
, ADMITS TO SUICIDE IDEAS, ADMITS TO PAST SUICIDE ATTEMPTS, ADMITS TO PROBLEMS
WITH ALCOHOL, HAS HAD A CHANGE IN JOB OR MARITAL STATUS
***** THERE IS NO WAY TO COMPLETELY ASSESS SUICIDE RISK. THE MORE OF THE ABOVE
FACTORS THAT ARE POSITIVE, THE GREATER THE RISK.*****

IV. MANIA SYMPTOMS:

PATIENT HAS NO SYMPTOMS OF MANIA

V. PSYCHOSIS SYMPTOMS:

PATIENT ADMITS TO DELUSIONAL IDEAS

VI. ALCOHOL USE:

PATIENT ADMITS TO USING ALCOHOL 2-3 TIMES PER WEEK, ADMITS TO PROBLEMS WITH
ALCOHOL, ADMITS TO SYMPTOMS WHICH MAY BE DUE TO ALCOHOL DEPENDENCE, HAS BEEN
ADVISED BY A PHYSICIAN TO STOP DRINKING

VII. ANXIETY SYMPTOMS:

PATIENT ADMITS TO SYMPTOMS OF ANXIETY (PANIC) ATTACKS. THESE SYMPTOMS NEED
INTERPRETATION IN LIGHT OF THE MEDICAL HISTORY, ADMITS TO SYMPTOMS OF ANXIETY

VIII. DRUG USE:

PATIENT DOES NOT USE NON-PRESCRIPTION DRUGS
PATIENT ADMITS TO TOBACCO USE, ADMITS TO PROBLEMS WITH TOBACCO USE, ADMITS TO
CAFFEINE USE

IX. SOMATOFORM DISORDERS:

PATIENT HAS FREQUENT HEADACHES, HAS HAD SURGERY, ADMITS TO UNUSUAL MEDICAL
COMPLAINTS. THESE SYMPTOMS MAY BE SEEN IN A VARIETY OF MEDICAL AND PSYCHIATRIC
DISORDERS AND NEED INTERPRETATION IN LIGHT OF THE MEDICAL HISTORY
```

*Figure 9–6. Final report generated by psychiatric history-taking program.*
```

MEDICATIONS

WHICH OF THE FOLLOWING MEDICINES DO YOU TAKE REGULARLY?
  1) YES   2) NO

MIDOL
  1) YES

EMPIRIN
  1) YES

BUFFERIN
  1) YES

ASCRIPTIN
  1) YES

ANACIN
  1) YES

TYLENOL X-TRA STRENGTH

MEDICATIONS

WHICH OF THE FOLLOWING MEDICINES DO YOU TAKE REGULARLY?
  1) YES   2) NO

SINUTAB
  1) YES

SINE-OFF
  1) YES

QUIET WORLD
  1) YES

PERCOGESIC
  1) YES

ALLEREST
  1) YES

ANACIN-3

MEDICATIONS

WHICH OF THE FOLLOWING MEDICINES DO YOU TAKE REGULARLY?
  1) YES   2) NO

EXCEDRIN
  1) YES

CORICIDIN
  1) YES

DATRIL
  1) YES

DRISTAN
  1) YES

VANQUISH
  1) YES

SINAREST

Figure 9–7. *Medication portion of general medical history program. Precise documentation of nonprescription medications taken can provide surprising results.*

question and then look to see the examiner jot a brief note or two. This is anxiety provoking and might influence later answers. This may be particularly true in adolescents who are constantly reading the examiner and observing the examiner's response to their answers. Sometimes even a twitch of an eyebrow or the trace of a smile on the examiner's face could indicate approval or disapproval of the patient's answer. The results are difficult to record and certainly they must be dictated or written by hand, both somewhat time consuming.

In our staff training we were all exposed to great variability in patient history between the medical student, intern, resident, and attending physician. This would indicate either a poor reproducibility of information, wide variability in the questioning skills of the examiners, or the patient thinking about their illness and previous answers before responding to the next examiner. Often the solo practitioner succumbs to the temptation of scribbling cryptic notes, not reproducing them in typed form owing to the expense of an office practice, and much of the data are sometimes lost to other observers who wish to review the chart.

Written Questionnaire

This is a self-administered time-saving device that has been available in various forms for many years. Certainly, it has benefits over the written history, and the data is automatically recorded as the patient fills out the questionnaire. It is a standardized approach that allows the same questions to be asked of each patient. Brodman and associates described the Cornell questionnaire, which contained 195 questions.[3]

This format, unfortunately, does not allow easy individualization of the questions and branching is either cumbersome or nonexistent, depending on the type of questionnaire. The patient must have good reading skills and must be motivated enough to fill out what might be a frightening selection of questions. Questionnaires are not easily reviewed each time a patient returns to the office, and no clear-cut synthesis exists except in the handwriting of the examiner or through dictation. It certainly represents a step toward time-saving; probably most clinicians have employed or developed some type of questionnaire to meet their individual needs.

Coddington and King[5] used the computerized questionnaire as a screening test to identify children who require psychiatric evaluation. They provide a very good argument for computerized histories as a means of screening patients.

Automated Interactive Histories

This would represent the "state of the art" approach to data collection from a patient. Qualification and quantification of each positive

```
                        PERSONAL HABITS
=======================================================================
CHOOSE ONE:
  1) I CURRENTLY SMOKE CIGARETTES
  2) I USED TO SMOKE BUT QUIT
  3) I NEVER SMOKED AS A HABIT
```

```
                        PERSONAL HABITS
=======================================================================
HOW MUCH DO (DID) YOU SMOKE?
  1) LESS THAN 1/2 PACK
  2) 1/2 TO 1 PACK
  3) 1 TO 1 1/2 PACKS
  4) 1 1/2 TO 2 PACKS
  5) 2 TO 3 PACKS
  6) 3 TO 4 PACKS
  7) GREATER THAN 4 PACKS
```

```
                        PERSONAL HABITS
=======================================================================
HOW MANY YEARS HAVE YOU BEEN SMOKING?
  1) LESS THAN ONE YEAR
  2) 1 TO 5 YEARS
  3) 5 TO 10 YEARS
  4) 10 TO 15 YEARS
  5) 15 TO 20 YEARS
  6) 20 TO 30 YEARS
  7) 30 TO 40 YEARS
  8) 40 TO 50 YEARS
  9) GREATER THAN 50 YEARS
```

Figure 9–8. Use of the branching logic to provide precise quantitation of personal habits.

symptom are possible, and branching logic can be employed. Figure 9–8 demonstrates the branching logic for a smoking history in A. K. Olson's "general medical history." Other examples of automated history taking are described by Slack and associates,[20, 21, 22] as well as by Brodman and Van Woerkom.[3]

BENEFITS IN COMPUTERIZED HISTORY TAKING

Time Efficiency

Kanner[12] described the use of his PMH (programmed medical history). He stated that he spent an average of 80 minutes per history and physical examination prior to the use of a computer. By employing the automated system, he was able to save 20 to 25 minutes per patient. He felt that most of the time was saved by reading the printout rather than having to acquire all the information by interview. The patient spent approximately 40 minutes completing the automated history, and the patient was then interviewed after the physician reviewed the printout. He wrote that the patients improved their verbalization after seeing text regarding their chief complaints and that they were already exposed to "ample self-expression," and he felt that he was eventually able to almost double his work capacity in new patient assessments by utilizing his automated system.

Private practitioners in the United States are faced with certain economic pressures that require higher efficiency and reduction of expenses such as typing. Computerized history taking would be a logical solution to that problem. Reproducibility of a review of systems and histories is good, utilizing a standard set of questions, and although patients may well change their answers when confronted with the verbal interview, the physician benefits from the patient having already spent time thinking about the illness in these terms.

The use of "expert histories" should be mentioned at this point. One could imagine a scenerio in which a family practitioner in the midst of a busy day is faced with a patient in a 10-minute time slot who perhaps has three new complaints. If the patient were first questioned by a small portable computer, a great deal of information would be available to the practitioner during their short interview. It might uncover a good deal of clinical information, which could lead to a longer visit, hospitalization, or even the initiation of testing or referral based upon historical features. We don't anticipate that these expert histories would circumvent the specialists, but they might uncover information earlier in the course of illness, avoiding more advanced disease and expensive medical work-ups. The reviewing of such printouts could even be considered "a cognitive service" and perhaps might even be reimbursable eventually by insurance companies.

Comparison to History By Dialogue

Simborg and associates[19] in a review argued that computer histories were superior to those acquired by individuals. Slack and associates[20] compared the histories of allergy taken by computer and manually and concluded that the history was superior when taken by a computer. Martin and associates[15] compared symptoms recorded from computer versus dialogue or record. Lapin and associates, in testing their program in a psychiatric setting, noted that their computerized history always asked the relevent questions and produced legible, reproducible reports.

Leviton and associates[14] applied a behavioral history to children with headache and several advantages were described, including the following:

1. The questions were structured and aroused less suspicion in the children who thought the questions were aimed only at them.

2. It asked essential questions.

3. It identified areas requiring in-depth questioning by the physician, nurse or psychologist in a further interview.

4. It made the patient think more about the issues in order to be ready for the human interview.

ACCEPTANCE BY PHYSICIANS

H. B. Wright, in a letter to *The Lancet*,[29] described the need, in this age of technology, to acquire a "real time history." He was impressed with the delegation of sophisticated tasks to nurse practitioners in the United States and developed a history-taking program which he then tested in London. The physicians in his center eventually accepted the printouts and found them to be quite helpful. Richard B. Friedman[10] pointed out that automated histories were useful for obtaining standard family history, past medical history, occupational history, and review of systems, and he felt that they would free the physician for more productive interpersonal interaction with patients. Bana and associates[1] tested their program with six internists and one neurologist. They found it helpful to review the printout prior to the interview and perceived that 85 per cent of their patients liked the program. The physicians felt that their program provided information not otherwise available to them in the personal history of the patient. They felt that the patients were better prepared for their human interview after they went through the program. It would therefore seem that the automation of medical histories is quite acceptable to many patients and physicians who comment.

All technologic advancements have their detractors, and we are sure that airplanes, penicillin, and television all had their critics. From the author's personal experience, as well as a careful review of the literature, it appears that patients and physicians alike welcome this new technology as a means of improving patient care and making better use of the physician's time.

FEATURES OF A GOOD COMPUTERIZED HISTORY PROGRAM

User-Friendliness

The phrase "user-friendly" has found its way into the jargon of computer and noncomputer persons alike. What it describes is a program that can be operated easily by the patient or the physician's assistant and will not require any amount of training. There might be some anxiety on the part of office personnel, nurses, or even some physicians regarding the use of a computer, and certainly no formal computer training is necessary to operate a "friendly program." One would not expect to take a course in electronics before purchasing a television or radio, and certainly no other training would be necessary to operate an easy program.

An important decision in automating histories would regard the type of patient being interviewed. In certain settings such as pediatrics or dementia evaluations, the patient cannot be expected to input the data directly. Often a family member would be asked to answer the questions on the screen. In setting up a dementia screening clinic several years ago, the author found it necessary to develop a standard questionnaire. This eventually took the form of a computerized history program designed for family members. Data from the family member then became part of the data base and provided a printout that allowed the physician to make decisions regarding the need for placement, workup, and so on. In most settings, however, the patient would be entering the information, and this is quite acceptable to most patients.

One may consider the issue of direct versus indirect data entry. By direct data entry, we mean that the patient or a family member would sit directly at the keyboard and input the information. This would eliminate the need for a keypunch operator or input personnel, would reduce the possibility of transcription error and most likely would represent the most efficient means of interrogation. There have been programs over the years requiring the patient to fill out a form or questionnaire, and the information is then entered into the computer. The latter system obviously does not offer the advantage of branching logic when the system machine is unable to interact with the patient.

In selecting a good patient history program, one should look at the language on the screen to be certain that it is not technically frightening to the patient or unnecessarily "cute." Several years ago it was considered fashionable for the computer to call the subject by their first name and to make "cute" comments throughout the program. With a more sophisticated public, this is unnecessary and perhaps is even insulting to some people. Plain dialogue, utilizing lay language and putting technical terms in parenthesis or at least followed by explanations, is the most effective means of communication.

Complexity of the questions must also be considered. Certainly it would be very time consuming for the patient to manually type in complete words or sentences as answers to each question. This would defeat the purpose of the branching logic, for the program would be unable to branch based on verbal input. The most effective format, in the author's experience, is that of the simple "yes or no" or multiple choice formats. It is sometimes useful to give the patient a "none of the above" or "skip it" option to avoid embarrassment. This would indicate uncertainty in an area that can be pursued in more detail by the human examiner. There are some questions for which free text entry is unavoidable, and there is a blank space where the subject types in the answer. For example, a question asking about current medications would require that the drug names be typed in. Multiple choice questions are the easiest, and certainly not all multiple choice questions will fit the need of every patient. It is essential for the patient to correct input errors before the final report is printed, and a good program would allow either the opportunity to go back one question or to go back at the end of each section in the history to make the appropriate changes.

The Printout

The format of the printout determines how the data will be used. Figures 9–1, 9–2, and 9–4 show sample printouts of general medical history, back history, and headache history. The information is gathered and processed in such a way that the diagnosis might be quite apparent but the diagnosis is not actually made. It will be foolhardy for clinicians to accept medical software that pretends to make the appropriate diagnosis "most of the time." Such programs will be available in the near future, although appropriate testing validation would be necessary before these programs could be trusted.

Another useful application of the printout would be to give the patient an actual copy of the printout so that the patient can become aware of the history, symptoms and perhaps even habits not previously thought about. Some physicians even ask the patient to sign a copy of the printout to prove that appropriate questions have been asked.

Content of the Program

A good program is balanced somewhere between a concise practical series of questions and a massive time-consuming body of information, which might be of more help in an academic rather than a clinical setting. Over the years, programs have been developed for research purposes which require a great deal of patient time in inputting and a great deal of the physician's time in reading the results. There should be a happy balance, and in experience, 15 to 30 minutes of patient time seems to produce a very detailed history and does not succumb to short attention spans. Just as the overly detailed history of the medical student is somewhat cumbersome for an attending physician to evaluate, an overly detailed medical history program might be more of a hindrance than a help.

Decision Making Versus Data Gathering Programs

A word is necessary in differentiating these two types of programs. Artificial intelligence technology is advancing, but even in large mainframe computers, a practical substitute for a clinician's judgment is not yet available. While current history-taking software cannot be imbued with true attributes of "artifical intelligence" and still remain practical for the office setting, even simple programs can spot patterns and associations that might otherwise be missed. For instance, as the result of a patient response, a program might generate a printout that tells the physician that a patient is on potassium-wasting medications and reminds him to check serum potassium levels.

Storage of Information

Perhaps one benefit to automated history taking is the collecting of data, which can be accessed at a later date for the sake of correlation or research. In a practical office setting, this is not a necessary feature but would be a useful capability in a microcomputer program. One must keep in mind that even though some programs can be "stored to disk," one must ask whether one can simply recover the printout from the storage form or whether each fact can be taken out and correlated. This would require extensive and expensive programming to sort through data bases. It is fashionable for "computer consultants" to give lectures on office automation and the computerization of medicine, and many of these speakers will advise the audience to have "database capabilities." The physician must simply determine what tasks need to be performed by the program and then choose the appropriate program. In this author's experience, magnetic storage of each patient's history serves no clinical purpose whatsoever, because the printout is the working record. Also keep in mind that the printout from the program is discussed and reviewed with the patient, and physician notes are then added. Any stored data would be lacking these notes and some of them are quite important. While we have found the paper printout to be most useful, on line storage of the history becomes invaluable when the data can be assessed electronically from remote locations.

Patient Acceptance

Mayne and associates[17] used an early version of the automated medical history and found good patient acceptance and physician acceptance in 159 patients at the Mayo Clinic. Bana and associates[1] interviewed 40 patients following a computerized interview, and the patients found their interview to be thoughtful, interesting, and considerate. Most of their patients like the program very much.

Present-Day Pitfalls

Pre-existing software on the market is somewhat sparse at this time because the market is just developing. There are "cottage industry" software vendors selling programs for "wellness" assessment, patient billing, or specific laboratory applications. One must inquire carefully about the software authors themselves. Athough most physician software authors are probably quite skilled in their respective medical fields, there is no guarantee that they are skilled computer programmers. One must look to the vendor to be certain that professional programming personnel were involved in the development, design, and testing of these programs. Although all programs have "bugs," the more professionally developed programs have fewer " bugs" and will offer appropriate support when needed.

Most pre-existing software is "author determined," in which the questions are built into the program as determined by the expert author. One should not be dismayed by a fixed set of historical questions, as no two physicians practice medicine alike, and certainly one must expect to ask some "pet questions" at the time of the person-to-person interview with the patient. The next stage in development will be a user-definable history-taking program that allows the individual physician to construct a custom patient history. This system offers the user blank question "trees" that may be linked in any sequence to produce output in the form of an individualized report.[30]

Several of our associates have demonstrated their programs to other physicians, only to be greeted with such comments as, "It seems so easy, I think I'll make one of my own." This is a wonderful idea for a hobby if one is willing to commit several hundred hours of time and accept the frustrations that can occur. Good history-taking software should not begin at the keyboard but should be the product of many months of planning and testing questions on selected patient populations.

SUGGESTIONS FOR USE TODAY

Incorporation of the Computer into the Office

Once the office staff has gotten over any initial paranoia of being "replaced by a computer," each will probably have an idea for new applications of the computer in your office setting. Training of personnel to operate the computer for patient histories should be minimal, and your software vendor should provide either a "hands-on" training session or a good tutorial disk or manual in its place.

Location in the Office

The patient history is best taken in a quiet part of the office. We have employed a "computer room" for several years that is essentially a small examination room dedicated to this purpose. A small desk, a comfortable chair, a computer and printer are all that we place in the room and the patient is able to quietly go through the program at his or her own speed. We find that the room is best located in an area where help can be easily obtained from nurses and other personnel if needed. An extra chair or two for family members and medical personnel is also helpful. We have found that the patients do quite well by themselves, but some patients require the reassurance of the nurse being present at least at the beginning of the interview. We employ a nurse clinician in our practice setting, and she usually sits with the patient, types in the initial information, and observes the patient while he or she is taking the history. When she is satisfied that the patient is comfortable and capable of completing the program, the patient is left alone, but we reinforce the idea that someone will be right outside if needed. Some physicians find it helpful to briefly stop by the room to let patients know that they are not being processed impersonally. Some physicians will assure the patient that this is not taking the place of their interview but will help the physician get more information about the patient.

Use of the Data

The printout is best utilized as a guide or framework for the actual person-to-person interview, as we have noted throughout this chapter. We cannot stress enough the need for personal contact with the patient because much of the data must be verified and sometimes expanded upon. Supplemental information is noted on the page, and this would then become part of the permanent patient record.

In conclusion, we feel that microcomputers have a proven place in the acquisition of patient histories, and the medical community as well as the lay public are quite receptive to the use of automated history taking. We also feel that the computerized history represents a non-threatening way to more efficiently meet the challenge of health care in the 1980s.

REFERENCES

1. Bana, D. S., Leviton, A., Swidler, C., et al.: A computer-based headache interview. Headache 85–86, 1980.
2. Bana, D. S., Leviton, A., Slack, W. V., et al.: Use of a computerized data base in a headache clinic. Headache, 72–74, 1981.
3. Brodman, K., and Van Woerkom, A. J.: Computer-aided diagnostic screening for 100 common diseases. J.A.M.A., 197:179–183, 1966.
4. Chun, R. W. M., Van Cura, L. J., Spencer, M., and Slack, W. V.: Computer interviewing of patients with epilepsy. Epilepsia, 17:371–375, 1976.
5. Coddington, R. D., and King, T. L.: Automated history taking in child psychiatry. Am. J. Psychiatr., 129:52–58, 1972.
6. Deykin, D., Balko, C., Slack, W. V., and Slack, C. W.: Patient-computer dialogue. N. Engl. J. Med., 286:1304–1309, 1972.
7. Francis, J. H., Pennal, B. E., and Wadsworth, W.: Development of a computer-assisted headache diagnostic and treatment system. Headache, 35–38, 1984.
8. Freemon, F. R.: Computer diagnosis of headache. Headache, 48–56, 1968.
9. Friedman, R. B., Huhta, J., and Cheung, S.: An automated verbal medical history system. Arch. Intern. Med., 138:1359–1361, 1978.
10. Friedman, R. B.: Mechanized history-taking. Arch. Intern. Med., 139:714, 1979.
11. Grossman, J. H., Barnett, G. O., McGuire, M. T., and Swedlow, D. B.: Evaluation of computer-acquired patient histories. J.A.M.A., 215:1286–1291, 1971.
12. Kanner, I. F.: Programmed medical history-taking with or without computer. J.A.M.A., 207:317–321, 1969.
13. Klein, M. H., and Greist, J. H.: Advantages of computerized psychiatric history taking. J.A.M.A., 220:1246–1247, 1972.
14. Leviton, A., Slack, W. V., Masek, B., et al.: A computerized and behavioral assessment for children with headaches. Headache, 182–185, 1984.
15. Martin, M. J., Mayne, J. G., Taylor, W. F., and Swenson, M. N.: A health questionnaire based on paper-and-pencil medium individualized and produced by computer. J.A.M.A., 208:2064–2068, 1969.
16. Maultsby, M. C., and Slack, W. V.: A computer-based psychiatry history system. Arch. Gen. Psychiatr., 25:570–572, 1971.
17. Mayne, J. G., Weksel, W. D., and Sholtz, P. N.: Toward automating the medical history. Mayo Clin. Proc., 43:1–25, 1968.
18. Metz, J. R., Allen, C. M., Barr, G., and Shinefield, H.: A pediatric screening examination for psychosocial problems. Pediatrics, 58:595–606, 1976.
19. Simborg, D. W., Rikli, A. E., and Hall, P.: Experimentation in medical history taking. J.A.M.A., 210:1443–1445, 1969.
20. Slack, W. V., Hicks, G. P., Reed, C. E., and Van Cura, L. J.: A computer-based medical-history system. N. Engl. J. Med., 274:194–198, 1966.
21. Slack, W. V., and Van Cura, L. J.: Computer-based patient interviewing. Part I. Postgrad. Med., 68–74, 1968.
22. Slack, W. V., and Van Cura, L. J.: Computer-based patient interviewing. Part II. Postgrad. Med., 115–120, 1968.
23. Slack, W. V., Porter, D., Witschi, J., et al.: Dietary interviewing by computer. J. Am. Dietet. Assoc., 69:514–517, 1976.
24. Slack, W. V.: A history of computerized medical interviews. M.D. Computing, 5:52–59, 1984.

25. Slack, W. V., and Van Cura, L. J.: Patient reaction to computer-based medical interviewing. Computers Biochem. Res., 1:527–531, 1968.
26. Stead, W. W., Heyman, A., Thompson, H. K., et al.: Computer-assisted interview of patients with functional headache. Arch. Intern. Med., 129:950–955, 1972.
27. Toole, J. F., Brady, W. A., Cochrane, C. M., and Olmos, N.: Use of computerized questionnaire in the etiologic diagnosis of headache. Headache, 73–76, 1974.
28. Witschi, J., Porter, D., Vogel, S., et al.: A computer-based dietary counseling system. Research, 69:385–390, 1976.
29. Wright, H. B.: History-taking by computer. Lancet 1:983–984, 1975.
30. Javitt, J. C.: A user-defined computerized history-taking program. Wilmer Symposium on Computers in Ophthalmology, 1986.

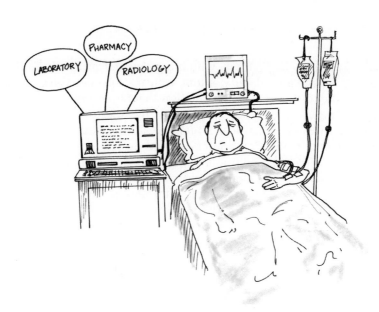

TEN

Software for Patient Management

Paul L. Marino, M.D., Ph.D.

Computer technology can provide an aid to physicians in many different areas of medicine. Office management systems, which have introduced many physicians to the capabilities of the computer, can provide an invaluable aid to the business aspects of medical practice.

Hospital Information Systems, which are devoted primarily to reporting laboratory tests and related patient information, can save physicians valuable time in retrieval of information that is pertinent to patient care. Finally, computers can aid physicians by suggesting diagnoses and therapy in individual clinical situations. This latter area of computer implementation, called "computer-assisted decision-making," represents an attempt to use the computer as an "expert" in clinical problem-solving situations. This chapter will cover some of the more practical applications of computer-generated information and diagnostics in patient management, with particular reference to the use of microcomputer-based mathematical calculations as an aid in clinical problem solving.

CLINICAL COMPUTING TASKS

The computer is concerned primarily with performing operations on input items (data) to make these items more meaningful. Information is defined as a collection of items that has meaning, and therefore, the computer can be viewed as an information system. The type of information generated is dependent on the manner in which the input data are processed. The basic types of data operations are as follows:

Data Classification. This type of data operation places input data into predetermined categories, such as storing lists of patients according to disease category. This represents one of the most basic forms of data processing, but it does little to aid physicians with actual clinical problem solving.

Data Calculations. The computer is adept at performing mathematical calculations quickly and reliably. It can play an important role as an aid in the calculations needed in managing patients with certain clinical problems (such as hemodynamics, fluid and electrolyte disorders). This type of data operation goes one step beyond data classification as an aid to physicians in clinical problem solving. However, calculation-based systems are limited in the sense that there is no attempt to interpret the calculated data to generate specific suggestions for patient cure.

Data Interpretation. This type of data operation is geared to interpreting the input data to arrive at specific diagnostic and therapeutic conclusions. This can be accomplished by applying established "rules" to the data being processed, such as a simple system that operates on "if, then" logic (for example, *if* the MB isoenzyme of CPK is > 5 per cent, *then* the patient is likely to have an acute myocardial infarction). This type of approach is designed to mimic the actual reasoning of physicians in clinical problem-solving situations, and thus represents a real attempt at computer-assisted (or computer-generated) problem solving.

A number of relatively sophisticated "expert" systems have been developed to offer advice based on the accumulated knowledge in specific areas of medicine. One particularly ambitious program of this type is Internist-I,[18] a program designed for computer-assisted diagnosis in general internal medicine. This is a particularly large scope program, containing a knowledge base on over 500 individual diseases and 3550 manifestations of disease. Although programs such as this one are innovative and ambitious, these large programs are currently impractical because they require larger mainframe computers to operate and are not available for general use. In the last few years, more practical "limited domain" programs have been developed for the more accessible microcomputer, and this chapter will focus on these latter programs and their potential value in patient care.

COMPUTER-ASSISTED PATIENT CARE

Because the computer is capable of performing the most sophisticated mathematical calculations with relative ease, computer implementation has focused on areas of medicine that rely heavily on calculations of clinical and laboratory measurements. These areas include (1) hemodynamics, (2) acid-base disorders, (3) fluid and electrolyte disorders, and (4) nutritional therapy. The remainder of the chapter will present some of the available microcomputer applications in these areas.

Hemodynamic Problems

One of the most common problems encountered in intensive care units is altered cardiovascular function (such as heart failure, clinical shock states). The advent of the pulmonary artery flotation catheter has allowed hemodynamic monitoring to become a routine and valuable tool in assessing hemodynamic problems in the critically ill patient. These catheters permit measurement of right and left ventricular filling pressures and of cardiac output (Q) by the thermodilution technique. Using these measurements, along with the mean arterial blood pressure, it is possible to calculate systemic and pulmonary vascular resistances, and the stroke work of the right and left ventricles. If this profile is combined with calculations of the oxygen content in arterial blood (Cao_2) and mixed venous blood ($C\bar{v}o_2$), it is possible to calculate O_2 delivery rate (O_2 delivery $= Q \times Cao_2$), O_2 consumption ($Vo_2 = Q \times [Cao_2 - C\bar{v}o_2]$) and O_2 extraction ratio (O_2 extraction $= Vo_2/O_2$ delivery). The sum of these measurements provides a relatively comprehensive physiologic approach to altered hemodynamic function.

A number of programs are available that will generate a series of hemodynamic calculations (called hemodynamic "profiles"). These pro-

Parameter	Value	Normal Range
BSA	1.93	
CI	* 1.8	2.4 - 4
SVI	* 20.1	36 - 48
LVSWI	* 18.8	44 - 56
RVSWI	* 6.6	7 - 10
SVRI	* 3583	1200 - 2500
PVRI	* 531	80 - 240
O2 DELIVERY	* 226	520 - 720
O2 CONSUMPTION	* 93	110 - 160
O2 EXTRACTION	* 41	22 - 32

Press ANY KEY to continue

Figure 10–1. Example of patient hemodynamic profile.

grams are available for larger microcomputers[5, 14] as well as pocket computers.[13] The user is simply required to enter input data when prompted and can edit the input for any errors in data entry. Once this is accomplished, the calculations are performed rapidly and are displayed on the screen. An example of a hemodynamic profile[14] is shown in Figure 10–1; these profiles can usually be printed for permanent copy if so desired.

Although hemodynamic profiles contain valuable information, the physician is still left with the task of interpreting the data that are generated. To minimize any problems that may arise from requiring physicians to function as experts in hemodynamic interpretation, a program has been developed that is capable of both interpreting hemodynamic profiles and suggesting therapy to correct the identified hemodynamic problem.[14] The program is called Hemodynamic Expert and is written in BASIC for the Apple II series and IBM personal computers. There are three main sections of the program: the first section generates hemodynamic profiles (the profile shown in Figure 10–1 is from this program), the second section interprets the major hemodynamic problem,

```
                    -- PROFILE INTERPRETATION --

             SUMMARY: HIGH PCWP / LOW CI / HIGH SVRI

INTERPRETATION:  CARDIAC DYSFUNCTION

POSSIBLE CAUSES:
 1. MYOCARDIAL DYSFUNCTION
    A. Ischemia or Infarction
    B. Toxic - Metabolic (eg. Late Sepsis / Severe Acidemia or Alkalemia /
         Hypothyroidism / Hypocalcemia / Hypophosphatemia / Drugs)
    C. Chronic Cardiomyopathy (eg. Amyloid)
    D. Significant Dysrhythmias

 2. ENDOCARDIAL DISEASE (eg. Mitral or Aortic valve dysfunction / Myxoma)

 3. PERICARDIAL DISEASE (eg. Tamponade)

 4. PRIMARY INCREASE IN AFTERLOAD (eg. Hypertension)


                   Press ANY KEY to continue
```

Figure 10–2. Computer interpretation of hemodynamic profile depicted in Figure 10–1.

and the third section suggests specific therapy to correct the identified problem.

In Hemodynamic Expert, the profile interpretation is based on the relationship of three variables in the profile: (1) The pulmonary capillary wedge pressure (PCWP) used as an index of left ventricular preload, (2) the cardiac index (CI) used as an index of ventricular pump function, and (3) the systemic vascular resistance index (SVRI) used as an index of left ventricular afterload. Each variable is categorized as low, normal, or high so that there are 3^3, or 27, possible combinations of the three variables. Each combination represents a unique hemodynamic problem. When the hemodynamic profile is generated, the computer selects the three variables from the profile and matches the combination to the appropriate interpretation. An example of a computer interpretation is shown in Figure 10–2, which is an interpretation for the profile in Figure 10–1. Each interpretation contains a summary of the three variables used for interpretation (seen at the top of the figure), a statement of the hemodynamic problem (cardiac dysfunction in this case), and a general list of disorders to be considered. (Note that the pulmonary capillary wedge pressure is not shown in the profile, as it is a measurement and is not a calculated parameter.) Once the interpretation is obtained, the suggested therapy for the specific problem is displayed. The therapy for the problem in Figure 10–2 is shown in Figure 10–3. Note that there are general therapeutic suggestions, along with more specific information (for example, drug doses), if needed.

```
              THERAPY FOR CARDIAC DYSFUNCTION
              ------------------------------
A. Administer the following types of drugs:
   1. POSITIVE INOTROPIC AGENTS (eg. Dobutamine may be the drug of choice
      for low cardiac output states without hypotension; if hypotension
      is present, Dopamine may be preferred.)

   2. AFTERLOAD REDUCING AGENTS (eg. Nitroprusside)

   3. PRELOAD REDUCING AGENTS (eg. Sublingual Nitroglycerin) - Preload
      reduction should be reserved only for cases of severe pulmonary
      edema (i.e., pure preload reduction may DECREASE cardiac output)

B. If drug administration results in a decrease in pulmonary capillary
   wedge pressure (PCWP) to ± 20mmHg, then INFUSE VOLUME until the
   PCWP = 20mmHg or is equal to the plasma colloid osmotic pressure.

      Press the number of your choice and press the RETURN key.
   1. Drug Info. - Positive Inotropes      4. Principles of Volume
   2. Drug Info. - Afterload Reducers          Infusion
   3. Drug Info. - Preload Reducers         5. None of the above
                                   ?
```

Figure 10–3. Computer-suggested therapy based upon hemodynamic file depicted in Figure 10–1.

Hemodynamic Expert thus represents an attempt to develop a comprehensive decision-making program based on accepted guidelines or "rules" of hemodynamics. It is thus a simple example of how an "expert" system developed for the microcomputer can be used as an aid in patient management.

Acid-Base Disorders

As demonstrated in the section on hemodynamics, any area of medicine that has a relatively well defined set of rules for data interpretation will lend itself to computerized interpretation of input data. Another example of such an area is acid-base derangements, in which identification of the type of disorder is dependent primarily on the relationship of three measurements: arterial P_{CO_2}, arterial pH, and the serum bicarbonate concentration.

A number of programs have been developed to interpret acid-base disorders. Bleich[2, 3] was the first to develop a comprehensive program on acid-base disorders. This program was written for a larger mainframe computer but required a random access memory (RAM) of less than 1 million characters. The program not only identified the type of acid-base disorder (such as primary or mixed metabolic or respiratory disturbance) but generated an evaluation note that included (1) a review of the pathophysiology of the disorder, (2) possible etiologies, (3) calculated electrolyte therapy, (4) suggestions for further tests to narrow the diagnosis, and (5) pertinent references. Goldberg and associates[7] followed this with a program (also developed on a mainframe computer) that was capable of generating the most likely diagnosis of an acid-base problem using additional clinical and laboratory information to narrow the list of differential diagnoses. More recently, Weiner and associates[21] have developed an inference-based program that is capable of generating a status report on patients that includes the input data, the acid-base diagnosis, and the suggested therapy for the identified problem.

Less comprehensive, but possibly more useful programs have been developed for the microcomputer. Martin and Jeffreys[16] have designed a program for the IBM PC-XT that can be used to generate arterial blood gas interpretations when the computer is interfaced with a blood gas machine. After the blood gas machine determines the desired measurements, the data are automatically transmitted to the computer for data interpretation and data storage. Such interfacing alleviates unnecessary time spent with data acquisition from the blood gas machine and data entry into the computer. Programs for acid-base interpretation are available for small hand-held computers.[7, 17] Maxwell and associates[17] have developed a program for the first generation pocket computers (such as Radio Shack TRS-80 PC-1 or Sharp PC-1211, each with only 2K bytes of memory) that is capable of calculating various measures of gas exchange (for example, arterial/alveolar Po_2 ratios) as well as interpreting acid-base status. Although such programs are limited in their scope by the memory limitations of the smaller pocket computers, their real value lies in the fact that they do not require expensive, sophisticated computer systems to operate.

Fluid and Electrolyte Disorders

Another area of medicine that requires mathematical calculations for patient care, and is thus well suited to computer implementation, concerns disorders of fluid and electrolyte balance. Despite the obvious suitability of computers in this area, surprisingly little has been done to develop software for this field of medicine. Bleich[2] expanded his original acid-base program (mentioned in the prior section) to include evaluation of various electrolyte disorders (for example, disorders of sodium balance). The format of the program remained the same as for the acid-base program, with data entry leading to an evaluation note that contained specific recommendations for diagnosis and therapy of the problem. Although comprehensive, the usefulness of the program is limited by the requirement for a larger mainframe computer to operate the program.

A microcomputer program has recently been developed to evaluate

```
- LOGIC FOR CORRECTING HYPERNATREMIA -

  1. Correct sodium for elevated blood
     glucose

  2. Calculate free water deficit

  3. Identify type of fluid lost and
     estimate or measure sodium in lost
     fluid

  4. Calculate sodium deficit and fluid
     deficit

  5. Estimate or measure ongoing sodium
     and water losses

  6. Add deficits and ongoing losses


  7. Construct intravenous therapy using
     total sodium and fluid requirements
```

Figure 10–4. Computer logic sequence for the correction of fluid and electrolyte imbalance.

problems in sodium and potassium homeostasis. This program, called Fluid and Electrolyte Expert,[15] not only is capable of aiding in the diagnosis of various fluid and electrolyte disorders but also can create specific treatment regimens that are tailored to an individual patient. An example of the capabilities of such a program can be demonstrated in the section of the program that deals with hypernatremia. In this section, the user is first asked to determine if the intravascular volume is low, normal, or high. Therapy in each volume situation can then be tailored to correct the specific problem in sodium and water balance that is characteristic of that situation.

In Fluid and Electrolyte Expert, the sequence of logic steps used to determine therapy for hypernatremia with a low intravascular volume is shown in Figure 10–4. The serum sodium is first adjusted for any increase in serum glucose. The patient's usual weight is then entered, and the free water deficit is calculated and displayed. The user is then asked to identify the type of fluid lost (for example, diarrhea) from a list of available choices. Using the estimated (or measured) sodium concentration in the lost fluid, the program will then calculate and display the sodium deficit and the adjusted fluid deficit. These deficits are then used

```
                        Fluid Therapy

Fluid deficit :                 2737 Mls
Sodium deficit :                 136 Meq
Basal daily fluid requirement : 2050 Ml  assumes patient afebrile
Basal daily sodium required :    175 Meq


  The patient needs the following therapy :
    486 Meq Na and 6837 mls of water over the next 48 hours.
  This may be approximated by giving :
  Normal saline @   111ml/hr for 4 hours to relieve intravascular volume deficit
  followed by 1/2NS at 142 ml/hr X  8 hrs.followed by 1/4NS at 142 ml/hr X   8 hrs.
  followed by 1/2NS at 142 ml/hr X  8 hrs.followed by 1/4NS at 142 ml/hr X   8 hrs.
  followed by 1/2NS at 142 ml/hr X  8 hrs.followed by 1/4NS at 142 ml/hr X   8 hrs.


  Avg. =  61 Meq Na/l at 142 ml/hr X 48H. Check electrolytes periodically and revi
  se fluid therapy using this program.

                  No allowance made for oral intake.
  Press  <P> to print recommendations  or <ANY KEY> to return to main menu:
```

Figure 10–5. Therapeutic approach suggested by computer based upon the system shown in Figure 10–4.

to construct a regimen of intravenous therapy using commonly employed salt solutions (such as 0.9 per cent sodium chloride or 0.45 per cent sodium chloride). The therapy protocol is designed for a 48-hour period so that ongoing sodium and water losses must be accounted for; these losses either can be estimated by the program or can be measured and entered by the user. Once the deficits and ongoing losses are determined, the program will display (and print, if desired) the actual intravenous solutions to be used and the recommended rate of infusion. An example of the therapeutic suggestions that can be generated by such a program is shown in Figure 10–5. At the top of the figure are the calculated deficits (sodium and volume) and an estimated daily fluid requirement. Following this are the specific suggestions for intravenous therapy, including the type of intravenous salt solution to use and the recommended rate of infusion. Note that volume deficits are corrected quickly (in the first 4 hours) but free water deficits are corrected more slowly (over 48 hours).

This is an example of how a calculation-based system can provide practical information for individual patient management. Fluid and Electrolyte Expert also has sections that deal with problems in potassium balance and hypovolemia, with each section capable of generating specific recommendations tailored to the individual patient.

Nutrition

Recent awareness of the high incidence of protein and calorie malnutrition in hospitalized patients has lead to a flurry of interest in

```
                                          1/1/85
EST. KCAL - 2311
EST. GM. PROTEIN - 83

SUGGESTED FORMULATION -

370 CC OF 50% DEXTROSE
630 CC OF 7% AMINO ACIDS
AT 79  CC/HR X 24 HR.
710 CC 10% LIPID (30 CC/HR X 24 HR)

THIS FORMULATION WILL PROVIDE -

TOTAL KCAL/DAY          2308 (38 KCAL/KG)
GR PROTEIN/DAY          84   (1.4 G/KG)
VOLUME/DAY (CC)         2606 (42 CC/KG)
% KCAL AS PROTEIN       14
% KCAL AS DEXTROSE      52
% KCAL AS FAT           34
% NONPR KCAL AS FAT     40   (1.2 G/KG)
NONPR KCAL/G N RATIO    148
FINAL DEXT. CONC.       18 %
```

Figure 10–6. Specific nutritional recommendation for hyperalimentation based upon calculation of basal caloric need.

nutritional therapy, particularly parenteral nutrition. Constructing an appropriate nutritional program for the individual patient requires a well-defined set of determinations. First, an assessment of the present nutritional status (for example, visceral and somatic protein stores) is performed. Second, ongoing nutritional requirements (such as daily caloric needs) are determined. Finally, a specific regimen is constructed (using available enteral or parenteral solutions) that will correct any nutritional deficits and satisfy ongoing needs. Many of these determinations require mathematical calculations; thus, nutritional therapy is an area that is particularly well suited for computer implementation.

A number of microcomputer programs have been developed to aid physicians in the nutritional therapy of individual patients.[1, 8, 9, 12] These programs vary widely in their scope and complexity. The more basic programs, such as the Automated Metabolic Profile,[1] can aid in nutritional assessment by performing simple calculations of ongoing nutritional needs (daily caloric and protein requirements) and by graphically plotting both input data (such as serum albumin) and calculated nutritional parameters (such as creatinine height index) to generate a comprehensive profile of an individual patient's present nutritional status. The more sophisticated programs, such as those developed by Edwards[8] and Krasner and Marino[12] go one step further and use the nutritional assessment to generate parenteral nutrition regimens that are tailored to individual patient needs.

An example of the type of specific recommendations that can be generated by nutritional software is shown in Figure 10–6. This display was generated by a program developed in BASIC for both the Apple II series and IBM personal computers.[12] This program first estimates basal caloric needs using standard formulas (the Harris-Benedict equations) and then adjusts daily requirements for the patient's present condition. The user can then enter the type of parenteral nutrition solutions to be used, along with the maximum volume that can be tolerated. Using this information, the program then constructs a parenteral regimen similar in format to the example shown in Figure 10–6. As shown, the upper part of the figure presents the actual solutions to be used and the rate of infusion, and the lower portion of the figure documents precisely what the designed regimen will deliver. This type of highly specific nutritional prescription contains information important to the pharmacy (concentration of substrates in the solutions), nurse (infusion rates), and physician (total number of calories provided) and could literally be used to substitute for the nutritional order sheet. This type of printout is a good example of how calculation-based software can provide valuable, practical information for the physician.

THE COMPUTER AND PHYSICIAN PERFORMANCE

The ultimate utility of computer-assisted decision support lies in its ability to improve physician performance in three areas: (1) physician response to acquired patient data (for example, recognizing an abnormal laboratory test and determining how to act on the information), (2) the efficiency of the decision-making process (the amount of time consumed in arriving at a decision), and (3) diagnostic accuracy (the frequency of false positive and false negative diagnoses). Although few studies have been performed to evaluate the effects of computer aids on physician performance, the available evidence suggests that computer assistance can enhance physician performance in the clinical setting.

The potential role of the computer in altering physician responses to abnormal patient data is suggested by studies of physician performance based on arterial blood gas data. Although many physicians feel capable of interpreting arterial blood gases without assistance, Broughton and Kennedy[4] reported a 33 per cent prevalence of inappropriate therapeutic decisions by physicians in response to severe abnormalities in reported blood gases. Hingston and associates[11] reported that 70 per cent of physicians in a university teaching hospital felt that computer assistance in blood gas interpretation was not necessary. However, the same study group (which did not include pulmonary specialists) could correctly answer only 40 per cent of the sample questions on the topic generated by a computer program based on the principles of arterial blood gas interpretation. Studies such as this one suggest that physician performance in interpretation of laboratory data can be enhanced with computer aids.

The influence of the computer on the efficiency of the decision-making process has not been studied extensively at present, but the role of the computer in this area seems obvious. For example, Thorp and associates[20] found that the time required by house staff physicians to write parenteral nutrition orders was significantly reduced with the use of a computer program (a mean time of 14.8 minutes per patient without the program and 5.2 minutes per patient with the program). Indeed, in any area in which numerous calculations are performed, the computer should play an important role in minimizing the time consumed and the risk for error.

The ultimate goal of computer-assisted decision making is to improve the diagnostic and therapeutic accuracy of physicians. Although there are few studies comparing computer and physician accuracy in an actual clinical setting, the results of the available studies are encouraging. DeDombal and associates[20] developed a computer program to diagnose causes of acute abdominal pain and compared the accuracy of their program with that of staff physicians in an emergency room setting. In the 304 patients studied (all of whom underwent laparotomy), the computer program had a diagnostic accuracy of 92 per cent compared with 65 per cent for the physicians. Since 50 per cent of the patients in this study were found to have nonspecific findings at surgery, the computer program may have spared unnecessary surgery in some cases.

As indicated previously, physicians frequently are inaccurate in predicting the cause of acute abdominal pain. This is also the case with chest pain, particularly predicting the likelihood of myocardial ischemia as a cause of chest pain, because 50 per cent of patients admitted to coronary care units with the diagnosis of cardiac ischemia are inappropriately diagnosed.[19] In an attempt to improve this situation, Pozen and associates[19] have developed a computer program that uses stepwise regression analysis of seven patient variables to predict the probability of acute ischemic heart disease in patients with chest pains. When used by physicians in an emergency room setting, this program reduced the occurrence of false positive diagnoses (cardiac ischemia diagnosed but not present) from 55 to 33 per cent, while not decreasing the occurrence of false negative diagnoses (cardiac ischemia present but not suspected). Because a false positive diagnosis in this setting can result in an inappropriate hospital admission, the potential value of this type of computer aid becomes obvious.

In summary, it seems that computerized diagnostics can indeed improve physician performance in actual patient management situations. As physicians become more familiar with the microcomputer, and as diagnostic software becomes more refined with repeated use, it is very probable that computerized diagnostics will play an increasingly important role in improving patient care.

FUTURE DIRECTIONS: THE CONSULTANT SYSTEM

Clinical problem solving can be a complicated process involving a number of decision pathways. As such, diagnostic software should be versatile enough to include all possible pathways involved in the decision process. This often requires a memory capacity that exceeds the capacity of conventional microcomputers, and therefore, current versions of diagnostic software are often limited in scope and versatility. However, as microcomputers become more powerful, the ability of software to mimic the actual decision-making process will improve.

The accuracy of diagnostic software is dependent on its knowledge base, which must be furnished by the computer expert. Therefore, the ideal process of developing diagnostic software would be to combine the efforts of the foremost medical authority (or panel of authorities) in a field with computer experts who are adept in developing decision-making software. The situation does not exist at present. Rather, software is being developed by physicians who are familiar with computers, regardless of their expertise in either medicine or software development. Although the resultant software represents an advance in clinical decision making, this situation may not be optimal. What is needed is a collaboration between medical experts and computer experts to generate software that has a valid, comprehensive knowledge base and an effective design. The resultant software could form a "consultant" system. For example, a physician who wants a consultation on a patient with a particular problem might simply select a disk from a medical diskette library that contains the knowledge base of the foremost medical authority on the subject. In this setting, any physician would have easy access to the reasoning of the experts in any given field and could thus obtain a "consultation" from the experts in any given area. The implications of this are far reaching, in terms of both improving the quality of patient care and limiting the cost of consultations.

REFERENCES

1. Argawal, N. R., et al.: The automated metabolic profile. Crit. Care Med., 11:546, 1983.
2. Bleich, H. L.: Computer-based consultation. Electrolyte and acid-base disorders. Am. J. Med., 53:285, 1972.

3. Bleich, H. L.: Computer evaluation of acid-base disorders. J. Clin. Invest., *48*:1689, 1969.
4. Broughton, J. O., and Kennedy, T. C.: Interpretation of arterial blood gases by computer. Chest, *85*:148, 1984.
5. Cohn, J., et al.: Automated physiological profile. Crit. Care Med., *3*:51, 1975.
6. deDombal, F. T., et al.: Computer-aided diagnosis of acute abdominal pain. Br. Med. J., *2*:9, 1972.
7. Doyle, D. J.: A hand-held microcomputer system for anesthesiology and critical care applications. Proceedings of the Eighth Annual Symposium on Computer Applications in Medical Care. Washington, Institute for Electrical Engineers, 1984, p. 1021.
8. Edwards, F. H.: Computer assisted planning of parenteral hyperalimentation therapy. Crit. Care Med., *10*:539, 1982.
9. Giacoia, P., and Chopra, R.: The use of a computer in parenteral alimentation of low birth weight infants. JPEN, *5*:328, 1981.
10. Goldberg, M., et al.: Computer-based instruction and diagnosis of acid-base disorders. J.A.M.A., *223*:269, 1973.
11. Hingston, D. M., et al.: A computerized interpretation of arterial pH and blood gas data: Do physicians need it? Resp. Care, *27*:809, 1982.
12. Krasner, J. B., and Marino, P. L.: An analytical approach to creation of parenteral feeding solutions: Implementation on a microcomputer. JPEN, *9*:226, 1985.
13. Krasner, J. B., and Marino, P. L.: The use of a pocket computer for hemodynamic profiles. Crit. Care Med., *11*:826, 1983.
14. Marino, P. L., and Krasner, J. B.: An interpretive computer program for analyzing hemodynamic problems in the ICU. Crit. Care Med., *12*:601, 1984.
15. Marino, P. L., et al.: Fluid and Electrolyte Expert. Philadelphia, W. B. Saunders Co., 1985.
16. Martin, P. L., and Jeffreys, B.: A microcomputer based system for storing, reporting, and interpreting arterial blood gas data. Proceedings of the Eighth Annual Symposium of Computer Applications in Medical Care. Washington, Institute for Electrical Engineers, 1984, pp. 761–764.
17. Maxwell, C., et al.: Clinical application of the hand-held computer in respiratory intensive care. Crit. Care Quart., *6*:85, 1983.
18. Miller, R. A., et al.: Internist-I. An experimental computer-based diagnostic consultant for general internal medicine. N. Engl. J. Med., *307*:468, 1982.
19. Pozen, M. W., et al.: The usefulness of a predictive instrument to reduce inappropriate admissions to the coronary care unit. Ann. Intern. Med., *92*:238, 1980.
20. Thorp, J. W., et al.: Computer assistance to formulate, order, and evaluate parenteral nutrition solutions. Proceedings of the Seventh Annual Symposium on Computer Applications in Medical Care. Baltimore, Institute of Electrical Engineers, 1983, pp. 219–221.
21. Weiner, F., et al.: Computerized medical reasoning in diagnosis and treatment of acid-base disorders. Crit. Care Med., *11*:470, 1983.

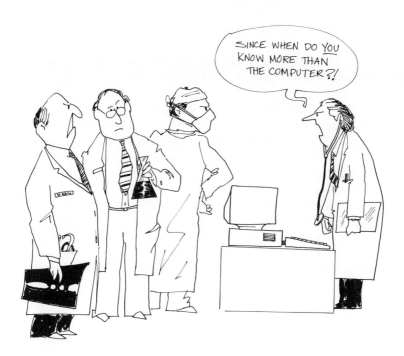

E L E V E N

Computer-Aided Diagnosis and Decision Making

James M. Fattu, M.D., Ph.D.

Edward A. Patrick, Ph.D., M.D.

Expert systems in medicine, put simply, are computer devices that accept findings about a patient and provide a differential diagnosis with a probability or certainty estimate. The source of the system's expertise is derived from a knowledge base, which is obtained from records of patients, from the medical literature, or from medical "experts." Expert computer systems are used to classify the findings (signs, symptoms, or laboratory tests) about a patient into a ranked list of diseases that are most likely for that patient. This differential diagnosis is based upon some threshold of diagnosis based upon probabilities, weights, or certainties (depending upon the system). Major differences are present in approaches to expert systems. Variations include systems that provide a single diagnosis as the output rather than a ranked differential diagnosis, and systems that provide actions such as treatments or testing procedures as the output. This chapter will explore the basis of expert systems, their use in medicine, their differences, their source of expertise (knowledge), and how this knowledge is learned or discovered.

WHAT IS AN EXPERT SYSTEM?

What Is an Expert?

A medical expert is a highly skilled individual with advanced training and knowledge in a particular field. The expert serves as a consultant to colleagues in difficult cases. Regardless of whether the situation involves a suspected intra-abdominal crisis or the diagnosis of a difficult anemia, the medical expert brings to the practice of medicine skills that advance the science and improve patient care. Human traits that the physician expert brings to diagnostic decision-making include (1) the ability to interact with other persons, (2) the technical skills necessary to do a physical examination or a diagnostic or therapeutic procedure, (3) the ability to acquire and use knowledge and to organize and synthesize information, and (4) the ability to apply clinical judgment.[1] Ben-Bassat, however, cautions that different experts may have different weaknesses in their problem-solving skills.[5]

What Is an Expert Computer System?

In contrast to the physician expert, a computer expert has a limited but powerful role. Although a computer system can interview patients for a history, it is poor at interpersonal skills. The computer cannot do a simple physical examination or perform a complex invasive procedure. The computer expert system can provide superb intellectual skills. It can process information to create knowledge, and it can be used to organize knowledge to produce a differential diagnosis, to recommend a testing procedure, or to recommend treatments. The computer system can help to find "holes" in our knowledge by recognizing and incorporating subtle diagnostic clues often overlooked by humans. Although no single system has achieved ultimate development, the diversity of approaches would appear to be beneficial to the study of artificial intelligence in medicine (AIM).

Expert medical computer systems are classification systems based upon a measure of how close the findings from a patient (signs, symptoms, laboratory tests) are to a diagnosis. A classification in medicine is based on the differential diagnosis in that it measures how close the findings about the patient are to the diagnoses considered. The interpretation of the classification depends upon some decision rule. Explanation of the decision (diagnosis) may be appended.

For example, consider a 60-year-old patient who presents with acute onset of hemiparesis and headache. The differential diagnoses presented by the expert system include subarachnoid bleeding, intracerebral bleeding, cerebral embolus, tumor, and so on. Each choice in the differential diagnosis may be provided with some probability, certainty, or weight (depending on the system). Based on a decision rule (perhaps some threshold of probability), the advice may be a final diagnosis or recommendation for further information, for example, to obtain a CT scan or magnetic resonance imaging (MRI) scan of the head. The result of this information may be added to the patient record, and a revised differential diagnosis can be obtained.

Components of an Expert System

Knowledge Base. The knowledge base in medicine for expert systems consists of either hard data (patient records) or softer knowledge obtained from literature review or "experts in the field." The knowledge base contains general relationships applicable to many presentations of the diseases. In production rule systems, the knowledge base contains the "if, then" productions and their weight or certainty of occurrence.

In statistical pattern recognition systems, the knowledge base contains the categories of disease, the features describing these diseases, and the relative frequency of diseases and features in diseases (probabilities). Relationships among features for a disease are carefully engineered mathematical expressions that resemble complex production rules.

Inference Structure. An inference structure, which contains a mathematical decision rule or a structure within which production rules are processed, is required to process patient findings using the knowledge base in order to arrive at some form of classification. In production rule systems, the inference is based upon a form of heuristic search—

comparing the production rules within the knowledge base to the findings. In a statistical system, the inference is based upon a mathematical formula. Parts of the mathematical formula may explain or describe a process otherwise thought of as heuristic.

Some expert systems based on production rules require a supervisor, sometimes called a *reasoning engine*, to call the production rules into operation. The supervisor itself is a production rule or set of production rules. Many expert systems designed around production rules (which can be thought of as packets of relationships) require the supervisor to put the packets together or to assign relationships among the packets. Use of the phrase "reasoning engine" gives the connotation of human behavior. However, this supervisory activity can be time-consuming and may in fact decrease performance over an approach that directly engineers knowledge.

Interviewer. An interviewer is a component of the expert system utilized to input findings (signs, symptoms, laboratory tests, radiologic procedures) about a patient into the expert system. The expert system, through the interviewer, can interact with the user by asking questions about the patient. For statistical approaches, the interviewer converts the questions into well-organized knowledge that can interact with the knowledge base.

Classification. The differential diagnosis (classification) about a patient is obtained from the knowledge base and the findings. Generally, this is the differential diagnosis in medicine. It is expressed in terms of some probability of occurrence or by weights or certainties (system-dependent). A classification may be modified by factors that incorporate loss or utility. The risks of a procedure, such as an angiogram, could be given a loss factor, or a very expensive procedure could be given a cost factor. The risks of missing a diagnosis, such as lung cancer, because a chest x-ray was not done would represent a loss factor.

Actions. Actions can be the direct conclusion of an expert system based upon the findings about a patient. Recommendations can also be made, depending upon the classification (diagnosis). An action may be another test to confirm a diagnosis; it may be a surgical procedure, such as biopsy; or it may be a treatment protocol.

Explanation. In a statistical system explanations may consist of probabilities of occurrence of findings for each disease considered. It can indicate features not in agreement with the highest ranking disease in a differential diagnosis. In a production rule system, an explanation includes the rules that were applied in order to arrive at a decision. Because a production rule system puts together its packets of knowledge, it has an added need to explain itself.

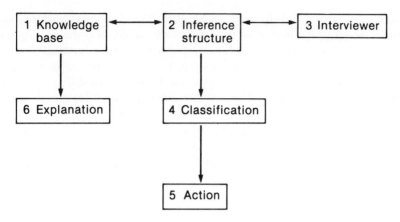

Figure 11–1.

Establishing the Medical Problem

The medical problem faced by developers of expert classification systems can be illustrated using the approach proposed by Patrick.[34, 35] In medicine, knowledge is collected in an organized, logical manner based upon anatomic, physiologic, and pathophysiologic findings. In each area of medicine, there are subsystems of interest, such as anemias, white blood cell disorders, thyroid disorders, chest pain syndromes, hypercalcemia, and so on. A subsystem has a definable number of disease categories within it. In any expert system, a definable number of final categories must be recognized. There may be combinations of these categories (called complex classes), and this will be discussed later. The signs, symptoms, laboratory tests, x-ray procedures, and similar findings, which describe the disease categories in the subsystem, are the features of the subsystem. Each feature will have accompanying feature values. A feature may be family history of cancer, with values of true or false; heart murmur may have values of systolic, diastolic, or laboratory values such as white blood cell count with values of <1000, 1000 to 4000, 4001 to 10,500, or >10,500 cells per mm³. For each disease category, a certain relative frequency of occurrence of each of the feature values can be identified. This requires expert knowledge, literature review, or samples from patient records (hard data). In more advanced systems, it is necessary to know the frequency of several features at the same time (features dependent upon each other) for a category. The frequency of feature values (with multiple features taken together) for a category is referred to as the "category conditional probability." In statistical pattern recognition, the set of all probabilities for feature values of a disease category is called the "category conditional probability density function."

In rule-based systems, the function is broken into packets of information called production rules. But knowledge stored in this format appears to have no unifying model for the disease under consideration. There is a relative frequency (incidence) of a particular disease within a patient population (a priori probability). This frequency of disease may be different at different sites and can be different during epidemics of disease, or similar situations. It has been incorporated in rule-based as well as statistical systems.

In expert systems, whether production rule or statistical, the preceding points must be considered to assure completeness. In later sections, we will discuss how these considerations are viewed by various authors.

Problems in Medicine to Which Expert Systems Apply

Expert medical systems have been under development for nearly two decades. Most of these have been applied to special, well-delineated areas of medicine that are consistent with the way physicians collect and process data themselves. For example, a subsystem of anemias would consist of all the causes of anemia and those signs, symptoms, laboratory tests, and ancillary procedures that would help to classify the anemias.

In medical diagnosis, areas that have been well studied include thyroid diseases, breast diseases, drug poisoning, electrolyte disorders, abdominal pain, neurology, interpretation of electroencephalograms, jaundice and liver dysfunction, ventilator management, pulmonary function test interpretation, infectious diseases, digitalis therapy, rheumatology, hematology, chest pain, ophthalmology, serum protein electrophoresis interpretation, and oncology, to name but a few. An enterprising effort to include all the field of knowledge of internal medicine in a single system has been attempted in Caduceus, formerly known as Internist.

BASIS OF EXPERT SYSTEMS

Expert systems have been defined as programs designed to represent and apply factual knowledge of specific areas of expertise to solve problems.[21] Popular descriptions of expert systems see them as being created using "rules" or heuristics that are obtained from experts (the knowledge of experts). Alternatively, knowledge may be obtained from samples from nature and repetition—hard data. No matter what the basis of the expert system, it must operate in the "real world." In evaluating its performance, one must distinguish between "human-like" behavior and "optimal" performance. An expert system best fits the real world when it provides diagnostic, therapeutic, or testing assistance and meets criteria of validity, reliability, and verifiable follow-up.

The development of expert systems historically has evolved in two major directions. The first has been to represent knowledge as symbolic data. It has been said of this form of expert system that the power of the expert system derives from the knowledge it possesses, not from the particular formalisms or inference schemes it employs.[18] Advantages of a production rule approach include the following:

1. Modularity—the storage of knowledge in independent rules. Thus, rules can be easily added or removed.

2. Knowledge acquisition by the system is simplified with the addition of rules without considering prior rule organization. This can also be a disadvantage in that no overriding model prevails.

3. Explanation of the rules used for an inference—this offers semantic advantage but is not unique. Statistical systems can explain their inference in terms of the knowledge of samples from nature (in medicine, patient records).

Some difficulties in rule-based approaches include the following: (1) rules do not organize diagnostic information as the physician intuitively does, and (2) there is difficulty in managing all the necessary context for rules, applications, and antecedent clauses (*if* facts).[8]

Rule-based approaches in recent lay literature have been equated to "artificial intelligence." However, the definition of AI may be in the eye of the developer, and there is no uniformly accepted definition of artificial intelligence.[8]

The other major approach to expert systems has been through statistical methods, particularly statistical pattern recognition (SPR). This is a science that deals with descriptions of patterns, such as diseases. Patterns are grouped by category, and the variability within a category is described mathematically. Uncertain knowledge in a category is accounted for by an inference function, called the category conditional probability density function. Procedures for learning this knowledge are studied in SPR.[30, 35] SPR has provided a rich mathematical framework by which we can learn the efficiency and deficiencies of expert systems for comparison.

Again, in evaluating or comparing forms of expert systems, we must be cognizant of whether the system is designed to simulate "human-like behavior" to the user or attempt to achieve optimal decision-making, therapeutic, and testing performance.

In Table 11–1 we summarize some important characteristics of selected systems.

Table 11–1. A Comparison of Expert Systems

Feature	Consult-I	Mycin	Expert	Caduceus	Help
Type of system	SPR and AI	Production rule	Production rule plus precedence	Semantic network	Bayesian and AI
Source of knowledge	Expert and records	Expert	Expert	Expert	Records and Expert
Method of knowledge storage	Features and probability	Production rule and certainty	Production rule and weights	Production rule and weights	Probability and rules
Decision rule	Likelihood and a posteriori probability	Heuristic search	Heuristic search	Heuristic search	Bayes
Concept formation of complex classes	Yes	No	No	Ad hoc method	No
Conditional probability	Yes, in c.c.p.d.f.*	Similar in C.F.†	Similar in weight	Similar in frequency	Yes
A priori probability	Yes	No	No	No	Yes
Dependence among features	Yes	No†	No†	No†	No (?)
Complex features	Yes			No	Yes
Feature selection	Yes, in actions	Necessary	Yes	Yes	Yes
Utility (risk/gain)	Physician to do	?	?	Yes, import value	Yes
Actions	Yes	Yes	Yes	No	Yes
Explanation	Yes, basic consulting	Yes	Yes	Yes	Yes
Generalizability‡	Yes	No	Yes	No	Yes
Microcomputer operation	Yes	No	?	No	No

Key: c.c.p.d.f. = category conditional probability density function; C.F. = certainty factor (a weighting factor).

†Dependence among features—it could be argued that production rule systems permit local dependence among features. This, however, is limited. It does not provide the rich dependence of a statistical system.

‡Generalizability of a system is meant to indicate that it can be used to create expert systems from many knowledge bases. It is adaptable, not "hard wired."

Rule-Based Systems

In the simplest form, rule-based systems progress from algorithms to production rules to frame systems and finally semantic network systems. The latter three have been referred to as artificial intelligence (AI) systems. In AI, there are five primary application areas for research. These are: (1) natural language processing, (2) problem solving and planning, (3) computer vision, (4) robotics, and (5) expert systems. This discussion considers only the fifth category—expert systems.

Algorithm-Based Systems

Algorithm-based systems are essentially computerized protocols. These protocols, for example, in oncology, involve procedures for selection of patients, treatment regimen, dose modification, study parameters, and evaluating criteria of response. These protocols are fixed; that is, binary answers are offered as yes or no. Such systems do not involve probabilistic information and do not provide relative probabilities of one disease to another. Also, they do not provide information about multiple diseases present at the same time.

Production Rule Systems

Production rule systems have been popular in the implementation of expert systems. These systems are based upon "production rules." Each of these rules has a premise and an action (an *if* statement, then *action* statement). A well-known production rule system, Mycin, has been applied to the area of infectious diseases.[37] A typical rule would be as follows:

if (1) The infection is primary bacteremia, and
    (2) The site of the culture is one of the sterile sites, and
    (3) The suspected portal entry of the organism is the gastrointestinal tract,
then there is suggestive evidence (0.7) that the identity of the organism is *Bacteroides*.[12]

The numbers used to indicate the strength of a rule (the 0.7 in the example) is termed a certainty factor. This is related to probability; however, the authors have gone out of their way to say that this is not a true probability. Indeed, Greenes has stated that such uses of certainties are surrogates of probability.[19] Decisions are made by search procedures in which all rules relevant to a goal must be reviewed. Once all relevant rules have been used, the total weight of the evidence must fall within some threshold value. If this threshold is achieved, a decision is said to be made. If not, the system must ask further questions of the findings about the patient. Explanation of such a system is in the form of the rules that were used. Actions are provided in the form of antibiotics of choice for infections. An outgrowth of Mycin is the system Oncocin[38] for oncology treatment. Oncocin is reported to have increased speed over Mycin, and has the ability to generate a hard copy of the patient progress report as well as the treatment protocols.

Frame-Based Systems

A system known as Expert (formerly called Casnet)[22, 23] has been called a frame system. The authors have described this as a production rule system containing precedences (for therapy). The frame system is "packet-oriented" with pieces of knowledge being stored about a disease category. The association of these packets of knowledge can be assembled as a causal relationship for a disease category. The Expert model presumes that a category is described by an accumulation of small pieces of knowledge. The Expert system allows for actions, for example, treatment of ocular herpes, and these are prescribed by both production rules and precedences. A precedence would be a sequence such as sickest > sicker > sick > healthy. The Expert system has been applied to eye diseases, rheumatology, and hematology. The Expert model allows for weights to be applied at each node in the decision process in order to conduct its search.

Semantic Network

A system called Caduceus (formerly called Internist)[27, 28, 36] has attempted to include much of the field of knowledge of internal medicine. It is a system allocating weights to feature values (called manifestations by the authors) and using a counting rule search procedure to come to a decision. The Caduceus system creates a master differential diagnosis (hypothesis) when the findings about a patient are presented. It then tests the differential diagnosis based upon the scores of the weights. The Caduceus/Internist system is trained with weights called evoking strength (given the finding on a patient, how strongly should the diagnosis be considered); frequency (an estimate of how often a patient with the disease will have the finding); and import (how important is the manifestation for disease). The authors state that the numbers used for each of these weights are "judgmental"—not probabilities.[27] The system also uses rules of search called pursuing rules, rule out rules, and discriminating rules. It does allow for the activation of interconnected subsystems in order to find complex classes (more than a single disease present at the same time in the patient). Caduceus includes over 650 diseases in its system knowledge base. It is reported to operate faster than its predecessor, Internist, partially by forming intermediate diagnoses (hypotheses) in its logic sequence.

Bayes Framework

Let us now reconsider the classification problem. A simplified approach will be presented here, trying to minimize any mathematical formalism. Nonetheless, this approach is sufficiently general to describe much about all expert systems. Let us assume that we were dealing with a subsystem of medicine, such as head trauma. A number of disease categories will be present and can be defined by experts. In order to express the probability of a disease for a set of findings on a patient (history, physical, laboratory tests, imaging procedure results), we can use an expression of probabilities known as Bayes theorem. In a simple form, we express the Bayes theorem[4] as:

$$P \text{ (Disease} \mid \text{Findings)} = \frac{P(\text{Findings} \mid \text{Disease}) * P(\text{Disease})}{P(\text{Findings})}$$

On the left side of the equation, **P(Disease | Findings)** states that we desire to compute the probability **(P)** of each of the diseases for that subsystem under consideration, given the findings for a new patient (the symbol " | " is read as "given"). This probability is computed from the right side of the equation.

The probability of the findings given the disease is **P(Findings | Disease)** also known as conditional probability. Much work has been done in the area of statistical pattern recognition on engineering this function.[30, 33, 35] Much criticism of Bayes theorem has been with regard to misunderstanding the construction of the conditional probability function. Much of that criticism is inaccurate in terms of present-day knowledge. Not only do we know the probability of a single finding for the disease, but we can learn complex probabilities, such as the probability of headache, and hemiparesis, and ... | disease, a dependent conditional probability. This learning involves records and repetition, that is, the knowledge can be acquired by collecting patient records (hard data).

The probability of the disease, **P(Disease),** is the frequency of that disease in the population. This is valuable information, which may fluctuate within a single community, such as at times of epidemics of infectious diseases. This probability can also be estimated from literature. The denominator of the right side of the equation is a normalizing factor. Bayes theorem has been used in a number of medical expert systems; for example, the relative risk of a patient having a coronary event, given certain risk factors.[15]

Utilities

In practice, the physician does not always choose the diagnosis with the highest probability. Consider the following example[2]:

Category	Probability
Malignant supratentorial tumor	0.45
Cerebral abscess	0.40
All other diagnoses	0.15

From the treatment standpoint, the second diagnosis (abscess) may have the best outcome and would, therefore, be the most operative. Thus, the probability of the diagnosis is not always sufficient for deciding treatment. It is often useful to incorporate the gain that the patient could expect from different treatments appropriate to the diagnoses. A utility provides the probability of the categories modified by some gain or loss factor; for example, the risk of doing a test because of an associated high morbidity rate.[10, 20]

Consult-I

A system, called Consult-I, has been developed which incorporates statistical pattern recognition with methods from artificial intelligence.[30, 33] Based upon a formal mathematical approach, the system provides a structure by which to compare other systems. A medical area for decisions, such as anemias, is called a subsystem, containing all the possible diseases under consideration. In addition, more than one type of anemia can be present at the same time—for example, pernicious anemia and iron-deficiency anemia. The system, Consult-I, has the capability for recognizing this presentation of two or more diseases at the same time (called a complex class). Characteristics of both diseases, such as signs, symptoms, and laboratory tests, are called features. Each of these features has feature values. For example, the feature hemoglobin has feature values of < 5, 5 to 10, 11 to 15, and so forth. An example of a nonordered, nominal feature is examination, with values of splenomegaly, lymphadenopathy, and pallor. The Consult-I system, in distinction from most statistical systems, can handle nonordered data and nominal data. The nominal data may include such information as hair color or eye color.

In Consult-I, presentations of diseases are stored as subcategories (Fig. 11–2). That is, a presentation of thyroid carcinoma may be medullary carcinoma (a subcategory) with a certain age and sex grouping as well as endocrine manifestations, while another subcategory of thyroid carcinoma would be follicular carcinoma with a different presentation. The entire subcategory presentations with their probability distributions of each feature are stored within the Consult-I framework. This is called engineering the category conditional probability density function (probability of the findings given the disease). The system, Consult-I, can be trained from textbook and expert interaction, but is ideally trained from hard data obtained from patient records using the Consult Learning

Category: Hemolytic anemia
 Subcategory: Hemolytic anemia secondary to drugs
 Subcategory: Hemolytic anemia secondary to prosthetic valve
 Subcategory: Hemolytic anemia secondary to autoimmune disease

Category: Thyroid carcinoma
 Subcategory: Follicular carcinoma
 Subcategory: Medullary carcinoma
 Subcategory: Anaplastic carcinoma

Figure 11–2. Example of categories and subcategories within CONSULT-I.

System. These records, with the ability to make probabilistic inferences, comprise the knowledge base.

Statistical systems have been criticized for failing to address the "combinatorial explosion" of possibilities of features and feature values for diseases. For example, if a system contains 100 binary (true/false) features, then there are ($2^{100} - 1$) possible combinations, an enormously large number. In Consult-I, the dimensionality of this problem can be reduced by the introduction of prior knowledge—in essence, expert knowledge superimposed on hard data samples. Thus, a solution to the combinatorial explosion of possibilities is the integration of AI with SPR.

Consult-I utilizes rules analogous to production rules within the probabilistic knowledge base.[17] A "can't" rule states that if a specified condition occurs in the findings about a patient, then a particular category cannot (can't) exist. For example,

 if the patient is not taking thyroid hormone,
 then the diagnosis cannot be factitious hyperthyroid.

Consult-I recognizes that hard data records as well as experts will have holes in their knowledge. The "insignificance rule" inserts some small probability into the knowledge base until an accurate probabilistic estimate or a "can't" can be supplied, using hard data. Thus, the category is neither missed nor enhanced if the findings about a patient contain an insignificant feature value. Other rules incorporated into the probabilistic knowledge base of Consult-I include rule-in rules, rule-out rules, critical, and noncritical features, and focusing rules. Dependence packets of knowledge comparable to frames (called minicolumns) contain dependent relationships about a disease, for example, the hypothalmic-pituitary-thyroid pathophysiologic relationships in a thyroid subsystem.

Action rules also are incorporated in Consult-I. For example,

 if the top-ranked category (in a posteriori probability) is hemolytic anemia, **and** the most likely subcategory is hemolytic anemia secondary to drugs,

then the action is to withdraw the offending drugs (list of offending drugs given).

Complex features in Consult-I include relationships such as ratios (BUN/creatinine) and other mathematical formulas. These have the benefit of reducing the complexity of the system. In addition, networking of subsystems to communicate with each other reduces the complexity of a single system attempting to contain this field of knowledge.

Consult-I utilizes certain fuzzy set operations[30, 44] in constructing sets of feature values and in implementing logical "and" and logical "or" operations.

Patrick's Framework

The inference operation in Consult-I is based upon a new theorem,[32] which allows deduction of new categories of disease never before seen by the system. This is accomplished using knowledge of records and repetition.[30] In addition, the system can explain its decisions from the probabilistic knowledge base; that is, it can show the subcategory presentations. This is appealing to physicians because it is how diseases are frequently described in textbooks. Decisions are made from optimal theory and presented as both likelihoods (when the prior probability of each disease is assumed equal) as well as what is called true a posteriori probability, that is, the probability of each disease given the findings including the frequency of those diseases in the population. Actions, based upon the probabilistic decisions, can be provided by Consult-I. These actions can be in the form of further laboratory tests in order to confirm a diagnosis or can be in the form of treatment protocols.

The Outcome Advisor

The Outcome Advisor (OA) is a system having some of the knowledge structure of expert systems such as features with feature values and categories. It stores patient records and creates knowledge by processing these records relative to the findings about a new patient. This means that the relationships among features are not determined until the findings are known. A production rule system may find it impossible to develop and store all possible productions for all possible findings. The Outcome Advisor does not store any productions; rather, it creates a complex production once the findings are presented.

Picker Consult System for Diagnostic Imaging

In 1984, Picker International incorporated the Consult Learning System and Consult-I as a module of the magnetic resonance imaging scanner. The Consult Learning System (CLS) allows the radiologist to define categories and features involved in imaging modalities. It permits the comparison of imaging modalities in terms of sensitivity, specificity, and cost (MRI versus CT versus other tests). The knowledge obtained from the CLS is incorporated into the probabilistic knowledge base for the expert system Consult-I. It can be used for patient triage, such as identification of the most sensitive and cost-effective imaging modality, can suggest scan sequences, and can suggest other medical tests to confirm a diagnosis. The system links subsystems that solve physical equations (including indices of time, contrast, signal to noise, and so on) with subsystems that include clinical information.[45] It can potentially be applied to trouble-shooting equipment and can allow creation of simulated conditions, which are useful for training radiologists and technicians.

Data Base Management Systems

Examples of well-known data base management systems (DBMS) are the Help system and the Regenstrief system. The Help system[41] has been implemented as a hospital information system that monitors patient care with patient prompts called Help sectors. The Regenstrief system[25] is a data base system with logic-driven protocols as physician reminders. It interacts with the physician, pharmacy, and laboratory. An example of a protocol is

if the patient is on digitalis, and if the ECG demonstrates more than two PVCs per minute,
then consider digitalis as the cause of the arrhythmia. The system will then give critical facts for review by the primary physician.

HOW ARE EXPERT SYSTEMS CREATED?

Rule-Based Systems

Artificial intelligence systems based upon production rules typically use rules such as the *if* (condition) *then* (action) pair previously described. A number of such rules are applied to a given disease category. These systems lack organized knowledge about that disease in comparison to the SPR model. The rules are typically generated by interviewing expert(s) in a field of specialty. Such a system then is tested and refined many times. Rules typically are given some weight or certainty. For example:

> **if** the patient has tachycardia and nervousness and a borderline T4 is increased,
> **then** the patient is hyperthyroid with a weight of 0.6.

It would appear to the observer that this weight, or certainty, is a probability of the disease occurring. However, many knowledge engineers argue that this is not the case. But because we now have the capability to develop knowledge bases from hard data, such a rejection of probability is not tenable.

Although production rules can represent the most common "if, then" combinations, it is impossible for them to cover all the possible presentations of disease. "Holes" in their knowledge will exist. For example, the developers of the system Expert for herpetic ocular diseases describe 30 categories of disease and provide for 51 therapeutic regimens. The authors, recognizing the extensive number of production rules necessary for a system of this size, have developed precedence rules to help limit the number of production rules needed.

Statistical Pattern Recognition

The area of statistical pattern recognition (SPR) provides an alternative organized approach to production rules for the development of expert systems. Using SPR, the developer defines a problem area, such as anemias, and guides the definition of categories of diseases, subcategories of diseases, features, and feature values (laboratory tests, patient history, and physical examination). A disease category is defined with its subcategory presentations. Each of these subcategories is supplied with the joint probabilities of the feature values occurring for that presentation. This is compatible with the way in which knowledge is collected in medicine. Furthermore, the collection of this knowledge can be facilitated by learning systems (such as The Outcome Advisor or Consult Learning System). As further knowledge is created from patient records collected in the learning system, the knowledge can be used to update the probabilistic knowledge base of the expert system (such as Consult-I).

The Source of Expertise (Knowledge) in Expert Systems

Most heuristic artifical intelligence (AI) systems are trained with knowledge of experts. It is well known that experts are inaccurate in their estimation of probabilities. For example, it has been demonstrated that experts tended to overestimate probabilities of the occurrence of feature values. No provision in production rule systems is made for training with hard data (records of patients). Statistical systems have this facility. It is advantageous for having accurate estimates as well to update the expert system. The system Consult-I has the facility for initial training from soft knowledge of experts and literature with the ability to be updated from hard data records.

Total System Versus Subsystem Approach

The vast majority of expert systems approach small subsets of medicine, such as thyroid disease, anemia, calcium blood levels, breast lump, infectious disease, rheumatology, and ocular subsystems. This differs from a system that tries to encompass multiple areas of medicine simultaneously, the best known being Internist/Caduceus. However, Feigenbaum[18] reported that it was impractical for knowledge engineers to create systems that encompass all fields of medical knowledge. He advocated, as have others, developing selected areas of application. Similarly, this is consistent with the approach taken by researchers in SPR. Models for interaction of one subsystem with others have been studied.[30, 33] The decision made by one subsystem can become the input to another system. For example, the diagnosis of hyperthyroidism in a thyroid subsystem can become a feature in a chest pain subsystem that in turn applies to the diagnosis of arrhythmia. The ability of one subsystem to activate another subsystem has been said to use an activation rule. Rules similar to these are used in the Internist system to form new hypotheses.

The Limitations of Expert Systems

Expert computer systems are not physicians. They are ancillary consultation devices that under the supervision of the physician can be used to enhance diagnosis, expedite laboratory testing, give advice for therapy, or determine parameters for a medical device such as an MRI scanner. The expert system cannot do a physical examination. It cannot do a medical procedure such as a biopsy. What it does provide is the ability to store knowledge of the past and a rich framework for arriving at a medical decision; but there are limitations to all systems. At present, some are difficult to use. It may require an extensive time period to obtain a consultation from the computer expert system. This is particularly true of production rule systems, which must use a search procedure and ask questions in order to enhance their ability to make a decision.

This search can be quite lengthy, lasting many minutes or even an hour. Physicians often are unwilling to sit at a computer keyboard, particularly for an extended period of time. The output of most expert systems as yet requires verification.

Hayes-Roth and associates[21] describe criteria for evaluating expert systems. They note that most systems have not been studied extensively enough. Another limitation is the extent of the knowledge that is placed in the system. An expert in one subarea of medicine may not be expert in all subareas. Furthermore, expertise that may apply to one regional area may not be transferable to another site. This suggests the need for data collection at multiple sites, using learning systems, once the expert system has been organized. These additional data must be used for updating and testing the system. Systems that cannot be updated by hard data are thus limited.

Statistical pattern recognition approaches allow hard data to be collected and utilized in systems. However, it is expensive to obtain valid, reliable, and verified hard data. In addition, if insufficient records are available for the knowledge base, then inaccuracies about some diseases are apt to be present. This can be circumvented to some extent by the combination of systems that utilize both artificial intelligence rules and statistical pattern recognition. The system Consult-I allows for expert training of the presentations of disease and the ability to update from hard data records. It has been our experience that this approach is superior to either approach (AI or SPR) alone.

The Limitations of Physician Users of Expert Systems

Feature extraction by physicians will significantly affect the performance of the expert system no matter how good it is in the hands of its developer. Physicians do perform differently when taking a history and conducting a physical examination, depending upon their training, interest, and field of specialization. For example, deDombal[13] reported in a study of 11,168 breast lesions, that there was high observer variation (on the order of 30 to 40 per cent) in regard to the presence or absence of axillary lymph nodes and size of the primary lesion. The quality of data being presented to the expert systems (the findings about a patient) will thus affect the performance of the computer expert system. Furthermore, the developer may use a different inherent classification of diseases than the user may be familiar with. The variability of findings is particularly a problem for arriving at a diagnosis from history and physical examination findings.

Data from the laboratory or radiology department are less subject to this variability. Systems must, however, be adapted to handle different laboratory ranges at different regional sites. A normal serum potassium at one institution may be 3.5 to 5.5 mmol/L, but at another institution, the normal range may be 3.8 to 5.8 mmol/L. The transferability of the expert system can be enhanced using the concept of "fuzzy sets."[30, 44] This concept allows us to describe laboratory tests as decreased, normal, borderline increased, increased, or very increased. The individual institution itself may then apply its own laboratory normal values and ranges. The advantage is that the knowledge base will apply the data at multiple sites with less need for modification.

Other limitations of physician-users include expertise in interpreting the expert system output. If the system is probabilistic, can the physician properly interpret a probabilistic differential diagnosis?

HOW DOES A PHYSICIAN USE AN EXPERT SYSTEM?

The physician consultant typically is asked to review a patient case when some characteristic(s) of the patient illness poses a difficult diagnostic or therapeutic management problem to the primary physician. The primary physician recognizes the advantage of obtaining an expert's opinion and skills to aid the patient's welfare. Typically, the primary physician requests the consultant to evaluate a specific problem, for example the diagnosis of a suspected endocrine abnormality such as hypercalcemia, or to assist in the difficult decision of whether to use medical or surgical management for a disease. The consultant then provides, after evaluation of the patient record, a recommendation for therapy and perhaps the skills to perform the therapeutic intervention.

Like a physician consultant, the computer expert system generally is applied to specific problem areas in practice. The primary physician may select a special area of medicine (subsystem) for consultation. Unlike the use of a physician consultant, the primary physician inputs the findings into the computer. This may be in the form of input to a computer keyboard or via some intermediary technician. The output of the expert system suggests a diagnosis or therapeutic intervention. It is up to the primary physician to judge the validity of this information and accept, modify, or reject it. The computer is available 24 hours per day. It can be less expensive to the patient, but it cannot do procedures, and it should not, without physician review, order laboratory testing or therapy.

The usefulness of an expert system was demonstrated by deDombal and associates[14] with a system for diagnosing abdominal pain. During the study the proportion of perforated appendices prior to surgery fell from 36 to 4 per cent, and the negative laparatomy rate dropped from 24 to 6 per cent. Six months after the study (using a checklist and the computer model), the rate of perforated appendices preoperatively rose to 20 per cent, and the negative laparotomy rate also increased. Many other studies also illustrate similar benefits to patient care.

Physicians can supervise a technologist in the use of an expert system while freeing themselves for managing diagnosis, treatment, hospital discharge, and follow-up care. For example, a MRI scanner is operated by a technologist under the supervision of the radiologist. However, the technologist must consider requirements such as patient condition, required signal-to-noise ratios, anatomic location for the scan, and so on. The expert system can offer expertise to the technician for optimal scanning in minimal time constraints. The clinical pathologist supervises numerous technologists to obtain laboratory data. Using the expert system, the pathologist can integrate the clinical findings and laboratory data, providing vital information to primary physicians.

SYSTEMS BASED UPON OTHER APPROACHES

In the literature, a number of decision-making systems have been based upon decision trees, weighting algorithms, regression analysis, multivariate analysis, discriminant analysis, conventional nonparametric testing, counting rules, and others. These systems have specific applications, but also greater limitations than the above-described expert systems for the medical classification problem of diagnosis. Let us now explore some of the characteristics and limitations of these approaches.

Decision Tree. The paths in a decision tree are fixed. Probabilities through the paths cannot be computed. This approach is a rigid, non-interactive system. It does not provide for dependence among features. It cannot allow for complex paths to be followed. There can be a very large number of paths. For example:

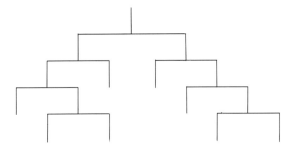

A decision tree generally is unsuited for use in an expert system because of the variability of disease presentations. Decision trees do have certain limited uses as production rules.

Weighting Algorithm. See previous discussion of algorithm approaches under Algorithm-Based Systems. A weighting algorithm does not allow for dependence among features. It is of limited usefulness in a classification system.

Regression Analysis. The standard formula for linear regression is

$$y = ax + b$$

The equation reflects the correlation between x and y. There are only two features (y and x). The feature values must be ordered (for example: 1, 2, 3, . . . , 10 or 10, 20, 30, . . . , 100). Events cannot be defined in a regression analysis. The mathematical model is linear.

Multiple regression is of the form

$$y = a_1x_1 + a_2x_2 + \ldots + b,$$

which measures the relationship between a particular dependent variable y and its multiple predictors. But y is restricted to being a linear combination of values of the predictors. It implies, for example, that as x_1 increases, then y also increases (if a_1 is positive), and likewise for x_2, and so on. Hard data can be used to estimate the parameters a_1, a_2, . . . b, but there is still the limitation of this linear model. Suppose that a_1, a_2, . . . actually depend on x_1, x_2, . . . in a complex way (perhaps in as many ways as there are combinations of x_1, x_2, . . .). We are perplexed about what model to propose if indeed there is a model. Systems that actually solve this problem are the Outcome Advisor and Consult Learning System. These systems store all the records and "wait" for the findings, x_1, x_2, ... Then they learn or estimate the probabilistic relationship between x_1, x_2, . . . for any y. There can even be more than one y (y_1, y_2, . . .).

Multivariate Analysis. Univariate analysis deals with one variable at a time. Multivariate analysis deals with many variables concurrently. It assumes a unimodal Gaussian probability density function. Experience has shown that most medical data are not unimodal. However, Gaussian constraints can be relaxed as the number of variables increases. Multivariate analysis measures the closeness of several findings about a patient to a category. The values of the features are assumed to be ordered. Its output includes (1) the variance of the categories and the events, and (2) the covariance between any pair of measurements in the data. It is cumbersome to interpret and therefore difficult to use for decision analysis compared to expert systems. In medicine, it has been useful for evaluating laboratory tests.

Discriminant Analysis. Ordinary discriminant analysis is a statistical procedure for maximizing the separation of two groups based on several measures. Multiple discriminant analysis is a procedure for maximizing separation of more than two groups on the basis of several measures. It is a form of multivariate analysis. The number of possible discriminant functions is one less than the number of categories (or variables), whichever is the lesser. It is rather difficult to interpret multiple discriminant analysis because one cannot be sure which discriminant functions apply. Hence, the usual restriction to two groups (categories).

Conventional Nonparametric Testing. Nonparametric testing would typically be used when conventional measurements are not available, (for example, when the data are nominal, such as eye color) or the data are only partially ordered. It can be applied to multiple categories and can also use ordered data. The limitations are that the tests of significance are usually not as sensitive to making discriminations as when parametric tests apply. This is in part due to the lack of rigorous error distribution functions for the nonparametric tests.

Counting Rules. A counting rule is a rigid classification technique with fixed numbers of events and categories. It is a form of nonparametric analysis. Weights are assigned to feature values, and these weights depend upon the category plus the findings. A decision is made by summing up the weights for each category, the highest sum being the category inferred. The counting rule does not take into account dependencies among features. It is rather inflexible.

KNOWLEDGE BASES

How Are Knowledge Bases Different From Data Bases?

Knowledge bases have been given many definitions, depending upon the viewpoint of the author. Knowledge from medical literature was extracted under the supervision of Bernstein and associates[6] for hepatitis. Although the hepatitis knowledge base was developed under consensus of a national panel of experts and provided a computer network, it was not designed for collecting patient records, computing probabilities, or direct interaction in an expert system.

In rule-based systems, knowledge consists of (1) the symbolic descriptions that characterize the definitional and empirical relationships in a domain and (2) the procedures for manipulating these descriptions.[21] In the Consult-I system, the knowledge base consists of features and feature values used to describe events (conditions and outcomes), including categories and subcategories. It includes the concept formation of categories not initially present or known. The system permits not only storage of category or subcategory presentations, but also deduction of new presentations never previously seen. Furthermore, this concept of a knowledge base implements higher order types of learning (see discussion on Learning Systems).

Systems that have been developed for gathering knowledge bases include SEEK (system for explanation with expert systems for the Expert system)[43] and Rx[9] for production rule expert systems. These systems

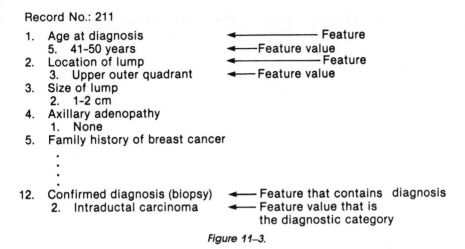

Figure 11-3.

analyze records looking for refinements for expert rules previously developed.

Consult Learning System and Outcome Advisor, previously described[30] can be used with production rule and statistical systems for updating the knowledge base or creating new knowledge.

In a conventional data base, the data are not organized for creating knowledge. A data base provides information, whereas a knowledge base provides not only information but organizes it to permit rapid access and the computation of inferences and classifications, and thus leads to the discovery of new knowledge.

The knowledge base for these systems is organized from records. It can be created by the organization and transformation of a data base. These records are systematically collected in an organized manner based upon the features, feature values, and categories. Records must be accurate. Quality control of records for any knowledge base is essential. This is costly, taking the time and commitment of collectors or supervisors. Once the records have been collected, the knowledge base allows the inferences of outcomes from conditions. An example record is shown in Figure 11-3.

Therefore, the knowledge base permits us to define logical combinations of feature values (pieces of knowledge) as conditions and logical combinations of feature values as outcomes. Logical combinations of events (conditions or outcomes) contain "ands" among features with "ors" between feature values. For example, in a breast lump knowledge base, after records of patients have been collected and stored, events could be defined as in Figure 11-4.

Condition: Age 30–39 OR 40–49 OR 50–60
                                        AND
                Lump in upper OR lower outer quadrant
                                        AND
                Positive family history of breast cancer
Outcome: Adenocarcinoma of the breast

Figure 11–4. Example of condition and outcome events in a knowledge base system.

The knowledge base will compute the probability of the outcome (adenocarcinoma) given the condition (age 30 to 60 years and lump in outer upper or lower quadrant *AND* positive family history of cancer). This illustrates a complex dependent relationship, one of a near limitless number of combinations of features that may be of interest to the practicing physician or researcher. Furthermore, this knowledge can be incorporated in an expert system in the form of a dependent probability.

Knowledge bases, separate from expert systems, can also be used for classification of multiple categories from hard data. That is, the user can pose a condition (simple or complex) and compute the a posteriori probabilities (probabilities after the fact) of all the potential categories under consideration. Figure 11–5 illustrates a knowledge base used for classification.

Using a closeness measure (how close the findings about a patient are to the records in the knowledge base), we can compute a classification even if records identical to the findings have never been seen before. In the Outcome Advisor or the Consult Learning System this is accomplished by a process using deduction, that is, proceeding from the general to the specific.

Benefits of a Knowledge Base

A knowledge base can provide the following benefits to practicing physicians:

Category	Probability of Category Given Findings (A Posteriori Probability)	Probability of Category (A Priori Probability)
1. Cancer 2. Fibrocystic breast disease 3. Fibroadenoma 4. Duct ectasia 5. Paget's disease		

Figure 11–5. Example of classification made from a knowledge base. The finding could be the condition in Figure 11–4. However, the probability is computed simultaneously for all categories in the differential diagnosis. This is Learning by Example (Patrick and Fattu, 1986), also known as "Induction Program" for converting data to knowledge (Hayes-Roth et al., 1983, p. 131).

1. An organization of the physician's knowledge of diseases in a medical area.

2. The ability to compare and collect records about patients for later retrieval.

3. The ability to make complex inferences about a new patient record based upon past experience. This can be useful for a medical practitioner trying to recall difficult cases or a medical researcher reviewing a cancer registry.

4. The ability to explore treatment outcomes. This will allow comparison of treatment outcomes for different disease presentations and selection of optimal treatment regimens.

5. A probability density histogram can be obtained for features. This is a display of the probability of feature values (signs, symptoms, history, laboratory tests, x-ray results) for given categories of disease. This has been particularly useful to pathologists for assessing the value of laboratory tests.

6. Multidimensional sensitivity and specificity of laboratory tests. That is, what is the sensitivity of two or more laboratory tests in combination for a disease?[7] Sensitivity is defined as the percentage of positive results of a test in patients with the disease. Specificity is defined as the percentage of negative results of a test among patients who do not have the disease. Multidimensional sensitivity and specificity may be extended to include signs, symptoms, and laboratory tests.[33]

7. The ability to synthesize hard data records into a useful form for training an expert system.

8. The learning of rules; that is, the relationships of diseases to findings and findings to findings.

How Can Physicians Create a Knowledge Base?

The creation of a knowledge base first requires the definition of the problem domain. A subsystem such as anemias may represent the problem area. The categories of disease must be defined. The taxonomy of disease and its degree of refinement should depend upon the purpose of the knowledge base. For example, an emergency chest pain subsystem may be concerned only with the presence or absence of chest pain due to coronary artery disease, while another research knowledge base may include pericarditis, myocardial infarction, angina pectoris, and chest wall pain. Once the problem domain and categories are defined, relevant features with their values must be selected. These features must be useful for defining the categories, the feature values must include reasonable ranges, the features must be collectable (extractable from records), and the features may require fuzzy sets (laboratory values such as increased, normal, borderline decreased, decreased, very decreased) rather than absolute values of the tests.

Several revisions of a feature list are often required for it to be useful. It is important to consider whether single or multiple site collection is proposed. An editorial board often is a preferred method for selecting the features and categories for a subsystem. The knowledge base of production rule systems is different. It consists of sets of rules about the subsystem composed of "if, then" clauses. These frequently are obtained by interviewing experts in a particular field.

Knowledge bases collected from patient records can provide much useful and needed information in medicine. However, the reliability and validity of records are essential. Reliability means *consistency* in observing whatever is measured or observed in a record. (In medicine we have referred to this as feature extraction.) Validity means the agreement of a panel of experts about the record among themselves and against individual physicians. Verification requires sufficient knowledge about the patient such that the diagnosis can be clearly distinguished from other disease categories. A "gold standard" must be maintained. In analyzing knowledge bases, we often discover new subcategories of diseases. We may, indeed, by such a process, be discovering new "gold standards."

What is a Learning System?

Learning is the process of acquiring knowledge or skill or the modification of behavior through training. Machine learning, such as used in Artificial Intelligence systems, takes several forms.[26, 30, 31] Two broad groups of learning are recognized: (1) learning with a teacher (supervised learning) and (2) learning without a teacher (unsupervised learning).

The first type of learning, learning with a teacher, uses records that are examples from known categories. In medicine, patient records with known diagnoses constitute an example of supervised learning. This type of learning is inductive learning, that is, it proceeds from examples to a trained system that can make inferences. This form of learning has been extensively studied in statistical pattern recognition.

A higher form of learning is learning without a teacher, or "learning by discovery," also known as unsupervised learning. Again, researchers in SPR have extensively studied this area since the 1960s. It is the learning of new categories or new subcategories of categories. A certain minimal amount of knowledge about the problem is required for this type of learning. Using it, we can take records and learn probabilities about categories where it is not known to which category a record pattern belongs. This has been called type 1 learning without a teacher.

A second form of unsupervised learning (type 2) allows us to generate what a complex class (two or more classes at the same time) would look like given patterns from only single diseases. For example, we may know what iron-deficiency anemia looks like alone, and what pernicious anemia looks like alone but we may not know what the two diseases look like when they appear together. A model of type 2 learning without a teacher would generate by deduction the complex class of these two diseases simultaneously without having seen them together before. Conventional artificial intelligence deals poorly with this concept.

A third type of learning without a teacher (type 3) is a process of learning how many and which features (characteristics about a disease) are correlated with other features for the findings about a patient. This is accomplished even if the findings are in an area where there is no previous training (feature values in previous records) for that particular disease. That is, the findings were never previously seen for the exact same disease category.

Systems that can learn by discovery are The Outcome Advisor and the Consult Learning System. These systems accept records of patients and help us to discover new knowledge, as described in the preceding concepts of learning. Learning systems will be essential for helping us update expert knowledge in expert systems. Learning systems, in themselves, can act as expert systems.[30]

A learning system is designed for collection of records in an organized manner for purposes of inference and classification. The training of a learning system is from individual patient records (hard data). An expert system is trained from the knowledge synthesized from many records, either from hard data or expert experience. The latter can take the form of a literature review or an expert who has considerable clinical experience. The weights provided to a production rule system from an expert represent such an example.

In a statistical system, the category conditional probabilities and a priori probabilities must be learned. These may be obtained from a learning system. Thus, a learning system can teach an expert system. For statistical systems, the knowledge from a learning system can be directly entered to the expert system. In a production rule system, the inferences can be tested on a body of records, and this probability can be entered as the weight or certainty of a production.

A learning system becomes an expert system when the records entered come from experts or literature review. That is, a single record would become the expert's knowledge. The knowledge of several experts thus could be entered into a learning system for evaluation. Another way of looking at this is that a learning system could become an expert system based solely on hard data records. That is, when the learning system is designed to be a classification system (with the ability to define categories, and then provide probabilities of each category for a set of findings), then the learning system can act as an expert system.

CONCLUSIONS

Since Ledley and Lusted[24] suggested the application of decision analysis to medicine, there have been many statements of an anticipated revolution in patient care. But in the 27 years since their paper, we have seen more evolution than revolution of systems. As yet, expert artificial intelligence (AI) systems for computer-aided diagnosis remain largely experimental.

If we explore the evolution of systems, initial approaches were largely statistical and based upon Bayes' theorem. Many assumptions were placed on the use of this formula, and they laid it open to criticism. Other methods explored included decision trees, algorithms, regression analysis, multivariate approaches, and discriminant analysis.[34, 39, 40] These reviews emphasized the problems of medical diagnosis and led us to evolve new approaches. In the mid 1960s and the 1970s, researchers in statistical pattern recognition (SPR), an outgrowth of communication theory and information theory, helped us to better understand Bayes' framework and closeness measures in the classification problem. Their goal was to develop optimal systems based on formal mathematical approaches.[30, 33, 35]

In the 1970s, another approach to medical diagnosis, based upon symbolic logic, led to the development of "rule-based" systems.[3, 21] A number of approaches in this area included those that equated AI only with systems that parallel human performance or thought, those that incorporate or relate to symbolic logic, and those that dealt with "brute force," not emphasizing theory or method.[42]

Much overlap and interaction between AI and SPR research has occurred.[11, 30] Both approaches, production rule and SPR, have professed to be "artificial intelligence." It would appear that there is no one definition of artificial intelligence.[8] Artificial intelligence, as it is currently perceived, applies to natural language processing, problem solving and planning, computer vision, robotics, and expert systems. Although all these applications apply to medicine, this chapter has been devoted only to the last—expert systems. Thus, if we look at the development of AI systems, we see a great deal of diversity of opinion about the definitions and goals of artificial intelligence in medicine (AIM).

The Present

At present, most expert systems remain experimental or investigational. The reader must be cautioned that in evaluating "state of the art" current expert systems, it is important to distinguish between what is predicted and what is available for practical use. Some systems appear to have gained usefulness. Examples include outgrowths of the Expert system for identification of serum protein electrophoresis patterns and for the treatment of herpes ocular diseases. Oncocin, an outgrowth of Mycin, is in use for treatment protocols of breast cancer and lymphoma. Puff is available for the interpretation of pulmonary function tests. Consult-I is in investigational use for the laboratory diagnosis of thyroid disorders and anemias. The Picker Expert System (an outgrowth of Consult-I and Consult Learning System) is integrated into the magnetic resonance imaging scanner for collection of knowledge bases and development of expert systems for the radiology imaging department. Caduceus for internal medicine remains experimental.

The present is faced more with issues to be dealt with in expert systems. Hayes-Roth[21] suggested that current issues include (1) the need for objective standards of excellence, (2) concerns regarding biasing and blinding of testing, (3) the elimination of irrelevant variables, (4) the definition of realistic standards of performance, (5) the need for sensitivity analysis, (6) the problems of confounding interactions among knowlege sources, and (7) the need for realistic time demands on evaluators. To this list we must add criteria for completeness of systems. That is, when is a system reliable and useful such that it can be placed at multiple sites with confidence?

The Future

Present systems have formed the base for future growth of expert systems. Statistical systems can offer us optimal decision rules. Artificial intelligence approaches can help us to overcome the combinatorial explosion of knowledge necessary for statistical systems by imposing prior knowledge on the training of systems. It is anticipated that a solution to improved expert systems in the future will involve the integration of artificial intelligence rules with statistical pattern recognition.[30] In the future, we will see the development of new inference operations, which will be implemented to better handle complex classes (multiple diseases present in the same patient simultaneously), dependencies among medical data, and the interconnection of multiple subsystems of medicine. Confidence measures in the inferences of expert systems will be further developed.

The generalizability of systems will be refined. Early systems, particularly production rule systems, were "hard wired" (rules were programmed for the system). More recent production systems, such as Emycin and Expert, allow insertion of rules in the generalized structure. Consult-I is a generalized system that allows both insertion of statistical data as well as production rule–like training.

Expert systems may become important in the medicolegal arena. A record of the findings about a patient, obtained by the physician, will be processed with the considered differential diagnoses. In this way, the physician will be able to document both the patient findings (history and physical, laboratory tests, x-ray) along with the differential diagnoses considered. The physician can then show actions for further evaluation in the form of the work-up. Any such use of this procedure at this time, however, is investigational.

Expert systems will be used for trouble shooting of medical equipment, as has been suggested for the Picker Expert System in magnetic resonance imaging. Simulation systems for training of radiology or laboratory technicians, medical students, and physicians in training will further evolve by using expert systems.

Expert Systems Derived from Knowledge Bases

Learning systems will be formed, based upon editorial boards who establish the structure of knowledge collection as well as evaluate the quality of knowledge (records) collected. These collection sites will be interconnected into networks of knowledge bases. Editorial boards will review results of knowledge base collection in order to identify the most sensitive and specific features and categories for medical diagnosis.

Learning systems based on records will be used to perform the following:

1. Understand the distribution of normal feature values compared to those for disease.

2. Predict the next best test or the most sensitive tests, laboratory analysis, or x-ray. Multidimensional sensitivity and specificity of tests will assist in learning the next best and least expensive combination of tests to obtain a diagnosis. It will allow us to develop complex diagnostic protocols that dynamically change as information is obtained about a patient. These can be integrated into the expert systems of the future.

3. Predict the best treatment for a patient.

4. Predict length of stay based on complex combinations of patient disease, severity of illness, treatment, past medical history, and laboratory tests.

5. Predict patients who are at high risk on presentation to emergency rooms.

6. Predict minimum cost (financial and morbidity) of screening tests.

7. Assist in quality assurance.

8. Select the most sensitive features for expert systems.

9. Learn knowledge for expert system training.

10. Create histograms of knowledge about findings and laboratory tests for diseases. A histogram presents the values for each feature for each disease based upon patient records. It has been found valuable, for

example, in clinical pathology in understanding the use of laboratory tests.

11. Provide basic consultation about diseases for conventional forms of learning. That is, the knowledge from learning systems can be converted to conventional texts of medicine.

Like prototypes such as Bionet, a national computer system for molecular biologists, learning systems will collect and disseminate medical knowledge for researchers and practitioners. Although prototype learning systems, such as the Hepatitis Knowledge Base,[6] show the technique for editorial board review for development of a knowledge base, those of the future will be organized with features, features values, and categories such that probabilistic information on records can be obtained.

Although expert systems of the present largely depend on literature and expert physician training, those of the future will be updated if not created from hard data knowledge bases.

REFERENCES

1. American Board of Internal Medicine: Clinical competence in internal medicine. Ann. Int. Med. *90*:402–411, 1979.
2. Asselain, B., Derouesne, C., Salamon, et al.: The concept of utility in medical decision aid: Example of an application, MEDINFO 77, Proceedings of the Second World Conference on Medical Informatics, Amsterdam, North Holland Puslishing Co., 1977.
3. Barr, A., Feigenbaum, E.: The Handbook of Artificial Intelligence, Vol. 2, Wm. Kaufmann, Inc., Los Altos, CA, 1982.
4. Bayes, T.: An essay toward solving a problem in the doctrine of chance. Philos. Trans. R. Soc., *53*:370, 1763.
5. Ben-Bassat, M.: Expert systems for diagnostic support. Proc. AAMSI Congress *83*, p. 69, 1983.
6. Bernstein, L. M., Siegel, E. R., Goldstein, C. M.: The hepatitis knowledge base. A prototype information transfer system. Ann. Intern. Med., *93*:165—222, 1980.
7. Blomberg, D. J., Fattu, J. M., and Patrick, E. A.: Learning sensitivity and specificity of laboratory diagnosis of thyroid disorders using Consult Learning System—An example of euthyroid sick syndrome. Proc. Eighth Symposium on Computer Applications in Medical Care, I.E.E.E., pp 35–40, 1984.
8. Blum, B.I.: Why AI? Proc. Eighth Symposium on Computer Applications in Medical Care, I.E.E.E., pp 3–9, 1984.
9. Blum, R.L.: Discovery, confirmation, and incorporation of causal relationships from a large time-oriented clinical data base: The RX project. Computers Biomed. Res. *15*:164–187, 1982.
10. Card, W. I., Good, I. J.: The estimation of the implicit utilities of medical consultants. Math. Biosci. *6*:37–44, 1970.
11. Chen, C. H.: Pattern Recognition and Artificial Intelligence Proceedings of the Joint Workshop on Pattern Recognition and Artificial Intelligence, held at Hyannis, Mass., June 1 to 3, 1976. New York, Academic Press, Inc., 1976.
12. Davis, R., Buchanan B., Shortliffe, E.: Production rules as a representation for a knowledge-based consultation program. Artificial Intelligence *8*:15–45, 1977.
13. deDombal, F. T.: How "objective" is medical data? In deDombal, F. T., and Gremy F. (eds.): Decision Making and Medical Care. North-Holland Publishing Co., 1976, pp. 33–37.
14. deDombal, F. T., Leaper, D. F., Horrocks, J. C., et al.: Human and computer-aided

diagnosis of abdominal pain: Further report with emphasis on performance of clinicians. Br. Med. J. *1*:376–380, 1974.

15. Diamond, G., and Forrester, J.: Analysis of probability as an aid in the clinical diagnosis of coronary artery disease. N. Engl. J. Med. *300*:1350–1358, 1979.

16. Fattu, J. M., and Patrick, E. A.: Training CONSULT-I as an expert system. Proc. AAMSI Congress 83, pp 102–106, 1983.

17. Fattu, J. M., and Patrick, E. A.: Application of a new theorem of a posteriori probabilities of events to medical diagnosis. Proc. Seventh Symposium on Computer Applications in Medical Care, I.E.E.E., pp 844–847, 1983.

18. Feigenbaum, E. A.: The art of artificial intelligence: Themes and case studies of knowledge engineering. Proc. International Joint Conference on Artificial Intelligence, pp. 1014–1029, 1977.

19. Greenes, R. A.: A goal-directed model for investigation of thresholds for medical action. Proc. Third Symposium on Computer Applications in Medical Care, I.E.E.E., pp. 47–51, 1979.

20. Habbema, J. D. F., and Hilden, J.: The measurement of performance in probabilistic diagnosis—IV. Utility considerations in therapeutics and prognostics. Meth. Inform. Med. 20:80–96, 1981.

21. Hayes-Roth, F., Waterman, D. A., and Lenat, D. B.: Building Expert Systems. Reading, MA, Addison-Wesley Publishing Co., 1983.

22. Kastner, J. K., Weiss, S. M., Kulikowski, C. A., et al.: Therapy selection in an expert medical consultation system for ocular herpes simplex. Comput. Biol. Med., *14*:285-301, 1984.

23. Kulikowski, C. A., and Weiss, S.: Representation of expert knowledge for consultation: The CASNET and EXPERT projects. *In* Szolovits, P. (ed.): *In* Artificial Intelligence in Medicine. AAAS Selected Symposium 51, Boulder, Colorado, Westview Press, 1982, pp. 21–55.

24. Ledley, R. S., and Lusted, L. B.: Reasoning foundations of medical diagnosis. Science *130*:9–21, 1959.

25. McDonald, C. J.: Protocol-based computer reminders; the quality of care and the non-perfectability of man. N. Engl. J. Med. *295*:1351–1355, 1976.

26. Michalski, R. S., Carbonell, J. G., and Mitchell, T. M. (eds.): Machine Learning: An Artificial Intelligence Approach. Palo Alto, Tioga Publ. Co., 1983.

27. Miller, R. A., Pople, H. E., and Myers, J. D.: Internist-I: An experimental computer-based diagnostic consultant for general medicine. N. Engl. J. Med. *307*:468, 1982.

28. Myers, J., Pople, H., and Miller, R.: Internist: Can artificial intelligence help? *In* Connelly, et al. (eds.): Clinical Decisions and Laboratory Use. Minneapolis, University of Minnesota Press, 1982, pp. 251–269.

29. Nilsson, N. J.: Principles of Artificial Intelligence, Palo Alto, Tioga Publishing Co., 1980.

30. Patrick, E. A., Fattu, J. M.: Artificial Intelligence with Statistical Pattern Recognition, Englewood Cliffs, Prentice-Hall, Inc., 1986.

31. Patrick, E. A., Fattu, J. M.: Mutually exclusive categories statistically dependent during concept formulation. Proc. Eight Symposium on Computer Applications in Medical Care, I.E.E.E., pp. 100–106, 1984.

32. Patrick, E. A.: A Theorem of a posteriori probabilities of events. *In* van Bemmel, J. H., Ball, M. J. and Wigertz, O. (eds.): MEDINFO 83, Proceedings of the Fourth World Conference on Medical Informatics, Amsterdam, North Holland Publishing Co., 1983, pp. 454–456.

33. Patrick, E. A.: Decision Analysis in Medicine: Methods and Applications. Boca Raton, CRC Press, 1979.

34. Patrick, E. A., Stelmack, F. P., and Shen, L. Y. L.: Review of pattern recognition in medical diagnosis and review of consulting relative to a new system model. I.E.E.E. Trans. Syst. Man Cybern. SMC 4:1–16, 1974.

35. Patrick, E. A.: Fundamentals of Pattern Recognition, Englewood Cliffs, N.J., Prentice-Hall, Inc., 1972.

36. Pople, H. E.: Heuristic methods for imposing structure on ill-structured problems: The structure of medical diagnosis. *In* Szolovits, P. (ed.): Artificial Intelligence in Medicine, AAAS Symposium 51. Boulder, Colorado, Westview Press, 1982.

37. Shortliffe, E. H.: Computer-Based Medical Consultation, Mycin. Amsterdam, Elsevier Scientific Pub. Co., 1976.
38. Shortliffe, E. H., Scott, A., Bischoff, M., et al.: ONCOCIN: An expert system for oncology protocol management. Proc. International Joint Conference on Artificial Intelligence, pp. 876–881, 1981.
39. Wagner, G., Tautu, P., and Wolber, U.: Problems of medical diagnosis—A bibliography. Meth. Inform. Med. 17:55–74, 1978.
40. Wardle, A., and Wardle, L.: Computer aided diagnosis—A review of research. Meth. Inform. Med. 17:15–28, 1978.
41. Warner, H.: Computer-Assisted Medical Decision-Making. New York, 1979.
42. Weiss, E. A.: The fifth generation: Banzai or pie-in-the sky? Abacus, 1,2:56–65, 1984.
43. Weiss, S. M., and Kulikowski, C. A.: A Practical Guide to Designing Expert Systems. Totowa, N.J., Rowman & Allanheld, 1984.
44. Zadah, L. A.: A theory of approximate reasoning. In Hayes, J. E., Michie, D., and Mikulick, L. I. (eds.): Machine Intelligence 9. New York, Wiley, 1979, pp. 149–194.
45. Gangorose, R., Patrick, E. A., and Fattu, J. M.: Magnetic resonance imaging scan setup and scheduling using artificial intelligence. Radiology 157:321, 1985.

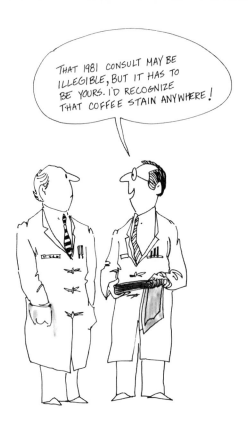

TWELVE

Computerized Medical Records

Frederick R. Jelovsek, M.D.

William W. Stead, M.D.

CAN COMPUTERIZED MEDICAL RECORDS IMPROVE PATIENT CARE?

You are familiar with the thick folders containing a patient's hospital record. Even some office medical records can be bulky for patients who have chronic problems. If all of a patient's medical facts were in one location, the chart could exceed a set of encyclopedias in size. Most people, however, have their medical records scattered throughout different institutions, offices, and geographic locations. What we gain from a compact disseminated medical record, we lose in access to pertinent medical facts that patients themselves do not remember or have not ever been aware of.

Even when we are fortunate to have the thick, encompassing medical chart, its lack of index and instant summary discourages us from reading it as thoroughly as we should. Knowing the computer's forte of search and retrieval at electronic speeds, a major benefit of computerization, in theory at least, should be to provide an easy-to-use index for quick retrieval of pertinent medical facts. This is important, for the record may contain *hard* data, such as biopsy reports, as well as *soft* data such as follow-up letters.

Another benefit might be to have the computer constantly analyze and abstract medical data so that at the push of a button, a physician could view a summary of the patient's medical history containing a one-page summary (or one video display terminal [VDT] screen) of past medical events which might influence a patient's health management today (Figure 12–1). Automatic data abstraction, however, is only the first step. Important data varies with each new treatment prescribed, finding elicited, and laboratory result received. One needs the search and logic capability of a computer to examine each possible combination of medical data elements and report all possible conflicts or interactions. At the same time, display of that data should be focused independently of the algorithms that check for interaction. Rules governing data relationships are likely to change, but the data itself will not.

Finally, a computer should help analyze and display data to illustrate physiologic trends and comparative health status with other patients. In other words, it should be able to take data and produce "information" about one or more patients. This is the quickest route to the best patient care possible.

Can computerizing a patient's medical record really produce such benefits? Yes, different software programs have been written to perform all these functions to varying degrees. Does any one software package have enough of these features to be practical and still improve patient care? Yes, several do. How much more development is needed to maximize the benefits of improved patient care which is attainable by computerizing medical records? A lot!

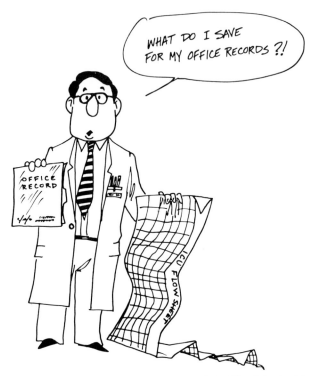

Figure 12–1. Medical data reduction and abstraction. It is difficult to decide which data is important to save if the patient has had an intensive hospital course resulting in numerous studies and laboratory values. Computerization of records permits storage of all data and abstraction or display of data subsets on demand.

There are still critical questions which are unanswered:

1. Should you supplement or replace the manual chart?
2. What data are important?
3. Should word processing data storage be used, or should the data be encoded?
4. How should the data be organized?
5. What report formats are necessary?
6. Should the user interact with a VDT or paper printout?
7. Should the physician capture data directly from the patient?

Not only are these questions unresolved at the present time, but it is likely that eventual answers will vary, depending upon the type of medical practice and resources available.

Table 12–1. Direct Benefits of Medical Record Computerization

- An automatic index by time, diagnosis, medication, procedure, and study result
- An automatic summary of important past and current medical history
- Reminders about possible conflicts in therapy or scheduled tasks
- Transformation of data to produce new insights into a patient's health
- Legible, available records
- Multiple display formats

BENEFITS OF COMPUTERIZED MEDICAL RECORDS

Before we struggle with critical issues, let us look in more detail at the potential benefits of computerized records (Table 12–1).

Indexing

Handwritten or typed medical charts never come with a table of contents or an index. Medical data is gathered in chronological order, and each word must be read to find specific occurrences of a diagnosis, for example. Actually, to index the record, we wouldn't even have to codify each data element. In a computerized medical record, we could merely collect and store the narrative document produced at a physician's visit in a "word processed" file. If we did this, however, and later wanted to find the occurrence of "diabetes," we would have to ask the computer to find all instances of letters that match the following:

DIABETES
diabetes
Diabetes
Diabetes Mellitus
D.M.
DM
D M
D. M.
abnormal carbohydrate metabolism

Computers need to be given all the rules about capitalization, punctuation, abbreviations, synonyms, idioms, and so on. The very nature of computerization—defining each element that is entered—provides the indexing feature as a by-product. An index is nothing more than the name and the electronic location of a topic (variable), and these must be fully defined in order to be stored electronically in the first place.

If *diabetes* is codified at the time of initial data entry, the retrieval process is made much easier; without codification, there are problems not only with synonyms but also with abbreviations, shorthand, misspellings, and inappropriate terminology. Thus, in order to achieve the indexing benefit of a computerized medical record, one must define tables (or dictionaries) of all the possible diagnoses, procedures, therapies, subjective features (symptoms), and physical findings (signs), and so forth. In addition to defining elements, some form of data organization must be superimposed. With medical records, this usually is the date and time of occurrence.

In the early days of organizing records, actual structure of the code was important because data analysis was performed by simple sorting and counting programs. Today's software has powerful text processing and subgrouping capabilities that can analyze virtually any data situation. The remaining sole function of coding is standardization of meaning and efficiency in storage. Moreover, it is desirable with today's software that code sets governing storage should be as uninterrupted as possible. Codes should not have meaning embedded within their structure because interpretive meanings change. If the interpretation is embedded in stored data, there is no way to recover the original data. Rather, assessment should be applied at the time of report generation so that all old data can be validly interpreted by new rules. For example, the presence of retinal hemorrhages and exudate should be stored as such, not as class 3 retinopathy. One should store the exact findings of cancer spread, rather than a diagnosis of stage II, because next year it is possible that stage II will be reclassified or divided into substages A and B. The original extent of a disease must be recorded more explicitly than by a staging diagnosis, or it will not be possible to retrospectively determine a patient's prognosis by current concepts.

Highlighting Important Medical Data

Computers can retrieve and emphasize pertinent data elements.[9] This capability, however, is more a task in defining what is wanted rather than difficulty in programming the software. If the patient is pregnant, a history of a stillborn infant is essential in any medical summary, but if the patient is being seen by an ophthalmologist for a 'cataract, the reproductive history would be inappropriate for an instant, highlighted computer summary. Some elements are universally important (such as allergies), but most depend upon specific data values.

In the manual record, certain structures currently fulfill the role of highlighting. The problem list, a relatively new introduction to medical records,[14] prevents overlooking prior abnormalities and provides a total health picture of the patient so that current complaints can be evaluated in context. As a *highlight*, it avoids the tendency to prescribe a treatment for each of a patient's problems without reviewing the total therapeutic program. In one study,[13] patients on hemodialysis were found to be

```
999-99-9911 PATIENT, VERY SICK

NO.  ONSET  RESOLVED       PROBLEM LIST

  1. ??/??/??              HYPERTENSION-DIASTOLIC
  2. 05/21/80-06/20/80     RECURRENT HYPERTENSTION-MALIGNANT
  3. 11/??/77                RENAL INSUFFICIENCY
  4. 07/14/80-07/20/80     DRUG EFFECT - ? HCTZ
  5. 07/14/80-07/20/80       HYPONATREMIA
  6. 03/??/79                HEART FAILURE
  7. 04/??/80-05-20-80     THROMBOPHLEBITIS
  8. 01/12/81-01-30-81     FRACTURE - L WRIST
  9. ??/??/??              FAMILY HX - HBP,DM
```

```
999-99-9912 PATIENT, VERY SICK

NO.  ONSET  RESOLVED       PROBLEM LIST

  1 01/12/81-01/30/81      FRACTURE - L RADIUS-SIMPLE
  2 04/??/80-05/20/80      THROMBOPHLEBITIS
  3 ??/??/??               HIGH BLOOD PRESSURE
  4 11/??/77               RENAL INSUFFICIENCY
  5 03/??/79               HEART FAILURE
```

Figure 12–2. Problem lists by different specialty physicians. A, The nephrologist's problem list, containing a detailed classification of hypertension and mention of fracture. B, The orthopedists' problem list on the same patient containing more detail on the fracture and listing certain diagnoses as separate entities rather than as secondary to hypertension. The computer as a diagnostic tool should permit these differences in practice patterns and not force providers to use models designed for others.

taking up to 16 different medicines; a computer listing of these medications forced physicians to carefully choose which medications to continue because most patients could not realistically follow such a complicated schedule. After computerization, many patients had drug regimens reduced by almost 50 per cent. Highlighting pending laboratory results reduced duplicate laboratory study orders.

Time-oriented data prevents overlooking health trends that have not yet reached abnormal limits, and encounter-orienting data shows the logic of what was done on a given day. If data are arranged according to problem, all the supporting evidence for a diagnosis is together. Many times these structures are placed at the front or back of a manual chart, disrupting the original chronological order of a medical record. Computerization should produce highlighting on demand without the worry that some chronologic data have been overlooked.

The rules to create highlighted medical summaries have not yet been well identified in any medical record system, computerized or not. The on-line, interactive problem list that a nephrologist creates will always have a different content and format than the one produced by an

```
VISITS:   87 (7):   86 (10):   85 (9)
-----------------------------VISIT PROFILE -------------------------------------
                           YEAR:   <---------87---------><-----86------>
                           MONTH:  10  7  6  5  3  2   1 12 11 11 11 10
CODE           PROBLEM     DAY:    23  6  6 15 15 23 21  3 26 24 19 23
--------------------------------------------------------------------------------
6221  VAGINITIS NOS                        33    33 33    33
 401  HYPERTENSION,UNCOMPLICATED           33             33 33 33 33
 460  ACUTE URI                               29       33
 461  SINUSITIS                                            33
 Y70  TESTS                                                            33
--------------------------------------------------------------------------------
      TYLENOL 3                                    *
      HYDRODIURIL                                                         *
```

Figure 12–3. Time series of medical events. A visit profile with the most recent encounters at the left showing the dates of diagnosis and treatment as well as the provider (number) who saw the patient.

orthopedist seeing the same patient. The best feature that computerized medical records currently provide is to allow the physician to construct his or her own summary (Fig. 12–2) and secondly, to display routinely all recent visits with corresponding diagnoses and laboratory results.[3] It is this most recent series of events that is likely to contain the highest proportion of important medical data (Fig. 12–3).

Computer Reminders

Using computers to constantly analyze data and raise red flags according to preset rules may be one of the greatest impacts this technology will have on patient care.[7] Unfortunately, our minds are not perfect at remembering every possible drug-drug, disease-drug and drug-laboratory study interaction. Not only do we forget some of these relationships, but often we fail to learn about them in the first place. Computers can serve as alarm clocks and flag raisers if we give them the rules by which to function.[8, 10] In order to benefit from the identification of possible drug-drug interactions one must not only record the prescriptions written for the patient but also record the names and doses of any other medications the patient is taking, both prescription and over-the-counter drugs. This is often more of a logistics problem than one of computerization. Some current computerized medical record systems provide for flagging these interactions if one defines which medications they apply to (Fig. 12–4). Comprehensive pharmacy systems will often include an electronic form of interaction flags, but even recent textbooks on drug interactions are not specialty-specific nor fully up to date because this is a constantly evolving knowledge area.

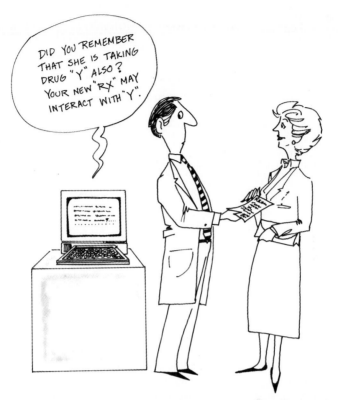

Figure 12–4. Drug interaction warmup. A major advantage of computerization is the ability to program into the computer reminders about drug interrelationships that may not be appreciated at the time of the patient's visit.

In addition to reminders about adverse interactions, preventative health maintenance, including immunizations, can also be scheduled to remind the physician. This may range from a simple time schedule such as *date of next tetanus shot is one year from today* to more complicated logic such as *if rheumatic heart disease is present, and if any surgical procedure is scheduled, if not currently on prophylactic antibiotics, then flag prophylactic antibiotic warning.*

Prospective data collection can also benefit from a computer's reminder algorithms. If a group of physicians want to conduct clinical research, the computer can prompt for findings and add to already gathered patient data, assuming that the Computerized Medical Record (CMR) software has the feature to allow nonprogrammers to define new data elements.

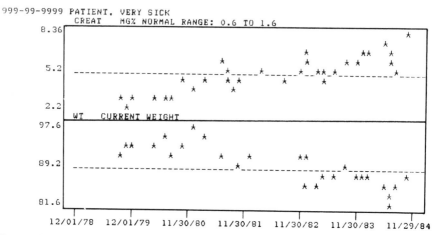

Figure 12–5. Patient data display. Serum creatinine concentration rises with an increase in production, an increase in muscle mass, or a decrease in clearance from impaired glomerular filtration rate secondary to renal disease. This graph of a patient's increase in serum creatinine level with a simultaneous linear decrease in weight illustrates how the renal disease is progressively worsening.

Data Transformed to Information

The medical record is basically a time series of data, but because it is so tedious to find and plot each data element on graphs, patients hardly ever benefit from their own data being examined in relation to their own personal norm. For many years we have known that patients should serve as controls unto themselves. Computerization can permit new insights into how a patient's health status is progressing. A major improvement in health care can take place just by the graphic display of a patient's own data (Fig. 12–5). If physicians add to this the comparison of that patient to similar patients in their own practice settings, physicians can be much more certain about a patient's health status because they don't have to rely only upon textbooks or journal articles about patients who may not be the same as theirs.

If all patients in a physician's practice have computerized medical records, that physician gains from the ability to assess areas of personal experience, determining complication rates and successes with various diseases. Recollection of our experience is often very different from our actual experience, and yet, we behave according to what we think our experience has been.

SIMPLE DATA BASES VERSUS THE COMPUTERIZED MEDICAL RECORD

Whether academic and research-oriented or in practice and patient care–oriented, most physicians will at some time want to follow a specific

Table 12–2. *Differences Between Simple Files for Clinical Research versus an Entire Medical Data Base for Patient Care*

Item	Simple Files	Medical Data Base
Nonmedical data	Minimal or absent	Moderate amount of administrative data
Data structure	Different, unique variables	Similar variables (arrays) linked by time
Number of parameters	Limited choices	Multiple branching variables, lists
Parameter type	Transformed variables	Original variables

type of patient in detail. We may want to record comprehensive data, looking for new discoveries in the disease process. We all have the clinical research fever somewhere within us. To accomplish this, we design data sheets containing a dozen to several thousand variables and then computerize the forms, looking forward to the time when all data has been entered so we can "play" with it. This process has gone on for decades, and 90 per cent of medical journal articles present the results of analyzing these simple data bases.

How do simple data bases differ from a fully computerized medical record? Table 12–2 itemizes some general differences. Simple data bases contain minimal amounts of administrative data, but medical records for patient care must include extensive documentation.[6] For a small research project one might be interested in a laboratory test only if there is a result for it. In a medical record one will want to record the fact that the test was ordered (as a separate data element from the result itself) to have a reminder to seek out the result should its value not be returned in a timely fashion. The next scheduled appointment, type of insurance coverage the patient has, or the next of kin are all administrative elements that are needed in the medical record for patient care but would not be put in a simple research data base.

The style and structure of the data elements themselves will vary between simple data bases and computerized medical record systems. In a specific study, two elements might be defined, indicating pretreatment and post-treatment lesion size, but in a medical record one element, lesion size, is recorded, along with a date and time. The reason for this is the knowledge that many more occurrences of this finding are likely. It is more manageable to have one variable recorded in a time series than it is to have multiple identifiers such as lesion size pretreatment, lesion size post-treatment, lesion size at third visit, and so on.

The style or type of variables will also vary between original data elements and transformed data elements. In a medical record one would normally record the birth date and use the present date to calculate age, but in a simple data base one would only record age, assuming that age change over the course of the study is not likely to influence the findings. In a medical record one would be more likely to record the time of labor onset, delivery, and placental expulsion because these events may need to be related to other timed events such as fetal distress. In a simple study data base, you would likely transform the data and record only length of first stage of labor, length of second stage of labor, and presence or absence of fetal distress.

Another difference between a simple data base and a fully computerized medical record has to do with the vast numbers of possible values a variable can take. For a small research project, the presence of hypertension (yes or no), diuretic use (yes or no), and major complications (yes or no) might be sufficient to answer the questions that a simple data base is designed for. For patient care, however, actual diagnoses or treatments are needed; it is better to create a long list of possible diagnoses, the categories of *diagnosis one, diagnosis two, diagnosis three*, allowing them to take on any one of 300 to 500 different values, rather than having 300 to 500 variables with a potential yes/no result.

Finally, a major difference between simple data bases and computerized medical records stems from the multiple branching nature of medicine. In continuing patient care, a finding may elicit a whole new set of data elements, which must be recorded to clarify appropriate health management. Most simple data bases are designed to collect a fixed set of data on all patients and cannot handle the changing number of collected variables (and thus length of the record), but this is mandatory for patient care. Therefore, variable-length formatted records are more necessary for medicine than they would be for the banking industry, for instance.

WHAT GOES INTO THE MEDICAL RECORD?

As we gather many different data elements for the computerized medical record, we know we will want to tie those elements to the time, location, and source of data collection. Are there groupings of data elements that will have similar structure for collection and display? If there are, we should create those groupings with similar characteristics so that one software subroutine can be applied to that entire group. Otherwise, computer programmers would have to write a different set of instructions to handle each of the thousands of possible variables we might choose to collect. We could be naive enough to think that each element has basically a name and a value, and therefore, one data entry routine would handle all possible choices; but in practice, there are groupings of data variables having such similar attributes and being different from the other groups whose classification can benefit software design.

Diagnoses do not usually require range checking for upper and lower numerical limits as do many laboratory tests, but they do require a designation as to whether they are acute or chronic, whether the problem is temporary or permanent and which diagnosis-related group (DRG) they belong to. Medications have a value (dose) and a type (capsule, injection), like laboratory studies (serum, urine), but they also have a number dispensed, a frequency administration, and refill designation. Procedures don't usually have results, just a record of their occurrence, or if they do have results, it is textual in nature and not easily coded, as are laboratory results. Procedures are often linked with consumption of supplies (intravenous trays, intravenous solutions, clean-catch urine "prep" trays) and don't require association with a dose or a permanent versus temporary status. Supplies (but not devices) are important administratively but lose medical significance quickly and need not be carried in the data base for long. Diagnoses and subjective and physical findings are not billable items, as are studies, therapies, and procedures, and thus do not need the whole financial processing overhead as do potentially billable items.

What, then, are the generic categories of medical data elements? If we use the medical management model in Figure 12–6, we can see that the computerized medical record architecture must be able to accommodate subjective findings (patient history, symptoms), physical findings (signs), and study results all in a very iterative process and then, subsequently, procedural and medical therapies administered, a diagnostic assessment of the entire process, and comments. If we assign a date and time, place of occurrence, and provider (source) with each array of data elements, we have a systematic method of recording a patient's medical history in an electronic form.

Are there other generic relationships among medical data categories? Yes, several relationships that are common, especially ones that are more managerial than medically important. Most medical data groups need pointers (indexes) to administrative reporting categories. For some reports concerning diagnoses, you might want to look at DRGs all cancer, all infectious disease, or all hypertension-related diagnoses. You might want to report by ICD-9-CM codes, ICHPPC, or SNOMED codes. Procedures might need to be reported by class (surgical, physical therapy, diagnostic) or code (ICD-9-CM, CPT). Thus all the atomic elements that are important for patient care have different reporting categories in which the possibilities are limited only by imagination and bureaucracy.

Another generic relationship that is administratively important is *association*. The individual test components of laboratory panels, the physical findings to be followed for disease X, the known medications that can produce spurious results in this laboratory test, or other diseases that can be manifestations of this diagnosis are a few of the hierarchical (one to many, many to one) relationships present in the medical record.

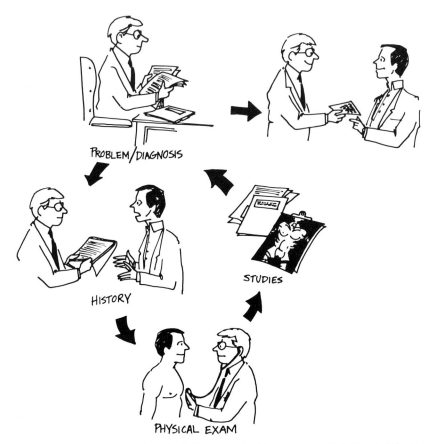

Figure 12–6. Medical record content. The period of the content of medical data spans from birth to death. At each encounter, the physician uses an iterative process that includes problem definition, history and physical exam, and further diagnostic studies until a plan of treatment (or nontreatment) is formulated. At each visit this process is repeated. The medical record is a permanent repository for all these findings, assessments, therapies, and comments.

Those relationships must be superimposed or *linked* in order for us to go beyond a mere duplication of the manual medical record in electronic form.

In spite of inherent classification and relationships, *noise* frequently accompanies medical data. Should data be stored just because it is available? If a plasma glucose sample is drawn from a vein with intravenous dextrose running in, and it measures 300 mg per 100 ml, should the result be discarded or stored and flagged as erroneous. Should normal laboratory ranges be stored along with the result in order to handle the problem of changing analytical techniques? What are the electronic rules by which data entry errors are flagged so that they do not continue to display in highlighted scenarios or time series graphs, while still being retained for medicolegal purposes? These and many other questions remain to be answered, although the lack of answers should not prevent utilization of electronic records.

HOW ARE DATA ENTERED INTO THE MEDICAL RECORD?

The logistics of collecting complete, accurate medical data are often much more difficult a task than the design of the computer system. Actually information flow logistics and design of a computerized medical record are very interrelated.[4] The appearance or position of a variable on a data sheet can influence its missing data rate. Agreement or perception as important will improve an element's chance of being collected, although the complicated, nonroutine patient is likely to have a higher percentage of data go unrecorded.

Data entry for a simple data base system can often take place efficiently by having a clerical assistant enter data sheet elements the evening or day after the form is completed. A computerized record for patient care, however, has the most potential benefit if data entry is performed in close proximity to time of data collection. In order to warn of a drug-drug interaction or questionable allergy, it would not be as useful for a red flag to wave two days after the physician saw the patient and wrote the prescription; the reminder for a pneumococcus vaccination does little good when the physican has just seen the patient and told her to return in 6 months.

To improve patient care significantly, the computerized medical record should exist as a "real-time" system, with data entry occurring while the patient is being seen, not as a batch system with data entry occurring after the fact. Numerous advantages affordable by computerization are lost if patient data is not entered in real time.[5] Benefits that ensue from data collection in the patient's presence include the following:

1. Improved data quality including completeness, accuracy, timeliness, and pertinency to the patient's problems.

2. Less volume of clerical work performing repetitive transcriptions, manual report collation, and the manual control process for verifying transaction recording.

3. Financial benefits due to fewer missed charges and improved cash flow of receipts.

These benefits can be lost, however, if software design or hardware performance adversely affects patient flow or provider data collection behavior. Patients will not wait in line at an office check-out while an assistant takes 15 minutes to enter 30 data elements, nor should system design require five different screens to enter data from one office visit. It must not take 60 seconds to retrieve a patient's appointment record when the patient is calling long distance, and it must be easy to update mailing addresses or enter insurance information, for these are frequently occurring demographic changes.

After spending 1 hour with a patient who has a complicated problem, it is reasonable to spend five minutes in interactive data entry to ensure medical accuracy. If the physician or nurse sees patients for a 5-minute weight and blood pressure check, it is not reasonable to ask them to double their visit time in order to enter medical data. Entering batches of laboratory results just sent from the laboratory on many patients should be as easy as entering an individual result on a single patient. Data flow logistics have higher priority in system design than most people would suspect.

Physician habits can also have a major impact on how data get to the record. One experience with computerized medical records illustrates the interface between unstructured recording habits and the requirements superimposed by computerization.[11] After the computerized record had been in place for 10 months, the physician's staff using the new system met to solve difficulties they encountered while trying to take care of patients by using the computer-generated record. A major complaint was that the pre-encounter report, a highlighted summary with space for new data entry, was restrictive and discouraged recording a complete medical work-up. Most internists have been trained to record a complete history and physical examination when they first get to know a patient. Instead of being all-inclusive, the system prompted for a focused set of symptoms and physical findings based upon a patient's problems and findings as designated from prior visits. Because physicians seeing the patient for the first time had not participated in recording the medical data in front of them, they felt uneasy without the ability to record general thoughts about a patient's condition and diagnostic or therapeutic alternatives. When a patient initially presents with a chief complaint, it is often difficult to narrow the problem to one specific diagnosis. With a paper record, during a physician's first encounter with the patient, it is more comfortable to indicate that there are several possibilities and that the appropriate diagnostic work-up will be done. However, the physician hesitated to record diagnostic possibilities until they were confirmed, because the computer record seemed so permanent and formal. Physicians wanted to indicate the logic by which they arrived at a specific conclusion. Narrative notes were not allowed in the system to any great extent, and although no objective data about the patient was being lost, the physicians were unable to emphasize or underline the pieces of information critical to their assessment.

In an experiment to determine which information would be recorded by a physician in a paper chart, but not on the computer report, the investigators attached blank progress note paper to each computer report and told the physicians to make notes whenever they felt the computer record was inadequate. For 11 per cent of the next 194 encounters, physicians wrote traditional notes. Two thirds of those notes were on patients being seen for their initial visit, and a complete review of systems was recorded. Other notes included information such as remarkable family histories, unproven diagnoses, and negative findings; however, the traditional notes never contained information that could not have been recorded on the computer report.

HOW ARE COMPUTERIZED FILES AND RECORDS ORGANIZED?

We've said the medical record is basically a time series structure of data elements that are variable in size and number because of the multiple branching nature of medicine. Organization for data storage will depend, to a large extent, on the manner in which we plan to use the data and the resources (hardware and software) we have available. Different structural classifications exist for data storage, depending upon the method by which each element is accessed (random, sequential, indexed sequential, binary-tree) and the manner in which the data are related to other elements (hierarchical, relational, inverted). These classifications apply to both simple data files and complex computerized records.

Different components of the computerized medical record may use multiple access methods, all within the same software. Patient records might be stored in random access or binary-tree files; the data dictionary (which defines elements to be collected), in an indexed sequential file; and textual results (such as operative notes or narrative comments) in sequential files. The choice of organizational structure depends upon performance requirements as perceived through the eyes of the software designer.

In a random access file, the index contains or can quickly calculate the exact physical location of a record so that only two disk accesses (the index and the record) are necessary to retrieve the data. In a sequential file, each element or record must be looked at to see whether it is the one wanted. In a 1000-record file this would mean 1 to 1000 disk accesses (average, 500) to retrieve a record, depending upon where it was in the sequence. Both binary-tree and indexed sequential structures minimize the number of attempts necessary to find the correct record by indexing them in such a way that the computer can narrow the possible disk locations in which it will search for the record.

Perhaps more important than access method is the method of relationships used in organizing the data. Traditionally, we are familiar with the hierarchical record structure in which all data pertinent to that patient's medical history are stored in one file folder. If we want to know anything about that patient, we pull up their one record. Admittedly, we may have to hunt for specific data within the record, for the chart itself may be quite thick.

Conversely, if we were responsible only for the laboratory and wanted to keep track of creatinine results, it would be extremely efficient to calculate laboratory norms if we had to pull only one record containing all creatinine results on all patients. This record structure is called an inverted file and is commonly used for small data sets (less than 100 variables) to optimize statistical analysis involving only a limited number of interrelationships among variables in a homogeneous group of patients.

A third form of data relationship, which currently receives much attention, is relational form. The best way to conceptualize this format is to imagine a very closely related set of data treated as an individual record and stored in its own file cabinet (Fig. 12–7). In this way a patient who had renal failure, underwent hemodialysis, and subsequently developed an abnormal cervical Pap smear secondary to immunosuppressive therapy would have records in at least three separate record files. If you wanted to treat the patient, it would be awkward to get all three records in a timely fashion, but if you wished to report your hemodialysis experience, it would be faster to go to the hemodialysis file and count your experience while looking through each *thin* medical record.

In general, a hierarchical record structure is used if the primary objective is to take care of the patient. With a simple, topically oriented patient data base for clinical research, a relational data structure will facilitate browsing through the records and will be much faster in producing fifty different reports looking for new disease or treatment relationships (Fig. 12–8). For a full-scale medical research project that uses multivariate mathematical relationships to predict the outcome of one disease, arranging the data in an inverted file relationship would minimize the amount of computational time necessary to analyze the data.

HOW ARE DATA DISPLAYED AND ANALYZED?

The display and analysis of a patient's or population's medical data are limited only by our imagination and the available software tools. These tools can present predefined comparisons and allow creative data manipulation (Fig. 12–9). Unfortunately, the majority of developmental effort in computerized medical records has had to be in defining what data, in what format, we wish to collect. Display and analysis functions are in their infancy. Although graphic display and statistical analysis software are highly developed in their own right, the integration of these packages with computerized medical records has not yet taken place to any great extent.

Actually, enhanced patient care can take place using relatively

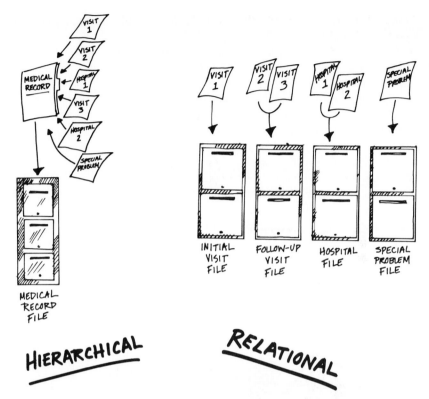

Figure 12–7. *Data storage in hierarchical and relational files. In a hierarchical file, all data pertinent to that patient are accumulated in one folder. In a relational data base, patient data are stored in many different files with similar data from other patients.*

simple graphics and statistical analysis that does not go much beyond cross tabulations and comparison of means. Just the ability to have data in electronic form so that a patient's actual study values can be plotted over time is a major step forward. If one adds the ability to compare one patient's findings with those of similar patients in an electronic data base, one really has transformed data into information (Fig. 12–10).

When information in the patient record has been carefully coded, the computer data bank can be used to define the natural history of a disease process and to identify deviations from expected outcomes. Unlike the human, a computer record system can review its *clinical experience* without placing increased emphasis on the last patient seen or the patient that responded unusually well or poorly to a regimen. The program can focus on a well-defined patient population, allowing determination of the normal values for very abnormal people.[12]

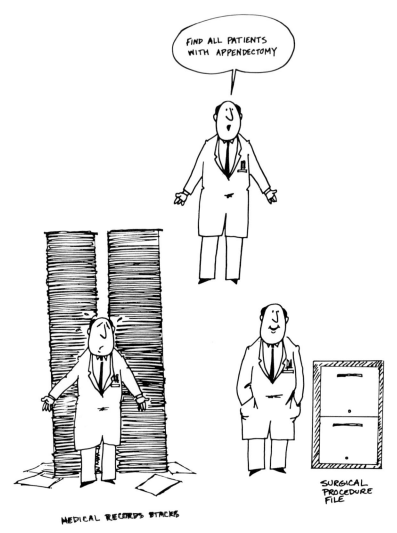

Figure 12–8. Data retrieval in hierarchical and relational files. Using hierarchical data storage, a very thick medical record must be reviewed in order to find a small amount of data concerning a surgical procedure, for example. With a relational data base structure, a much smaller record file is looked at and therefore it should take less work and time to produce reports.

PROTECTING THE PATIENT'S MEDICAL DATA

Privacy, confidentiality, and security from theft are all issues that must be addressed concerning patients' medical records.[1] The potential for abuse is as great or greater for manually recorded patient data as it is

```
Scattergram requested for Hematocrit versus Creatinine

     DX = ALL
     PCAT = RENAL - INSUFFIENCY

What date ranges would you like plotted?

1.   ALL DATA
2.   DATA FROM TEH PAST 100 ENTRIES
3.   DATA FROM CURRENT HOSPITALIZATION
4.   DATA FROM TODAY
5.   DATA FOR A SPECIFIED PERIOD ENDING TODAY
6.   DATA FOR A SPECIFIED PERIOD STARTING WITH A SPECIFIC DATE



Enter # or <CR>!
```

Figure 12–9. Software tools for generating reports can significantly enhance computerized medical records if the data in the record are accurate and relatively complete.

for electronic records. There is, however, one major difference between electronic and handwritten records. Depending upon the circumstances, abuse of electronic records can take place at a site physically separate from the actual location of the records. The desirability of computers to permit medical record access from different locations simultaneously also opens a new area of potential abuse problems. If the electronic record is in any way connected to telephone lines via modems or if telecommunication of medical data takes place over wire, cables, or radiowaves, then wire tapping can take place.

At the geographic location of the electronic medical record, security of data can actually be increased beyond that possible for the traditional medical chart. Password protection and well-defined user privileges can help improve the confidentiality of a medical record. Software trace subroutines can be implemented to record who is looking at what parts of the record. Data encryption methods for both transmission of files to distant computers and coding data for storage at one's local site (to protect against *wandering eyes*) have been well worked out. It must be remembered, however, that every technique to increase data security also increases the effort to access data by authorized users. The more you protect data, the harder it is to get to them under normal daily operations. There is no such entity as the totally secure computer system, just as there is no totally secure doctor's office filing system. The best that can and should be done is to provide a *relatively secure* system for medical databases.[2]

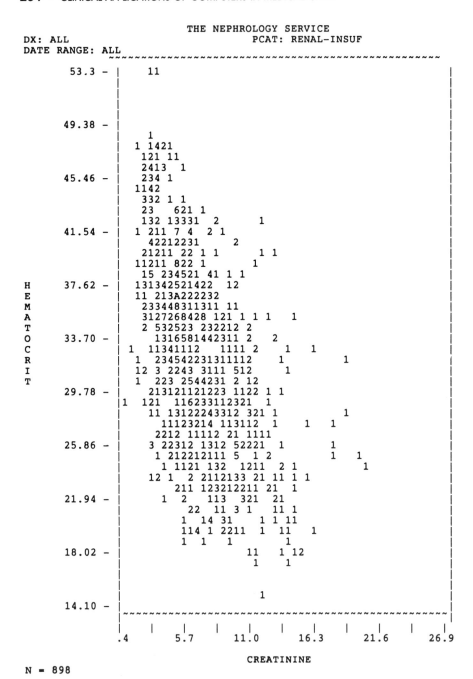

Figure 12–10. Hematocrit reading versus creatinine level for patients with renal insufficiency. When data are analyzed for interrelationships, new concepts are generated or old concepts examined more critically. Data are transformed into "information."

SUMMARY

Physicians in private office practice believe that medical data bases (in academic settings) are well developed and should be available *off-the-shelf*. What they want are medical systems that not only provide billing and financial functions but also help them to better take care of patients in the ambulatory setting, the largest arena of health care. Academic physicians believe that computerized office billing and management systems have become commonplace, but they want a clinical data base that doesn't have to be overhauled for every new patient with an infrequently occurring disease.

Medical data organization is a complex business. It is much more sophisticated in its relationships than a banking system or an airlines reservation data base. Health care providers must realize the work yet to be done to arrive at a push-button computerized medical record system.

REFERENCES

1. Covvey, H. D., and McAlister, N. H.: Computers in the practice of medicine: Volume II. Issues in Medical Computing. Reading, MA, Addison-Wesley Publishing Co., 1980, pp. 64–80.
2. Gabrieli, E.: Office computing and the right to privacy. *In* Oberst, BB and Reid, RA (eds.): Computer Applications to Private Office Practice. New York, Springer Verlag, 1984, pp. 121–126.
3. Hammond, W. E., Stead, W. W., Feagin, S. J., et al.: Data base management system for ambulatory care. *In* Blum, B (ed.): Information Systems for Patient Care. New York, Springer Verlag, 1984, pp. 218–231.
4. Jelovsek, F. R., and Hammond, W. E.: Formal error rate in a computerized obstetric medical record. Meth. Inform. Med., 17:151–157, 1978.
5. Jelovsek, F. R., Deason, B. P., Richard, H.: Impact of an on-line information system in the medical office. *In* Blum, B. (ed.): Information Systems for Patient Care. New York, Springer Verlag, 1984, pp. 322–329.
6. Kuhn, I. M., Widerhold, G., Rodnick, J. E., et al.: Automated ambulatory medical record systems in the US. *In* Blum, B. (ed.): Information Systems for Patient Care. New York, Springer Verlag, 1984, pp. 199–217.
7. McDonald, C. J., Wilson, G. A., and McCabe, G. P.: Physician response to computer reminders. J.A.M.A. 244:1579–1582, 1980.
8. McDonald, C.J., Blevins, L., Glazener, T., et al.: Regenstrief medical record system. *In* Blum, B. (ed.): Information Systems for Patient Care. New York, Springer Verlag, 1984, pp. 232–248.
9. Murphy, G.: The medical record summary, contents and utilization. *In* Oberst, B. B., and Reid, R. A, (eds.): Computer Applications to Private Office Practice. New York, Springer Verlag, 1984, pp. 53–67.
10. Shapiro, A. R.: SCAMP system. *In* Blum, B. (ed.): Information Systems for Patient Care. New York, Springer Verlag, 1984, pp. 249–259.
11. Stead, W. W., Hammond, W. E., and Straube, M. J.: A chartless record—is it adequate? J. Med. Syst. 7:103–109, 1983.
12. Stead, W. W., Garrett L. E., Jr., and Hammond, W. E.: Practicing nephrology with a computerized medical record. Kidney Int 24:446–454, 1983.
13. Stead, W. W., Hammond, W. E.: Computerized medical records: A new resource for clinical decision making. J. Med. Syst. 7:213–220, 1983.
14. Weed, L. L.: Medical records that guide and teach. N. Engl. J. Med., 278:593–657, 1968.

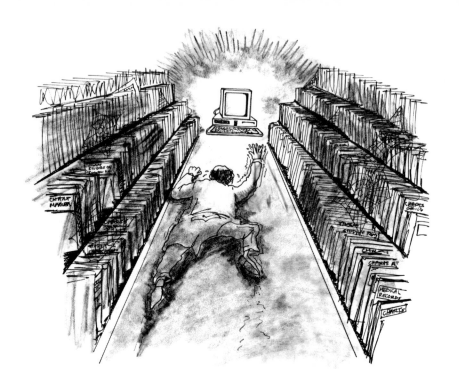

T H I R T E E N

Data Management Systems in Clinical Research

Chester King

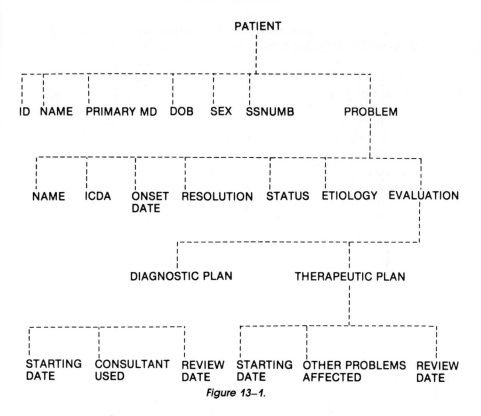

Figure 13-1.

Data management consists of everything that happens to data from the process of defining what is to be collected up to its output and analysis. Computerized data management implies facilities for entering, storing, and retrieving data in a variety of forms. Most data management systems fall somewhere between two extremes: file management systems and data base management systems (DBMS).

Traditional file management systems store data in unrelated files whose structure forces the user to be concerned with the physical layout of the underlying data storage system. Before data can be modified, or used in new ways, the physical details of the data storage system must be modified. This means the creation of redundant files, which leads to costly and error-prone data entry, update, or deletion.

Data base management systems have been recognized as efficient and cost-effective tools in scientific, commercial, and military applications for over a decade. There have been few medical uses in research or patient care because most DBMSs, which have been designed for commercial or scientific applications, have not been able to depict medical data in all its complexity. Most systems have also been difficult, if not impossible, for a nonprogrammer to use directly. They have been run on large, expensive machines, and they need the services of a staff of programmers to provide user interfaces for the nonprogrammers, interfaces geared to particular applications and requiring the services of these same programmers for any modifications. Microcomputer-based DBMSS tend, in varying degrees, to put these mainframe capabilities directly in the hands of the nonprogramming users.

A DBMS generally includes the following functions:

1. Describing the data items to be stored and organizing them into a data base structure (data base definition)

2. Entering values and checking their consistency with the item definition or the contents of the data base (data entry)

3. Editing previously entered values

4. Controlling access to data

5. Creating subsets of data objects, such as patients or patient visits, characterized by combinations of conditions of data elements such as height, weight, and diagnosis (querying)

6. Generating reports in a variety of formats (retrieval)

The DBMSs we review perform most of these functions. All the systems permit a programmer to write further programs beyond the prepared package, though with a great variation in ease and cost. We review three microcomputer systems based on the file management concept: SAS, RS/1, and dBase II. We also review the DBMSs that run on microcomputers: CLINFO, Clinical Data Manager, the VA File Manager, INGRES, ORACLE, SIR, MEDLOG, and FOCUS. Finally, we examine how systems oriented toward patient care can be used for research. For example, COSTAR is a file manager whose structure has been set up to handle medical records in a more predefined way than in a DBMS. These systems feature extensive user-oriented interfaces that help automate administrative, scheduling, supply, test ordering, and other functions as well as patient record keeping.

This review gives readers an idea of the capabilities of each system, enabling them to compare the systems and seek more information from the designers. For each system, we describe the file or data base structure, the data base definition process, the data entry, retrieval, analysis process, and the installation considerations.

We have not reviewed a number of mainframe systems, which require a large programming staff, such as TOTAL, DEC's DBMS, System 2000, and IDMS. We have also left out a myriad of systems that were designed for specific applications and are usually not portable to other sites.

The review is based on published articles, manuals, and discussions with users. We have had most of the system descriptions reviewed by users. However, this is no guarantee of accuracy: we have learned of errors in the 1980 survey, which was also submitted for review, long after that survey was in print. Perhaps this is inevitable when the subject matter is so rich and complex.

CRITERIA IN USING DATA MANAGEMENT SYSTEMS

Perhaps the most obvious difference between systems is how users interact with them: (1) through a command language, which supposes familiarity with the commands and how they are used, or (2) through a question-and-answer dialogue in English, which finds out what tasks the user wants done, explains how to do it, requests the needed information, and then performs the tasks. This dialogue method is far easier for inexperienced users and usually includes useful on-line documentation or help messages. It also avoids referring the user to a thick manual. Some systems incorporate the best of both worlds by using the dialogue method and a command language; experienced users can use the terser commands (see Table 13–5).

The command language found in most of the systems we review is termed nonprocedural. By contrast, procedural languages, such as C, FORTRAN, COBOL, BASIC, and MUMPS, are frankly programmer-oriented languages that specify to the computer what has to be done to perform a task rather than what task the user wants done. Thus, a nonprocedural command might be:

PRINT FILE1

whereas the procedural commands would involve a series of statements specifying how to do the output, how to go through the structure of FILE1, and how to format each line on output.

Nonprocedural languages generally do not contain typical programming constructs such as LOOP, in which the user-programmer specifies the steps that will iterate or repeat for each instance of a data item. Nonprocedural languages are meant to spare the user the details of how the computer actually does a task.

The term nonprocedural resembles the term data base management system in that there is no set distinction between nonprocedural and procedural, just as there is no set distinction between data base and file management. Systems that tend to the nonprocedural data base end of the scale tend to be easier to use. The appendix at the end of this chapter gives some examples of what is meant by procedural languages, nonprocedural languages, and dialogues.

DATA BASE MANAGEMENT AND DATA INDEPENDENCE

True DBMSs store data with a minimum of duplication and can use it for a variety of purposes by means of the general functions—searching, report generation, or statistical analysis—and through special purpose programs. The data can have varying degrees of independence from the functions or programs that process them. Systems whose data is stored more independently from the functions or programs that process them tend to be more flexible and easier to use.

At a minimum, users should not need to restructure their data for different uses, as they must in file management systems. Reference to data items by name, instead of positional location in a file, is another indicator of freedom from the complexities of physical storage structure.

In true DBMSs, changes in the data base structure, such as the addition of a new data item after data entry has begun, can be made without changing the programs that make use of the data. Experience with users in any clinical setting has demonstrated time and again that flexibility in modifying the data base is essential at all stages of a project or information system. No two users have the same conceptual framework; no predefined structure can satisfy the needs of all users. And most users' needs change with time; only actual experience shows what kind of data and what ways of organizing that data *really* best suit their needs.

Data independence permits the kind of unplanned interrogation and reporting of data that physicians need. Freedom from concerns with the underlying physical structure allows a more thoughtful approach in which users seek to represent their view of the world and not the computer's. Thus, users can get much closer to their data.

Data Base Definition

Once users decide how to organize data, they set up the tables in a file manager or enter the data base definition describing their view of the data into the DBMS. Such a definition includes the overall structure and the characteristics of each data item, such as maximum length, range of values, list of values, data types, and so on. The data type determines the kind of data that can be stored for a particular type of item—for example, integer, date, text, and so on. Systems differ in how natural the data types are. Some will have one type of integer; others will have several different types of integers based on the underlying operating system's characteristics, which are irrelevant to researchers' needs. Systems also differ in their ability to represent data—some lack dates or times, for instance. Table 13–1 compares what data types are found in a selection of the systems reviewed. Note: in this and other tables, the absence of a feature does not preclude programming it in; this depends on the efficiency of the underlying language and the state of the internals of the system (documentation, modularity).

Many parts of a DBMS use the data base definition to customize

Table 13–1. Data Types Supported by Representative Systems

Type	SAS	RS/1	MEDLOG	CLINFO	MISAR	CDM	SIR	INGRES	ORACLE	FOCUS	dBASE II
Number		X		X	X						
Integer	X		X			X	X	X	X	X	X
Real number	X		X			X	X	X	X	X	X
Text	X	X	X	X	X	X	X	X	X	X	X
List			X	X	X	X		X	X		
List + other						X			X		
Date	X	X	X	X	X	X	X		X		
Time	X	X		X	X	X	X		X		
Computed	X	X	X		X	X	X	X			

Note: Some systems differentiate between integers and real numbers; others represent both within one type. "List" refers to multiple choice list. "List + other" means that values that do not conform to one of the choices can also be represented, although systems differ as to the ease with which they manage this. The presence of a data type in a system does not necessarily mean the system can process data represented by the data type. This is particularly true of the text data type, for which RS/1, Prophet, MEDLOG, and CLINFO, among others, have no retrieval syntax.

Table 13–2. Data Checking Options

Type	SAS	RS/1	MEDLOG	CLINFO	MISAR	CDM	SIR	INGRES	ORACLE	FOCUS	dBASE II
Data type	X		X	X	X	X	X	X	X	X	X
Range	X		X	X	X	X	X	X	X	X	
Length			X	X	X		X	X	X	X	
Pattern						X			X	X	X
Duplicate			X		X	X		X	X	X	
Relational						X	X	X	X		X
Security									X		

Note: Pattern refers to pattern match, a check against a predefined pattern. Duplicate entry refers not to the entry of duplicate top-level cases, such as patients, which all system implementing data checks do, but to entry of duplicate lower-level items, which in MEDLOG is limited to visits. Security refers not to access to a particular data base, which all systems with any access controls implement, but rather to access to a particular case, which in a relational system means a row in a table and in a hierarchical one, a branch item.

their programs for the user's application. DBMSs differ in how easy it is for the user to manage this all-important data base definition; many create a number of the definitional characteristics through the data entry routines as part of validity checks. Users find that they have to keep track of far more elements with such systems; each time a new questionnaire is set up involving some of the same data items as in a previous one, great care must be taken to duplicate the same item characteristics or risk losing data consistency, validity, and integrity.

Such an "unintegrated" data base definition approach creates other problems, because the fine points of an item's characteristics are then unavailable to other parts of the system. For instance, during querying, the lack of an ability to check proposed queries against a full list of item characteristics reduces the system's ability to prevent nonsense queries, thereby taking up researchers' time. Statistical packages not tightly integrated with the entire data base definition have no way of knowing certain vital characteristics such as possible values and cannot therefore guide users in analyses.

The best data base definition is one that is used by all parts of the system and thus provides the most self-documentation in the system, as users can refer to it to find out an item's meaning no matter what task they are undertaking. This greatly reduces the memory burden on users. Such a data base definition can be called "fully integrated."

Data Entry

Users enter data through a data entry facility or through a user-designed questionnaire. Some systems only allow for programmers to create data entry questionnaires. The DBMSs perform varying degrees of data checks. Table 13–2 shows how some of the systems reviewed differ in this regard. Some systems offer screen-oriented data entry; these should be evaluated in terms of how integrated the data base definition is.

Systems differ in how much on-line assistance is offered the data enterer, in the user's ability to define how the system prompts for data entry, in whether questionnaires can branch to different questions based on the data enterer's responses, and in their data editing styles. Such branching is useful in the world of medicine, in which data is frequently sparse because no one patient has all diseases or is given all laboratory tests. Table 13–3 shows some of these data entry features for a selected group of the systems reviewed.

Retrieval

Retrieval is accomplished through programs that present varying amounts of user options for formating and selecting contents. These

Table 13–3. Data Entry Options

Type	SAS	RS/1	MEDLOG	CLINFO	MISAR	CDM	SIR	INGRES	ORACLE	FOCUS	dBASE II
Facility	X		X	X	X	X					X
Questions			X		X	X	X	X	X	X	X
Sequence			X	X	X	X	X	X	X	X	
Help			X		X	X	X	X	X	X	
Branching						X	X				
Work space			DB	DB	BR	LV	DB	BR	BR	LV	DB

Note: Facility means a standard data entry facility available after data base definition. Questions refers to a procedural language-based questionnaire. Sequence refers to control of promoting sequence: whether it can be modified. SAS has a forms package, which we do not review here. Help refers to an interactive help function to give a description of the item during data entry. Branching refers to branching logic, the built-in skipping of irrelevant questions based on previously entered data values. Work space refers to the size of the work space (locking granularity) that any one user can access at the same time (DB = data base, BR = branch item or table, LV = leaf value, value of an individual data item).

Table 13–4. A Comparison of Query System Features

Type	SAS	RS/1	MEDLOG	CLINFO	MISAR	CDM	SIR	INGRES	ORACLE	FOCUS	dBASE II
Equals		X	X		X	X	X	X	X	X	X
Less, greater		X	X	X	X	X	X	X	X	X	X
In range			X	X		X			X	X	
In string		X			X	X		X	X	X	
Pattern					X	X		X	X		
Alpha order						X	X				
First, last			X	X		X				X	X
Missing			X		X	X	X				
Dialogue			X	X	X	X					

Note: SAS has no query system. Less, greater is "less than" and "greater than;" in range is within range. In string, or string contains, asks whether a text item contains a specified string of characters. Alpha order means whether a string follows a given string alphabetically. Missing refers to a test for a missing value code common to all data types. All systems have a null, but one of the nightmares of biostatistics is distinguishing the null value from the missing value. Dialogue refers to whether an interactive dialogue is available.

abilities are important if the activities of the DBMS are to be integrated with those of patient care. Such integration is desirable in order to maximize the incentives users have to keep good quality data.

Data entry and sometimes retrieval can be characterized by the number of users who can have access to the data base at one time. A key consideration is the locking granularity, which is the granularity, or size, of the record unit from which others are isolated while a user works on it. The granularity ranges from the entire data base to the item value. Thus, there are systems that permit only one user to enter data for a data base at a time, others that permit one user for a certain section, and others that permit one user per data item. The locking granularity, or size of the work space, for various systems is compared in Table 12–2.

Analysis

Analysis is usually accomplished in two stages: first, the selection of subsets of the data based on logical criteria, and second, the analysis of such subsets via statistical programs. Systems vary widely in the ease and speed with which such queries are done. They also differ considerably in the richness of their query system, or how detailed and varied the questions they support are. Table 13–4 compares some query system features across systems. A key consideration for researchers and physicians is how easy such query systems are to use. Do they work through an interactive dialogue or assume knowledge of a query language (be it procedural or nonprocedural) and of the data base, which may be very complex and hard to understand, and perhaps have deficient paper documentation. Some systems have statistical programs or allow users to transfer selected data to full-fledged statistical packages such as SAS, BMDP, or SPSS.

Systems differ greatly in the ease with which they implement access control provisions and how extensive these are. The provisions range from control over users' access to capabilities and access into particular data items to ownership of individual cases within the same data base. These provisions are naturally of great importance in many medical environments.

No matter how powerful the nonprocedural language or how extensive the user interfaces, there will always be a need in more complex projects for procedural programming. The main issue here is whether the system possesses a built-in language, known as a data manipulation language, or whether a conventional high-level language such as MUMPS, BASIC, or FORTRAN must be resorted to. In the case of the built-in language, this usually implies symbolic reference, or reference by name, to data items, as opposed to reference to a file location, which implies knowledge of the system's internal structure. In the case of a high-level language, the costs involved are dependent on the programming efficiency of the language and how disciplined and well documented the system's internal structure is.

Installation considerations include the hardware and operating system requirements and the degree of support and documentation provided by the designers. Such considerations are affected by the systems' ability to manage sparse data physically on the storage media; some have to reserve space on the media for data that is not entered—for those diseases the patient doesn't have. Systems also differ in their ability to efficiently manage the storage space in case data is deleted. These types of disk management can require the costly on-going services of a systems programmer.

DATA BASE STRUCTURE

The data base structure is the user's view of how the system organizes and represents information. Most file management systems organize their data into tables whose rows or columns represent data items. Many DBMSs have either a hierarchical or a relational data base structure. The richness of the data base structure determines how accurately the stored data can represent reality and therefore how spontaneous, easy, and possible future investigations and reports can be.

Relational Systems

Relational systems organize data into tables, as do the file managers. However, they provide for ways of relating one table to another by means of "keys," or identifiers. Thus, one table might have patients' demographic data, and another might have the repeating visit data. The demographic table would have its repeating element (patient) identified by the patient's identification number (ID). The visit table would have its repeating element (visit) identified by both the ID and the visit number. For multilevel or multitable material designed to represent complex time relationships, the repetition of numerous keys can be a burden.

Patient Table

ID	Name	Sex	DOB	City	Phone
232	Paul	M	1956	Boston	732-0977
241	Mary	F	1950	Devon	980-7856
249	Scott	M	1934	Gary	345-9085

Visit Table

ID	Visit No.	Date	Weight	Temperature	Heart Rate
232	1	1/3/80	145	98.0	65
232	2	1/4/81	156	98.6	71
249	1	2/3/82	189	104.7	86

Tables are easy data structures to understand and fine for certain uses. In particular, tables are essential for depicting time-flow sheets, laboratory data, and so on. However, different systems with different data base structures can represent data in the same way; for example, both relational and hierarchical systems can represent time-flow sheets and other data in tabular format.

However, relational systems have trouble depicting complex relationships between tables without involving programmers. A mathematically complete way of describing and manipulating tables is known as the relational calculus. It has proved difficult to impart the full flavor of this calculus to nonprogrammers.

Relational systems are ill suited to hierarchical data; editing and deletion problems appear. For instance, if a patient is deleted from the patient table, his visits are not automatically deleted. Some relational systems allow users to set up links between tables on a permanent basis. However, the entire system may not work with these hierarchical structures. In particular, such linked tables can be virtual tables that are copied at the time of creation, so that any subsequent modifications to the data base will not be automatically reflected in the linked tables. If the linked tables are not updated when their base tables are, there may be update problems.

Even one link between two tables can cause awkward representation problems when the link creates a new table based on the first two. For instance, with the preceding patient and visit tables, the patient data would be repeated for each row containing visit data. The tables would become large and unwieldy and would suffer from query inclusion/exclusion problems. The complexities associated with these issues increase considerably in multilevel situations, such as patients who have hospitalizations, each with several procedures. The sparseness of medical data also creates problems; if there are several measurements of a data item, one column in the table must be reserved for each measurement. Typically, not all of these columns are filled in, and queries and reports may be awkward.

Hierarchical Systems

With all these drawbacks, you may ask, why is "relational system" the current buzzword among many computer scientists and software vendors? They are designed to solve business problems dealing with elements whose existence does not depend on each other—customer orders and inventoried parts, for example. Customer orders can exist in a data base without inventoried parts, whereas a patient's visit cannot exist apart from the patient.

Patient data are different from most business data; they depend on one element, a patient, for their existence in a system. The existence of the information below the top item PATIENT in a hierarchy depends on that item. If a patient is deleted, so are all his or her subitems' values—this is usually what you want to have happen. Because there is only one file, any editing of the data does not have to be reflected in multiple copies of tables. Medical data are patient-centered, and consequently, all the power (and complexity) of relational systems that deal with independent tabular representations is both unnecessary and overly complex.

What patient data lack in the way of cross-referencing complexity across different entities they more than make up for with internal cross-referencing needs. Hierarchies can reflect the complex interrelationship among all of each patient's data, as well as relationships across patients. Capturing these complex relationships is increasingly vital to both research and patient care.

The hierarchical systems differ in the number of branching levels they allow and in the way they are designed to appear to users. A number of them go to only three levels (CLINFO, MEDLOG, MISAR). This hampers efforts to represent complex hospital-based data in particular, such as patients who have multiple hospitalizations, and in each hospitalization multiple laboratory tests, x-rays, therapies, and operations, each of which might consist of different elements or events.

To represent such multilevel, repeating data at all in a three-level system, a tabular data format must be used to accommodate the maximum number of cases, but this runs into all the problems of a relational or tabular structure, as discussed previously. For example, when there are several possible instances of a measurement and associated comments, or when there are several associated measurements, the arrangements are as follows:

Example 1	Example 2
measure#1	1st set—measure#1
comment#1	1st set—measure#2
measure#2	1st set—measure#3
comment#2	2nd set—measure#1
measure#3	2nd set—measure#2
comment#3	2nd set—measure#3

The item names in such a set-up appear even if there is only one

Table 13–5. Types of System Interactions

Type	SAS	RS/1	MEDLOG	CLINFO	MISAR	CDM	SIR	INGRES	ORACLE	FOCUS	dBASE II
Medical research			X	X	X	X					
Data model	F	F	H	H	H	H/R	H	R	R	H	F
DBDEF drive			X	X	X	X					
DBDEF help			X			X					
Dialogue			DERQ	DERQ	DERQ	DERQ		EQ	EQ		DE
Command lang		X				X	X	X	X		
Data lang	X	X	X			X	X			X	X
Host inter	X					X	X	X	X	X	

Note: Medical research means the system was designed specifically for medical research. Data model refers to the way data are structured in the system. F stands for file, as in file manager, H stands for hierarchical, and R stands for relational. These terms are explained in a section on data base structure. DBDEF drive means the data base definition drives, or customizes, the standard functions in the system—functions present without programming once the data base has been defined. DBDEF help refers to whether the data base definition is used to generate data base–specific help messages in data entry, report making, or querying. The next four elements are arranged so that the ones requiring less training come first. Dialogue refers to whether an interactive dialogue is available to aid users through a question-and-answer session. D stands for data base definition, E for data entry, R for reports, and Q for querying. Command lang stands for nonprocedural command language, in which a request is formulated using a precise syntax without having to specify how the request is to be performed other than in general, user-oriented terms. Data lang refers to data manipulation language, a built-in programming language that refers to data base items by name and protects the programmer from having to know the internals of the system. Host refers to host language interface, the ability to use standard high-level programming languages, such as COBOL, FORTRAN, or MUMPS, directly with a data base.

measurement. Space is usually reserved for the maximum number of measurements anticipated. A multilevel hierarchy can better represent sparse medical data by only repeating as much as is needed.

An added problem with "shallow" three-level systems is that the unit of analysis for statistical purposes is frequently restricted to the top level (PATIENT) and possibly to the next branch item down, typically VISIT. This means that values for repeating data objects at lower levels, such as date of procedure for procedures within operations or size for kidney stones within interventions must be transferred to a fairly sophisticated statistical package with facilities for sorting and merging before they can be analyzed.

STATISTICAL ANALYSIS SYSTEM (SAS)

The Statistical Analysis System (SAS) is a sophisticated statistical package in which the file manager has been improved over the years. It runs most often on mainframe, IBM equipment in batch mode, although an interactive version is available under IBM's TSO or CMS operating systems. However, like a number of other products, SAS has been ported down to a microcomputer. The first port is to an IBM PC/XT 370, but this looks very much like the mainframe version, as it is clearly targeted to corporate (mainframe) users. A new release is due out in the fourth quarter of 1985 to run under IBM XT and AT DOS. We review SAS here because it is something of a standard, being widely used in academic research institutions and pharmaceutical companies. We review it in the expectation that the function of the DOS version will be similar, although there will doubtless be some restrictions over the mainframe version.

The best use of SAS in medical research is in the analytic phase, after the data have been sent over from a DBMS. We do not review several packages that have been added to SAS, including a data entry package and a graphics package.

File Definition. The files are two-dimensional tables in which columns have data item names as heads and rows refer to particular occurrences of those items. Files are defined through SAS programs. SAS programs are procedural and specify the step-by-step process of how the system does something. This differs from nonprocedural, or command oriented, languages, by which the user specifies what he or she wants. Users may need to have some awareness of the underlying physical structure. Tables can require specifications relating to the "block size" and the number of buffers, unless the system programmer has set the SAS up so as to handle large data sets. Each user can have any number of tables, but if the tables are to go on a disk, the number of tracks needed on the disk may have to be calculated in terms of the number of rows, block size, and row length. Tables do not handle sparse data efficiently, for empty cells take up as much space as those with values in them. Unused space is deleted by copying the file to another location.

Item names are at most eight characters long. There are five data types: character, numeric, date, time, and computed. Computed item values are derived from those of other items via an SAS program performing arithmetical operations on numeric items or logical operations on character items. Each data type can exist in a variety of specific formats. Numeric formats can specify the number of digits and include scientific notation, dollar format, fractions, floating point, fixed point, and other machine-readable formats. There are a variety of date and time formats. Character formats include fixed-length and varying length. The data base definition in a DBMS has, as we shall see, more possibilities for describing and restricting an item's values. This ensures greater data integrity through checks against the definition and allows various parts of the system to refer to the definition in order to tailor their actions to a specified data base.

Data Entry. Data can be entered from punched cards, magnetic tapes, or disks. There is no interactive data entry questionnaire. In order to prevent users from interfering with each other, only one user at a time is allowed to enter data in a particular table. There is a forms data entry package, but we do not review it here; it suffers from the not uncommon forms package problem of forcing users to define data item characteristics through the forms package for each form and not through the central data definition. This can lead to ambiguous and inconsistent data, as is discussed in the sections on the INGRES and ORACLE systems.

Retrieval. Reports can be generated through SAS programs for printing out tables. There are some formating options enabling users to do a line feed, label values, combine values with constant character strings or numbers, position values and constant by column, print sums, set the number of lines per page, and others. These options are incorporated into an SAS program.

Once data have been entered into tables, there are several commands that can be used to manipulate these tables. Users can delete columns or rows and reorder the columns. They can join two tables with the same data items and different values end to end. Tables can be joined side by side.

Users can sort columns alphabetically or by numeric values. These sorted columns can form composite keys, indexing the files. Tables can also be sorted by item values, creating a series of tables in which rows are segregated according to the values of one item. The subset command forms new tables by selecting those rows specified through a logical operator and a value. Character operators can be applied through PL/I, a programming language. The commands for rearranging tables by joins, sorting, and subsetting can be included in report programs. However, the only access to the files is sequential, and there are no rapid searches of indexed files.

Analysis. Before running the statistical programs, values are selected by performing table manipulations. SAS was originally designed as a statistical package and has a rich variety of statistical programs, whose description we will forego. It can be used as a statistical package for data managed on the other systems we review.

Installation, Support, and Costs. SAS is maintained and updated, and consulting questions are answered from 9 A.M. to 5 P.M.. SAS is favored by many pharmaceutical companies, as it provides reports in a format acceptable to the FDA. SAS is available from the SAS Institute, SAS Circle, Box 8000, Cary, NC, 27511.

There are numerous SAS installations. SAS has received considerable publicity and has been voted the number 1 package for 5 years in a row by a data processing association.

Differences between SAS and a DBMS. SAS may seem to organize data as a relational DBMS does—in tables. SAS programs can be used to implement some relational operators such as projection, restriction, set union, and set intersection. The join operations, however, are not equivalent to the join operation found in a relational DBMS. It is impossible to obtain the same data structures as in the relational DBMS.

There is no query system, and a program must be written for each different search of the files or each report, using the procedural SAS syntax. SAS files are accessed sequentially; those in the other systems we review are accessed in a more efficient manner. In addition, a DBMS usually has facilities for creating inverted files or other files optimized to speed up queries.

RS/1

RS/1 is a sophisticated file management system designed by Bolt, Beranek, and Newman for laboratory scientists. A new version of RS/1 features abundant on-line documentation and a menu-driven dialogue to facilitate entry into the system. RS/1 requires no knowledge of programming to use the English nonprocedural commands for creating tables, entering and retrieving data, and performing a variety of analyses and computations. RS/1 features a documented, PL/I-like programming language called RPL for applications beyond these commands, which can be included in RPL code. Like SAS, RS/1 is best used in clinical research during the analytic phase, with data extracted from a DBMS.

File Definition. RS/1 organizes data into tables made up of columns and rows; these can receive English names, but the user refers to them by position numbers, as "column 4" or "row 8." This requires attention to the physical layout of the tables because columns and rows can be inserted into existing tables. Any existing update routines must be modified after such insertions. Tables or parts of tables can be copied to make new tables. Data from one table can be copied to another. Tables can be transposed, rows becoming columns, and vice versa. Users can create an unlimited number of tables with up to 16,000 rows and 16,000 columns per table. This tabular structure mimics the traditional laboratory notebook.

A programmer is needed to build a table referencing other tables so as to store repeat instances of any groups of items. The ability to represent such repeat groups is more critical for the success of medical record applications than it is for laboratory ones. Tabular structures do not efficiently store the sparse data commonly found in medicine, as empty cells take up as much space as those containing values. This also poses logical problems for users in queries and reports.

There are four data types in RS/1: number, text, date, and time. Numbers can be represented in exponential, decimal, or integer notation. Text is enclosed in single quotes and can extend to several lines. There is no practical (32K characters) limit to the amount of text entered into a table cell, but only one line of 25 characters can be displayed without a special display program. All entered text is available for processing with logical and string expressions. A column or row can contain any of the types, including one type at one moment and another at another moment, which in a project requiring close control over data validity and integrity may cause some problems. A value can also be entered as an arithmetic expression. The result is computed and stored in the appropriate table cell. All cells are initialized to "EMPTY," the only value to represent missing, undefined, or null data. There are no security provisions beyond the operating system's file security and log-on procedure.

The data base definition in a DBMS has, as we shall see, more possibilities for describing an item's values. This ensures greater data integrity through checks against the definition and allows various parts of the system to refer to the definition for other purposes.

Data Entry. Data are entered into a table a column or a row at a time. Additional rows or columns can be entered at any time, as can individual items. To edit data, the item's row and column number are specified, and its value is replaced by a new one. No checks are performed on the data unless a programmer writes an RPL program. Care must be taken not to have more than one user access the same table simultaneously, particularly when both are entering or editing data, as no locking mechanism is available to prevent users from interfering with each other.

A SET command allows entire rows or columns to be set at the same value or to values computed from arithmetic or logical expressions, which can themselves involve entire rows or columns. For instance, one might "set column 4 to column 3 minus column 2."

Retrieval. Displays are made of (1) entire tables, (2) specified rows, columns, or combinations of rows and columns, and (3) individual items. A combination of rows and columns is called a table portion, for example, "columns 3 to 6 of rows 5 to 9" or "columns 3, 5, and 8 of rows 7 and 9." Tables can be displayed selectively according to criteria specified through the query system.

Analysis. The RS/1 query system functions by testing rows, columns, or table portions to see if they meet a condition formed by applying the standard arithmetic operators ($=$, $\neq$, $>$, $<$, $\leq$, and $\geq$) to specific values. Recently included is a string contain operator. Arithmetical, string, or logical operations can be performed on the rows or columns before they are tested, all in one expression of the sort: "display those rows where the difference between column 3 and column 2 is greater than 15." Several such conditions can be strung together by AND or OR. The RS/1 files are optimized for retrieval.

The SET command can be used in conjunction with the query system to set those cells that meet one or more conditions to a specified value or to values computed from values in other cells, as in "set row 5 of table 1 to row 3 of table 2 times row 4 of table 3."

Table rows or columns can be sorted according to text or numeric values in a specified row or column. Whether table portions are directly specified or derived by querying, they can be counted, added, and submitted for a rich variety of statistical and graphics procedures. These have been augmented in the VAX version of RS/1, particularly the graphics capabilities which make use of DEC's graphic interface. In addition, data can be sent to BMDP, which is a sophisticated statistical package. BMDP is not part of RS/1 and must be obtained separately ($700 for a 2-year license).

RPL programs written by Bolt, Beranek, and Newman (BBN) or by users are made publicly available.

Other Features. A File Transfer Program exists to ease transfer of data to other PDP-11s. A public-domain questionnaire and report generator, the "Data Entry Terminal (DET)," can be linked to RS/1. The DET features questionnaire formatting, data editing, and report formating in tables or in lists. Operating a DET requires a system manager familiar with the computer system and its text editor. Furthermore, the data item checks are not incorporated into a central data base definition file.

Installation, Support, and Costs. RS/1 runs on the IBM PC XT and AT, the DEC PRO 350 and 380, and the DEC Micro PDP-11 and the Micro Vax. RS/1 ranges in price from $3000 to $12,200, depending on whether it is being run on an IBM or a DEC PRO ($3000), a single-user Micro 11 or Micro-Vax ($6000), or a multi-user Micro 1 or Vax ($12,200). Support and updates are available for $200 per year on the IBM, 12 per cent of purchase per year on the DEC. Bolt, Beranek, and Newman is located at 50 Moulton St., Cambridge, MA, 02238.

CLINFO

The CLINFO system was developed under the sponsorship of the Division of Research Resources, National Institutes of Health, by a consortium consisting of personnel from the Rand corporation and four medical schools: Baylor, Washington, Oklahoma, and Vanderbilt. This group carried out an extensive requirements analysis to determine the needs of clinical investigators. CLINFO was first conceived as a tool for strictly defined research protocols in small intensive care units.

CLINFO runs on PDP-11s but not on the Micro 11. We include CLINFO in this survey despite the fact that they have no microcomputer version at present because CLINFO+, to be released in early 1986 on DEC Vax, will run on the Micro Vax II. CLINFO+ has kept the same data model and user interface as CLINFO, although a number of the limits will recede.

CLINFO is programmed in BASIC PLUS 2. CLINFO+ will be programmed in C. The system operates through a menu-driven dialogue. A system manager, a person with a programming background, is required to run various aspects of the operation of CLINFO, including merging data from the data entry files for permanent storage in the data base.

Data Base Definition. Investigators define a separate data base for each study. Users perceive CLINFO as having a three-dimensional data base structure consisting of patients, data items, and times of sample collection. The underlying data model is a hierarchy limited to three levels. The top level is "patients," the second level consists of branching items called panels, and the third level consists of the data items in each panel. A panel is identified by its name. A particular occurrence of a named panel is identified by the date and time of sample collection for the items it contains. Patients are identified by an ID up to eight characters long.

For each data item, investigators enter a name, a description, a data type, and some further characteristics based on the data type. The names of data items are at most eight characters long; their description is at most 20. There are six data types: text, number, character, date, time, and event. Text items can contain up to 70 characters, but cannot be searched; they record short comments. A panel containing a text item cannot contain any other kind of item. Number items contain real numbers and can be checked for data type and range. Character items are multiple choice, drawing their values from coded lists of up to 30 codes, each of which can be up to eight characters long. Character items are checked to see if a code belongs to the list. Longer lists of codes have to be accommodated through numbers, thereby placing the entire burden of managing codes and their meaning on the user. Date and time can be checked for data type and range. There can only be one searchable date per panel, which would seem to present restrictions on the representation of events associated with several dates (admission and discharge, for instance). Event items automatically take as values the data collection time entered for the panel containing a particular "controlling" item. An event can be defined to automatically take on a time value equal to the value entered at the data collection time when the controlling item takes on a first, last, minimum, maximum, or special value. Data items can be flagged as confidential but this has no programmed effect. There are no security provisions beyond the operating system's file security and log-on procedure. Once data entry has begun, the data base definition may only be edited in a limited way by the system manager.

CLINFO supports a total of 5488 patients per data base, 224 panels per data base, 1568 items per data base, and 30 items per panel. A data base is designed to support one research protocol. Data cannot be shared among data bases except by moving them through special files. The designer must specify the number of patients expected in a data base and the number of instances expected for each panel in order to optimize space allocation.

Data Entry. Data are entered into an UPDATE FILE. CLINFO requires that the system manager move data from the UPDATE FILE to the data base after verification. Users first specify a patient ID, a date and time of data collection, and a panel name. CLINFO then prompts for each item in the panel by name. The sequence of the prompts within a panel can be predetermined, but there is no branching logic based on user responses. If a number value is out of range, the system says so but allows the user to override it. Text item values cannot be checked for anything other than maximum length. Item values can be edited while entering data by replacing values. This replaces the previous value. There is no on-line help function within the entry facility to explain what values are expected for each item, in case the system rejects a value. Once a user begins entering or retrieving data or doing anything with a data base, the entire data base is made unavailable to other users. Machine-readable data can be transferred into the system.

Once in the UPDATE FILE, data can be edited by deleting and re-entering a panel. Once in the data base, the data can be examined panel by panel and edited but only by replacing item values. Data can be typed into worksheets directly or copied from the STUDY DATA FILE. They can then be analyzed or used for computations, and moved to the data base. Missing values, edited values, and out-of-range values are indicated in the data base by special codes.

Retrieval. Data can be moved from the data base to worksheets, where analyses are done, to the terminal for display, or to communication files, where the data can be processed by a program written in whatever language the operating system supports. CLINFO systems obtained through the NIH support BASIC 11. Data in communication files can be moved to another machine. Each data base may have 10 such communication files.

The rows and columns of the output table can be any two of the following dimensions: patients, items, or times. The third dimension is held constant in any one table. The user can specify the patient or patient subset, the items or panels, the time period relative to a time marker (an event or absolute date), and the time unit that determines the resolution of the retrieved data. The time period may be between two time markers, a list of time units relative to an event, or a range of units relative to a marker. The first, last, minimum, maximum, mean, or nth value can be specified within each unit so as to avoid retrieving more than one occurrence of an item per unit. The values retrieved can also be restricted through the same logical conditions as in subset creation. An event can serve to single out a particular occurrence of a data value so that its date and time act as reference points for the retrieval process. A display of all the events, their type, date, time, controlling item, and the latter's value is available. The retrieval process can be complex; thus, the user is presented with an updated list of the specifications after each new one is entered.

Analysis. Subsets of patients can be created and stored according to specified criteria. However, it is not possible to create subsets of panels, so that statistically, "patient" is the only unit of analysis. Subsets can be created by placing logical conditions on existing subsets. There are two kinds of conditions: number, date, and time items can be restricted to a range of values and character items to lists of values. It is not possible to create subsets based on text items. Subsets can be joined by "and," "or," or "not." The time period during which items must take on their required values can be specified, much as in retrieval. There is a set of graphics and exploratory statistical programs. Data can also be transferred to statistical packages.

Special Options. RESPONSE FILES provide the capability of automatically remembering a user's responses to CLINFO prompts so that any task can be repeated, regardless of its complexity. RESPONSE FILES can be edited to allow for variability in execution. BBN's File Transfer Programs and data entry facility, DET, are also available, as described for RS/1.

A system manager is required to open up new projects and grant access to a data base. There are no provisions for owning patients or restricting access to particular data items.

Installation, Support, and Costs. CLINFO runs on PDP-11s under the RSX-11M operating system or on the VAX under VMS. Because of the use of BASIC+ and an unmodular design, modifications to the system are very costly, and they have awaited the development of CLINFO+. However, the fact that CLINFO+ is not improving on the CLINFO data model will continue to cause difficulty to those who have a need for a deeper hierarchical structure or relational structures.

Clinical research centers may apply for special NIH grants to obtain CLINFO from BBN. This grant includes salary for a system manager with a programming background, which the designers feel is necessary to manage the system. CLINFO can be purchased from BBN for a $40,000 license fee, which includes training, installation, documentation, and 1 year of maintenance. Additional maintenance is available.

Clinical Data Manager

Clinical Data Manager (CDM) was designed by the Health Systems Project at the Harvard School of Public Health as a general-purpose DBMS for clinical and public health research and patient care. The design stresses the need to integrate the concerns of patient care and administration with those of research. Consequently, numerous reporting options are available, as well as a link to a word processor. The system has supported a variety of projects in the Harvard Medical Area since 1976 and has been disseminated since 1982 in a new release written in Standard MUMPS.

CDM is a user-friendly system based on menu-driven dialogue with on-line help available at every turn. CDM is designed for intensive use without the need for any professional programmer.

Data Base Definition. CDM's data base definition is fully integrated: all parts of the system reference this definition to provide each application its on-line help tailored to user-defined needs.

CDM has a hierarchical-relational data base structure. Any number of hierarchies can be related to each other in ways similar to the joins in relational systems; they are linked so that queries and reports can be run on more than one hierarchy at a time. This is useful in patient care applications that need separate hierarchy files to represent doctors or drug protocols without repeating the data on these for each patient, as would be done in a pure hierarchical system. Users define the top item in each hierarchy, as well as all branching and leaf items. A hierarchy can accommodate many levels of branching items, for a total of up to 1×10^{15} data items.

CDM's multilevel hierarchies are designed to represent subordinate groups of items which themselves contain logically related groups of items, a common situation in medical records. For instance, a patient might have a branching item "hospitalization," consisting in turn of a number of branching items such as laboratory tests, operations, and so on. An operation branching item might contain several procedure items for procedures performed during the same operation, each procedure being characterized by its own descriptors.

Users who do not program will define their data base an item at a time through a dialogue which provides help on-line and checks for logical inconsistencies. For each item, the user specifies a name and a short name recognized by all the system's facilities. The system will also recognize any unambiguous abbreviation of the name or short name. The data base definer can give a help description, which other users can view as part of help messages, and a description of unlimited length to describe the item and its purpose in depth. Also defined are the maximum number of occurrences, maximum length, and security classification.

Because CDM is written in MUMPS, users are spared the task of managing the physical structure of the disk in terms of allocating space before data entry and reallocating space after data deletion. Thus, the maximum number of occurrences is set only for data quality control reasons and, like any other definitional characteristic, can be modified at any time.

Each leaf item is characterized in a variety of ways, depending on its data type, which are set up in a natural way that is understandable to unsophisticated users. There are nine data types: integer, decimal, text, date, time, list, list/free text, yes/no, and computed. Date and time items can be used to time stamp branching items, as in VISIT and VISIT DATE.

List items represent any number of user-defined, discrete choices, each of which has a coded and an English representation recognized as equivalent by all the system's facilities. A special multiple choice type item, "list/free text," allows "other" values, which are not a part of the coded list. The "other" values are treated as string values, can be queried, and can be converted to newly entered codes at a later date. Thus, codes don't have to be fully established at the start, a common requirement in medicine.

Text, integer, and floating point items can have their values constrained to fit a pattern defined in terms of a sequence of the particular number of letters, numbers, or punctuation allowed. All items can have their values constrained to lie within a certain numeric or alphabetic range.

Leaf items can be defined as unique identifiers for any branching items immediately above them. The designer can also define leaf items so that they are indexed in inverted files at the time of entry. CDM is optimized for retrieval so that inverted files need only be used for data manipulation purposes, sparing the users the frequently time-consumming task of inverting items when they need to run a query.

Similarly, any text item can be made an alphabetic key so that patients can be identified by name simply by entering leading characters. In case of ambiguity, a dialogue offers users a list of choices. Any alternate key, primary or alphabetic, can be used in place of other identifiers at any place in the system's dialogue.

Each characteristic defining a data item can be modified through an editor, even after data entry has begun. The editor then displays the modified item definition for approval. Both leaf and branching items can be added or removed, again even after data entry and without regard for physical storage effects.

Data Entry. There are three ways of entering data: through a data entry facility, through a screen package, and through a questionnaire written in the system's applications language, AL. In all data entry modes the system answers requests for help with an English description of the item generated from the data base definition. The description includes the designer's short description, the maximum length, the overall range, the units, the pattern, and the list of values if there is one. The system recognizes codes for missing and null values. Automatic code translation occurs for multiple-choice items; several English values can be mapped to the same internal value, greatly reducing the need for precoding medical data and enabling specialists to map their individual vocabularies into a common scheme.

The data entry facility functions when the data base has been defined. It prompts the data enterer by tracing through the data base structure, checking each value against the item's definition. Special codes enable users to back up and edit, skip over branching items and their subitems, or quit the facility. The screen package requires some definition of screen lay-out and is closely integrated to the data base definition.

An amateur programmer can write questionnaires incorporating branching logic, control structures, and more complex consistency checking. Data is edited by replacing specified characters in item values referenced through the item name. In order to allow multiple users to enter and edit data for the same item, the item value a user is working on becomes the level other users are locked out from, as opposed to the branch level or, indeed, the data base level on some systems.

Retrieval. CDM has two levels of retrieval facilities. The more interactive, or conversational, one has a help function and builds up the nonprocedural display specification through a dialogue with the user. This dialogue ends by translating the specification into English for approval and into the more terse display specification as a learning aid. The second level of query recognizes the terse nonprocedural language. There are numerous options for specifying the form and content of reports. The two basic display formats are hierarchical and tabular. The hierarchical format follows the data base structure; the tabular one "flattens" it, displaying the leaf items on one level as columns. Leaf items are displayed along with the unique identifier for the top item they describe.

Any combination of leaf and branching items can be viewed. Any list of cases, or branching items occurrences, defined through the query system can be picked for display, as can cases listed through keys, including alphabetic keys, which means asking for patient reports using their name. Users can display the first, last, or nth entry occurrence of an item value. Reports can be given titles; items can be displayed in numeric, alphabetic, and other orders; and all specifications can be saved for later reuse. A columnar report generator provides for sorting down five levels in the hierarchy with accompanying counts, totals, and averages at each level. For example, this could be used to get average laboratory values for visits sorted by dates for patients sorted by name.

Finally, a link to a commercial quality word processor enables users to pass data into the text of articles and letters—for example, echocardiogram reports, catheterization reports, letters to referring physicians, recall notices to patients identified through the query system, and so forth.

Analysis. Analysis proceeds in two stages: first, a selection of values and, second, statistical analysis. The query system, like the display facility, allows two levels of use. The more interactive one builds up a list of conditions that the user is then asked to join logically, also by joining some to form another condition and then joining that one to others. An English translation of the final query specification is shown for approval, along with its representation in the query language as a learning aid. A browsing feature allows users to look around in the data base and gain an idea of the items' meanings from the data base definition.

The conditional operators include the usual arithmetic operators (<, >, =, and so on), string operators (precedes alphabetically, contains, MUMPS pattern-match), date and time operators (before, after), and operators used on any item (equals, between, not between). Quantifiers can be used to specify how many values should meet the condition.

The resulting subsets can be stored and automatically updated at user-defined intervals. The subsets are lists of occurrences of branching items and thus do not take up extra space through duplication of data. These lists can consist of any branching item, giving full freedom of choice as to the unit of analysis. Thus, analyses can be made on patients, on their visits, on procedures, and on any branch item unit without having to go through complex sort and merge operations, as you would in SAS or RS/1. Subsets can also be created through a powerful, procedural data manipulation language, which is described subsequently.

Subsets can be displayed in a variety of formats or put in tabular form with their associated data on a tape for transfer to a statistical package or a word processor, including those built into the system. Subsets can be manipulated through the use of boolean logic (intersection, union, difference, complement) and through the use of various options for editing and displaying slices and their contents.

CDM features a built-in statistical package for exploratory data analysis, which has the unique feature of understanding the multi-level hierarchy and thus enabling analyses with lower level branch items, such as visit and procedure, as the unit of analysis without sorting and merging.

Special Features. The AL applications language is designed to allow amateur programmers to access the data base for a variety of purposes without having to possess detailed knowledge of file designs or conventional programming languages. In addition to writing questionnaires, users can produce reports in good English based on information in the data base. Flexible formating commands are available. AL can also be used to process machine-readable data for storage. Occasional data maintenance tasks, which would otherwise require an involved programming effort, are made much simpler. These might include rearranging data after the data base has been restructured, carrying out periodic consistency checks, or changing a coding scheme such as ICDA.

An access control system protects data through passwords, assignment of capabilities such as querying, and definition of items to protect all or even selected individual values. CDM also is being linked to a Practice Management System to provide billing, scheduling, general ledger, and other management functions that are similar to what COSTAR provides.

Installation, Support, and Costs. The documentation consists of 10 manuals. CDM is available from Clinical Data, Inc., at prices ranging from $4000 for a four-user permanent license to $8000 for 12 users and

$10,000 for large VAX systems. The license includes training, documentation, and a 90-day warranty. Support and updates are available for $900 per year.

CDM runs on any machine with an ANSI Standard MUMPS operating system. These include IBM XT/AT, DEC Micro 11, Micro VAX, Motorola 68000, Plexus, AT&T 3B2, Convergent Technology microcomputers, Altos, and many others. Clinical Data, Inc., sells turnkey packages on the IBM PC AT, the DEC Micro-11, and the DEC Micro-VAX. Clinical Data, Inc., is located at 1172 Commonwealth Avenue, Boston, MA 02134.

THE VA FILE MANAGER

The VA File Manager was designed in the Veterans' Administration environment to answer the needs of MUMPS programmers who were designing systems and continually having to write similar programs for data management in operational situations: laboratory systems, personnel files, and so on. The File Manager makes an effort to present nonprogramming users with tools, but its basic orientation is to provide hooks for MUMPS programmers to write their routines. The system is in the public domain and maintained by the VA for VA users; the VA cannot sign contracts to support outside installations.

Database Definition. The File Manager (FM) features a multilevel hierarchy as a data model. The File Manager has procedures for linking several hierarchies to model data that are independent of data in other hierarchies. For instance, users might want to keep track of data about patients and doctors or pharmacies. These entities do not depend on each other for their existence, so the most natural way of representing them is by separate hierarchies.

FM allows nonprogrammers to describe or define a hierarchical data base through an English language dialogue. Data types include numbers, text, lists, and dates. Times are treated as an adjunct to dates under certain circumstances; otherwise, they have no independent existence. Multiple choice lists in the File Manager are restricted in the number of values an item can have without resorting to "pointers" to separate hierarchies storing other values, which have to be maintained. It is possible to write a MUMPS code to specify conversion to upper or lower case for free text items (a necessity in order to be able to search them); also programmable are pattern matching constraints for numbers, text, and lists.

Data Entry. FM has a data entry facility ready for use after data base definition; it checks incoming data against that definition. The File Manager facility allows questions to be recorded. If a user wants to skip questions based on answers to previous ones (branching logic), a MUMPS program is needed.

Retrieval. FM provides a query system to allow nonprogrammers to ask unplanned questions. Conditions include less than, greater than, string contains, equals, not equals, and MUMPS operators.

FM allows users to store the results of a search as a subset for further manipulation, such as printouts and further searches. Further manipulations of subsets, such as using boolean logic on several subsets, editing subsets, and so on must be done in MUMPS.

FM only understands subsets based on a collection of cases of the top-level item. Thus, a user can never say "those visits where such and such was true" (unless visit is the top level item)—only "those patients who had at least one visit in which such and such was true."

In order to place selection criteria on an item and have the search run with any reasonable speed, a user must have defined that item as an inverted file, which means that data is organized in order to put all the values of an item together, instead of in their standard place in an individual record. Secondary files increase storage requirements.

Analysis. The File Manager has some descriptive statistics. However, there is no provision for moving data off to a statistical package without programming in MUMPS.

Installation, Support, and Costs. File Manager is in the public domain and can be obtained at nominal cost. File Manager is recognized to have sparse documentation. A single user's manual (35 pages) is targeted to both programmers and nonprogrammers. A second manual, the technical manual (20 pages), allows MUMPS programmers to use the system's hooks for their routines, but does not describe the internal workings of the system or the relationship between routines. This would make it quite difficult for any group outside the VA to learn the system enough to provide support or maintenance. Making enhancements would be more difficult.

FM runs on most any standard MUMPS machine. These include IBM XT/AT, DEC Micro 11, Micro Vax, Motorola 68000, Plexus, AT&T 3B2, Convergent Technology microcomputers, Altos, and many others. The File Manager can be obtained from the MUMPS Users' Group, P.O. Box 37247, Washington, DC 20013.

INGRES

INGRES was created in a university environment and has now moved to the private sector through Relational Technology, Inc. A number of firms have taken the INGRES system and have done their own enhancements. INGRES was one of the first systems to incorporate the notion of a nonprocedural language (QUEL) to handle all aspects of data management, data entry, reporting, and querying. However, it is command-driven, rather than dialogue- and menu-driven, and lacks the ability to respond with help messages, except as noted.

Data Base Definition. Users create tables through the command language QUEL. There are two basic data types: character and numbers. A programmer must set up routines to deal with dates and times. There are five number data types according to whether they are 1-, 2-, or 3-byte integers and 4- or 8-byte floating point. Coded lists are treated as either numbers or characters so that there is no built-in way of translating codes into their English equivalent or of mapping multiple English text labels onto the same code.

Character items can be up to 255 characters long. There is limited data compression, and the management of variable length data requires programmer intervention. Because medical data are typically sparse— that is, not all data items contain data for each patient—there can be a fair amount of wasted storage space, particularly if any free-text comments are being stored. The addition of a column in a table requires unloading and reloading the table.

The characteristics of each data item, other than the maximum length, which is defined along with the data type, are defined through the integrity command, which is applied to tables once they have been initially set up. The integrity command takes as its qualification or descriptive statement the following conditional operators: $=$, $>$, $<$, $\geq$, $\leq$, and not $\neq$. This command can be applied after data have been entered; if there are data that violate the constraints, this is reported and such data are then identified through the query commands.

However, if this integrity constraint is violated during an update operation, that particular update is ignored but not reported. Constraints must be removed to be replaced in order to alter them. In order to remove a constraint, the constraint's identifying number is looked up in a table, and a destroy integrity command is applied to the table with that number.

Data Entry. The command-driven data entry procedure would be too cumbersome for operational data entry, though useful for updating numerous elements according to an algorithm in QUEL. INGRES features a Visual Forms Editor, which allows users to set up default screens automatically derived from tables they have created. These can then be modified according to a number of parameters, including location of data item name, data slot for the data, lines, instructional text, and so on. Relational checks, that is, checks against other data, can be accomplished but only with other incoming data, not with data in the data base.

Some further checks pertain to the data base definition, but are set up only through the forms editor, making for a less than fully integrated data base definition. As noted previously, this can lead to problems with data integrity if multiple forms are used to enter data for the same data items or columns. Such checks include character string checks against a partial pattern match and checks against a list of legal values. There is no automatic conversion of English to coded value. Other checks, such as the range and the maximum number of characters, can be respecified in the forms editor, but this may lead to some confusion over an item's definition.

Although the command-driven update procedure will not flag errors, these are flagged in the interactive forms-oriented package, and the user is given an opportunity to re-enter the data. There is a cursor-controlled back-up and edit capability. The data editor itself is very complex, consisting of a number of commands for locating the precise character to be edited through positional notations. The concept of the editor frequently found in MUMPS systems, in which one simply specifies enough of the characters to uniquely identify the ones to be changed, is lacking. The MUMPS editor can easily accommodate insertions, deletions, and changes, which require separate commands in the INGRES editor.

Once data on a screen are entered, they must be put into the data base through a CONTROL-Z command. There appears to be no provisions for data-dependent branching, which is of interest in the sparse world of medical data. Thus, the user must TAB over the appropriate number of times to the next field or screen for which data must be entered.

There are no provisions for special codes for missing values. Table cells are null until filled and null if skipped over. However, as we have seen, it is crucial in research applications to be able, at least for some items, to distinguish between values that are missing and will never be obtained, values that are missing and will be obtained, and perhaps other types of missing values or values that indicate that a data item was prompted for but no data was available.

Retrieval. The QUEL language can be used to obtain displays of tables or of particular columns and rows in tables.

The INGRES Report Writer allows the user to set up a default report and then edit it or to set up a report from scratch. Such reports allow the user to select data columns, sort the data at several levels, position the text on the page, print summary data at defined breaks, and otherwise manipulate tabular data. One drawback of the tabular format is that if there are more columns than the width of the page can accommodate, the report has to make use of some sort of wrap-around feature, a practice that can be avoided in hierarchically organized reports in which arbitrarily large numbers of data items can be accommodated vertically, repeating for each case with indentations to denote the various levels, the approximate hierarchical equivalent of tables.

Analysis. The QUEL language, which approximates the relational calculus, also serves as a query language. Thus, users have to learn a language—there is no interactive help or browsing facility. The syntax is nonprocedural and allows users to retrieve selected data into new tables through a qualifying statement of the form "where" followed by a set of conditions using $=$, $<$, $>$, and combinations or negatives thereof. Partial pattern matching is supported. Computations may be performed during retrieval, using arithmetic operators and a library of trigonometric functions and square root functions.

A simplified query procedure is present in the "Query by Form" user interface: users can call up the form screen used for data entry and put in query statements in place of data, but in most cases only one conditional operator can be accommodated per data item.

This technique presents the further drawback of causing investigators to look at their data querying in the same way they view their data entry. An important aspect of data base systems is to model a certain reality; the closer one comes to that reality, the more varied your ad-hoc querying can be. Yet forms may well diverge from the data model and vice versa.

Queries over data in multiple tables can be performed, but an extra condition must be included for the first additional table and perhaps more than one for additional ones, depending on the keys used to identify each table. Thus, with a patient table and a hospitalization table, the query on hospitalization data would have to include a statement such as Patient I.D.–Hospital I.D. to ensure that the data referred to the same patient. If there is a table for the multiple procedures performed during one hospitalization, it might be necessary to identify not only the patient I.D. in the procedure table but also which hospitalization it occurred in, leading to a string of these equality statements.

An alternative is to create large tables "joining" several such base tables, but in INGRES such tables, called "views," contain only the data as of its date of creation. Furthermore, they add overhead to the system's operation. Finally, they suffer from the problems of repeated data as discussed in the introductory section on relational systems.

Statistics. There are a very few statistical features: counts, means, minimum, maximum, and sums. These are applied to columns and can be incorporated into the computational syntax with arithmetic operators to produce such results as averages by column categories of column values.

INGRES provides access to its data bases from certain languages on DEC's Micro Vax-11. Thus, QUEL statements can be embedded into Vax C, FORTRAN, Pascal, BASIC, and COBOL. This would allow programmers to move data into statistical packages on the Vax or through the Vax to packages on other machines.

Installation, Support, and Costs. INGRES is available from Relational Technology, Inc., Suite 515, 2855 Telegraph Avenue, Berkeley, CA 94705. INGRES licenses cost around $2,000 ($200 per year for support and updates) on the following 68000-based microcomputers: Sun, Convergent Megaframe, NCR Tower, and the Elexi. INGRES licenses cost $15,000 for a supported license on the Micro Vax. Support runs to $4,000 per year. INGRES will be avilable under DOS, then under UNIX, on the IBM XT and AT by the end of 1985. An earlier, noncommercial version of INGRES can still be obtained from the University of California at Berkley for $200.

ORACLE

ORACLE is similar to the INGRES system, although ORACLE seems to have more functionality and enhanced throughput. ORACLE makes use of a command language very similar to QUEL called SQL. It is up to the applications specialist to generate menus.

Data Base Definition. ORACLE is a relational DBMS that supports the same data types as INGRES, in addition to date, time, and coded lists. Dates include the time of day in a date, which is noon by default if no time is specified. Time is supported only through the forms-oriented interface, as is a data type for money. Both date and time have a variety of formats, but they have to be predefined. A set of functions aid in manipulating dates and times in arithmetic expressions.

The coded lists in the SQL command language consist of one text value mapped to each code, which can only consist of integers—this is quite limiting in medicine, in which codes are frequently text or a combination of letters and numbers. The forms editor permits look-ups to a table of value without any code translation.

Like INGRES, ORACLE's data base definition process is command-driven, and the remarks on INGRES's data base definition process apply here, too. The SQL definitional characteristics include name, maximum length, and whether the values are unique or not for a given row. These characteristics are kept in the data base tables.

Other characteristics are defined through the Interactive Applications Facility, which defines screen-oriented input, query, and update routines. Thus, the classic data dictionary file, or data base definition, is in fact stored in two places: through the SQL commands and through the screen definition. If a different screen is set up, it is incumbent on the user to retain the previous definition. Similarly, if the same item appears in several screens, the user should ensure that the definition remains compatible. This can lead to severe data integrity problems, especially with less sophisticated users.

Data item characteristics defined through the data entry process include whether the item is mandatory, whether it has fixed length, its range check, some data types such as time and money, whether the value must exist in a table of values, whether values must be converted to all upper case or all lower case before storing, and a help message. If the user requests help, only this message is displayed, a possible drawback to the data enterer who may want to know which of the item characteristics has caused a value to be rejected.

Users pay an additional penalty with such a data base definition, as queries can be produced that don't match the item characteristics or its relationship to other items and reports generated on the basis of requests that would otherwise fail a test against the item definition either for item characteristics or for structural relationships between items in the query. There is no built-in way to decode a set of values into English equivalents, nor are there built-in units automatically associated with a column.

ORACLE employs data compression to reduce the usual problems tabular systems have with storage of sparse data. However, this is a physical technique, and users are still confronted with the empty cells of the table on the logical side with all that implies in querying and reporting. Some aspects of the physical characteristics of data on the disk must be managed, such as allocation of space, which periodically must be redone in a growing data base.

Unlike INGRES, a view can be updated directly. However, the view must be on a single table, so users are not relieved of the problem of data concurrency between base tables and the views they make up, if these are modeling hierarchical, patient care data.

Data Entry. ORACLE has a screen-oriented data entry and update applications generator, which is more sophisticated than INGRES's. Forms can be made to follow each other sequentially; data can be retrieved and updated, allowing the user to enter missing data at a later time more easily.

Data editing proceeds through these forms, and the editing commands are considerably simpler than in INGRES. Users can also use the command language to edit, but this is cumbersome, except in the case of multiple edits according to some algorithm, and may suffer from naming problems owing to the possibility of a difference between the screen prompt and the column name.

The maximum number of screens in a questionnaire is 31. Users can move back and forth sequentially according to the pre-established screen order, but there is no branching logic, which in a sparse data world may present some problems. The screens are defined through a sophisticated, nonprocedural applications generator, which proceeds through a dialogue to establish each item and its associated characteristics. Its complexity would seem to preclude use by unsophisticated users.

The locking granularity, like INGRES, is at the table level. Therefore, only one user can enter data into a given table at a given time without potential collisions.

Retrieval. Additions to the command language provide a rich command-driven reporting capability, involving numerous nonprocedural data manipulations prior to output. A report generator contains a complex set of commands, which include procedural statements, precluding its use by unsophisticates. There is no built-in step-by-step dialogue or on-line help in formulating reports.

Analysis. ORACLE provides the same query capabilities as INGRES and features additional string and date manipulation operators. ORACLE provides for fast retrieval on keys. However, it is suggested that only two to three items per table be made a key, as otherwise, update, insert, and delete operations suffer performance degradation. Thus, queries on most items run more slowly, unless an item is temporarily made a key and then unkeyed, which requires some judgment as to which items to key.

The use of clustering, another physical disk management technique, allows tables that are frequently referenced together through a join to reduce their duplicate join key through which the tables are linked to a single cluster key, the tables residing side by side on the disk. However, this would require sophisticated users to set up and manage.

Users can query through the forms package, as in INGRES, but this suffers from the fundamental limitations inherent in conceptualizing data from the data entry point of view. Ideally, one wants the data base definition to reflect the clinical reality as close as possible and have both data entry and querying independent of the definition conceptually so that a query does not have to depend on structures set up for ease of use in data entry. The more independent the data base definition, the closer it represents a reality, and the easier it is to ask unplanned questions. This query by form provides no interactive help based on the data base definition. It allows users one condition next to the items, then others at the bottom of the screen.

ORACLE contains the same type of limited statistical features as INGRES. Its richer command language allows for more easy construction of such displays as histograms than in a programming language. As in INGRES, data can be analyzed by exporting it to a formal statistical package.

Availability. ORACLE is available from Oracle Corporation, 7315 Wisconsin Avenue, Suite 1200 West, Bethesda, MD 20814. ORACLE licenses cost $6,000 for six copies (the minimum). Support is $1200 per year; updates cost $200. ORACLE runs on the following microcomputers: IBM XT and AT, the AT&T 3B2 and 300 (UNIX PC), the DEC Rainbow, Micro PDP-11, and Micro Vax, the NCR Tower, the TI Professional, the Convergent Technology microcomputers, the Compaq, and other IBM PC "look-alikes."

MEDLOG

Like some other systems we review, MEDLOG is descended from a mainframe forebearer, TOD, the Time Oriented Database, developed at Stanford University. MEDLOG runs on IBM XTs and ATs. By adhering closely to the TOD design, MEDLOG designers have implemented a research machine for time-oriented medical problems which former TOD users have been able to adapt to quite readily. MEDLOG is able to handle multiple data bases per copy and multiple users on each machine. MEDLOG handles up to 32,767 patients per data base, up to 65,535 encounters per data base, and up to 1000 items per data base, together with an additional 900 computed items. There is a limit of 25 data pages per encounter, which at 59 bytes per page, means a limit of 1475 bytes or characters per encounter.

Data Base Definition. MEDLOG's data model consists of a three-level hierarchy with one node at the third level: ENCOUNTER. Using this structure makes it easy to implement a variety of derived values (COMPUTE) options and options for sophisticated time-oriented retrieval. However, it does make it difficult to adequately represent time-related events, especially events that repeat in the context of other events, as discussed in the section on hierarchical systems.

With the DEFINE program, MEDLOG users define their data items as belonging to one of two categories: time-variant and time-invariant. Time-variant variables occur under the ENCOUNTER node and can be grouped into panels for data entry purposes, with up to 20 variables per panel. Only time-invariant variables can be text variables or numeric variables. All time-variant variables must be numeric.

The text variables for one data base cannot total more than 984 characters in length and are meant to record names, addresses, names of relatives, and other small bits of data not exceeding 40 characters each. Text variables cannot be searched or used for statistical purposes.

A built-in data type enables users to store up to 20 lines of 62 characters each for notes associated with a particular ENCOUNTER. This does not need to be predefined. For numeric items, users need to specify storage sizes, scale multipliers, and paging (which of 25 pages holding 59 bytes of data each that the variable is stored in); these are all related to physical storage characteristics. Such parameters are not needed for dates. There is no specific data type for time, as in the time of day an event occurs. Coded lists must have numbers as their stored values and are associated with text values for encoding purposes. The total length of all the code values for a particular coded item cannot exceed 125 characters, thus limiting the number of codes that can be stored for any one item.

Some aspects of the data base definition can be changed without damaging existing data, but many such changes may result in the need to re-enter previously entered data: there is no language or facility for converting old data to the new format. Such problems may arise when changing value codes, storage type, scale multipliers, and variable length. However, time-invariant variables can be changed to time-variant variables without difficulty.

Data Entry. Users select patients to enter data for through their last name, system key, or medical record number. Because data can be grouped in panels, each of which can continue into further panels, data can be conveniently grouped for entry purposes, though all are stored under the ENCOUNTER node. Thus, before any data can be entered, an ENCOUNTER with its encounter date must be entered for that patient.

Coded values are entered either through their numeric values or through the entire text equivalent, which must make for brief codes. Dates can be entered in American or International format, but must be entered as MM/DD/YY. The allowable precision for numeric data is determined by the scale multiplier.

Data are checked against the data base definition, and a variety of error messages can be returned if the check fails. Commands exist for moving the cursor, finding out the data base definition, quitting, and skipping to the next panel.

In order for the time-oriented features to work properly, encounters must be entered in the sequence in which they occur. If the encounters get out of sequence, a special program, FIXUP, is used to place the offending encounter back into sequence.

Retrieval. There are two flavors of reporting: (1) the Chart program, which displays all or part of a patient record, and (2) a separate, optional Report Generator, which produces group displays with formating and sorting. Chart allows users to select all encounters, the last four encounters, or encounters in a date or encounter number range. Individual variables or panels can be selected for display. Patients are identified by patient numbers, simple numeric tests on variables, or by membership in a group, established through the MEDLOG query system. The Report Generator provides custom reports for selected data sets.

Analysis. Analysis proceeds in several steps: transposition of the data into files optimized for searching and analysis, searching, and analysis. Transposition must occur prior to any querying or analysis. This is adequate for pure research use, but would make MEDLOG very cumbersome in any patient care application, in which one may need to query and report the data as soon as it is entered. Research and administrative uses would conflict, since a long statistical analysis would require that the transpose file remain unchanged, precluding the possibility of doing queries on fresh data.

MEDLOG provides a rich variety of computed item expressions used to derive new items from previously entered data. All the usual arithmetic operators are present, including logs and trigonometric functions. A variety of functions exist to aid in computing items when the entered values have to come from the previous encounter or some designated encounter. Date arithmetic is supported.

The MEDLOG query system (GROUP) has the usual arithmetic conditions and an interesting set of time-oriented conditions. Users can place conditions so as to compare values between different encounters selected in several ways: next encounter, last encounter, and encounter within a time period $+/-$ a time window. These are used to answer questions of the type "blood pressure $> \times$ within 6 months after surgery." Users can test for increases or decreases to a value (the same value for all patients being compared) or a range of values between encounters selected by these time criteria, as well as increase/decrease by percentage or by amount (the amount is added/subtracted to/from the initial patient value). You can test for the cumulative total, as in the total dosage of a drug. You can test for missing and entered values.

Once selected, groups, or subsets, can be manipulated in a variety of ways using the standard boolean logic. Groups can then be used to create reports and perform statistical analysis. There is a limit of 256 groups per data base, a somewhat low number for extensive analysis.

A rich set of exploratory data analysis techniques include bar charts, correlations, t-tests, MxN tables, anova, scatterplots with linear regression, Kaplan-Meier survival curves, and others. A COMMUNICATE program produces data sets for use in the major statistical packages: SAS, SPSS, and BMDP.

Availability. MEDLOG can be obtianed from Information Analysis Corporation, 201 San Antonio Circle, Suite 125, Mountain View, CA 94040. MEDLOG runs on the IBM XT/AT and sells for $7500 for the basic package. Options include Advanced Regression Analysis ($500), COMMUNICATIONS ($750), and Report Generator ($750). A multi-user, networked version sells for $9500 for the file server and first work station, costing $1,000 per work station thereafter.

SCIENTIFIC INFORMATION RETRIEVAL SYSTEM (SIR)

The Scientific Information Retrieval System (SIR) is a FORTRAN-based DBMS designed to meets the needs of the scientific research community, particularly those who are working with fairly large and flat data sets in a batch or quasi-batch environment. SIR runs on mainframes and large (32-bit) minicomputers. It is now being made to run on some 32-bit microcomputers, such as the Micro Vax, HP 9000, Sun, and Apollo.

SIR users proceed throughout the system via a command language. This becomes frankly procedural during retrieval. Users must take care to use commands properly, with the right syntax and in the right order.

Data Base Definition. SIR possesses an integrated data base definition, although because of its original batch orientation, there is no on-line documentation based on the definition. A sample SIR run in the User's Manual Appendix shows that it take 43 commands to set up a data base of 14 items.

SIR supports a network data model, which has features of a three-level hierarchy and those of a relational system because hierarchies can have many:many links (that is, doctors can have many patients and patients many doctors, if PATIENT and DOCTOR are two hierarchies).

Data types include integer, real values, text, list, date, and time. The format of the various data types is card-oriented, using columns and positional notation geared to batch entry. An interactive editor can be used to set up interactive entry with the same card-oriented commands used to specify the data type. Dates and times have to be entered in a specified format—none are built in. Lists can be automatically coded to integers, if the appropriate command is specified—this is to "save space." Another command specifies the list of valid values in a list. Still another command establishes labels for those values.

Users are encouraged to use integers rather than real values to save space. A separate command establishes the valid range of values. Missing values can be specified via another command. A useful feature is a command for establishing relational checks within the data currently being entered so that, for instance, the item sex has to be female if there are vaginal infections. However, this cannot make use of data already in the data base and has no provisions for taking a set action if one of the data is missing.

Data Entry. Users can readily set up through a series of commands a batch entry procedure of the type that would be used with off-line keypunch machines. Data thus entered is more error-prone. The same set of commands can be used with the interactive editor to set up on-line data entry. Checks can include range, list membership, relational, and data type.

Retrieval. A procedural, command-driven report generator enables users to produce hierarchically oriented tables oriented toward summary variables.

Analysis. SIR was written as a "front-end" data base manager for the SPSS statistical package. It makes a conscious effort to retain much of SPSS's syntax and facilitates the transfer of data from SIR to SPSS, although an interface to some other packages, such as SAS, is provided.

As always, analysis proceeds first through a query step, in which conditions are placed on the data and cases meeting those conditions are saved in a special file. SIR's query language is command-oriented—there is no interactive dialogue to take users through the query process on a step-by-step basis with on-line help. The language is procedural; the user has to explicitly state how the query is to traverse the records, using loop commands and pointer commands such as CASE IS and RECORD IS, PROCESS RECORD, END PROCESS RECORD, and END PROCESS CASE. There are commands for conditional testing, IF and ELSE IF, and for performing arithmetical operations during the retrieval. Some simple statistics are available in these programs: frequencies and plots. Data can be retrieved into variables and then manipulated.

Availability, Installation, and Costs. SIR runs on several 32-bit microcomputers: Apollo and Sun, for which it costs $10,000 + $1200 per year for support, and the HP 9000 and the Micro Vax, for which it costs $20,000 + $4000 per year for support. SIR is distributed by SIR, Inc., P.O. Box 1404, Evanston, Illinois 60204.

FOCUS

In the early 1970s a number of so-called fourth generation high-level languages appeared on mainframes, many of them emphasizing the "nonprocedural" approach to data base management. The RAMIS system (Mathematica, Inc., Princeton, NJ) was one of the first commercially viable packages available of this type. FOCUS (Information Builders, Inc., New York) was introduced a few years later and was based heavily on concepts in RAMIS but with many extensions. Both packages are still commercially successful and are very similar.

FOCUS has come out with a microcomputer-based version which presently encompasses a subset of the capabilities we describe. The builders have plans to make it fully compatible with the mainframe version, which is the one we describe. FOCUS was designed to be a complete applications development system to "eliminate programmers" by providing structured, English language facilities to create and maintain data bases and to generate reports and graphs from them. It is written in FORTRAN and IBM Assembler and runs in batch under IBM OS but is most effectively used interactively in the TSO and CMS environments. FOCUS contains powerful report generating capabilities and is well suited to the kinds of data processing needs found in the business community, and it is used in a wide variety of other areas.

Data Base Definition. The user first develops a data base definition, which describes the data base being used. The data base definition contains a name, alias, and format for each item and also contains the structural relationships between items, branching items ("segments"), and data bases. These may only be changed by dumping and reloading the data base using the REBUILD function of the system. This can be time-consuming and costly when used in an environment in which the structural and definitional requirements of a particular file change over time.

FOCUS is a hierarchical system. Related data items are organized into branching items, or segments. If any of the items in a segment exist, then all the space required by the segment is reserved. In order to avoid this problem, users have to segregate those items that variably occur into "unique" segments that have a one-to-one relationship with the primary segment but only take up space when the data are present. However, this can be time-consuming when the data set contains a large number of independent, multiple occurring fields under the same branching item. Such a data set is especially difficult to deal with in FOCUS and requires many more command lines in the data base definition and maintenance as well as creates major difficulties in retrieval.

In general, segments are used to describe data entities, and the standard way to relate segments to each other in FOCUS is in a multilevel hierarchy of up to 64 levels with any number of paths or branches of the hierarchical tree. In addition, any item at any level in a hierarchy may serve as a one-to-one, one-to-many or a many-to-one pointer into any indexed item in any other FOCUS data base or recursively into the same data base, providing some relational capabilities. Indexes are declared in the data base definition and are automatically maintained. In addition to those structures described in the data base definition, relationships may be created dynamically. The JOIN command allows standard relational data structures to be used (with penalties in performance) and the MATCH command allows the physical combining of data bases using a variety of relational operators.

The instances of each segment of a FOCUS data base are ordered according to one or more of the first items in the segment description. "Matching" upon these keys is necessary for the maintenance of the data base, thus leading to a reduplication of keys in a multilevel data base. A FOCUS data base can have a very large number of items (installation dependent), and a data base may be as large as 256 million characters under CMS. The internal data types available are integer, floating point, double precision, packed decimal, and alphanumeric (less than 256 characters). A large number of data item editing options may be declared in the data base definition. These are used at report generation time and include inserted commas, date translations, floating and nonfloating dollar sign, bracketed negative value, and translation of dates. No special data types such as date and time are available.

User access levels may be inserted into the data base definition at the item and segment level, and access may be restricted by data value as well. The Data Administrator Package (DAP) also allows the encryption of data, data base definition, and stored procedures.

Data Entry. Interactive data entry may be accomplished on standard scrolling type terminals through the PROMPT command or on terminals with cursor control and editing functions via the CRTFORM command. In the later mode, multiple screens may be defined for a single data entry sequence or for multiple functions within a single data entry session (for example, add, update, and delete screens with a menu screen). These data entry questionnaires are set up through the command language, which incorporates procedural (programming) notations at this point.

To check data for errors the user must set up a VALIDATE expression for each item within the data entry procedure. Validates may be performed on a single data entry transaction item, or they may involve several items including data base item from the hierarchical levels at and above which the data entry is taking place. The validate may also check the item against a list of valid values maintained externally to FOCUS. Invalid, duplicate, and accepted transactions may logged (copied) to separate external data bases for the purpose of providing an audit trail, for error recovery, or for other reasons.

Note that the data base definition contains only minimal information about fields. All data checking statements must be entered in each procedure needing data checking because there is no facility for storing these in the data base definition. This can cause extra time and effort where several different procedures are set up to enter or update the same data item. The same applies to the grouping and labeling of data values at retrieval time. Because of the limitation of the data base definition, these must be supplied at retrieval time.

As discussed previously, the maintenance of what is essentially data base definition characteristics in the data entry system makes for a less than fully integrated definition with its attendent data integrity and ease-of-use problems. Computational expressions may be inserted into the data entry procedure to derive new items from the entered data.

The entire data entry process is driven by the concept of the "matching" of keys of transaction (data entry) records to the keys of individual segments in the FOCUS data base. The user must pay special attention to the hierarchical structure so that data entry and matching proceed in parallel to the proper segments within the data hierarchy. Because of the grouping of data items under segments, or branching items, within each hierarchical level and path, this matching process can be extremely tedious to set up and manage for the type of complex or sparse hierarchical data produced by clinical research. When loading transactions from external data bases, processing speed is greatly improved if the incoming transactions are in order by their keys. In fact, if this step is not done, the time and costs of loading a large, out of order file are prohibitive.

Retrieval. Although the data entry language has some degree of procedurality, the reporting language is completely nonprocedural and allows the user to specify a variety of reporting options using commands.

The data that result from a query may be saved in an external character data base or in internal format as a "hold" data base for further processing using FOCUS. This involves using duplicate files. There is no feature available that allows the selection of subset of instances of branches of a FOCUS hierarchy. If data are saved in a hold file, the upper hierarchical levels are replicated onto the lower levels in the hold file. Thus, for each visit, demographic data would be replicated. Thus, users are led to redundantly store potentially a great deal of data, depending on the intensity and scope of their analyses.

Retrieval performance may be improved by using alternate data base "views" so that record selection is performed first on those segments requiring selection. The pointers to other levels in the hierarchy are then used to retrieve other segments, if required. Indexed items may also speed retrieval. Retrieval of individual cases is also fairly fast owing to the fact that the data for different segments are stored in different disk pages and the records are stored physically in the order received at data entry time. Based upon their key values, pointers are established to provide a logical (key) order to all the records in a segment. But where appropriate for a query, these pointers are not used and the records are read in physical order.

Analysis. The report generator can compute new items at the record level and report-column level. This is enhanced by a comparable graphics reporting capability using the same query language as the reporting module but with options to set axes, scaling, and other graph formating values. They are usually output on a printing terminal but may use a Diablo (daisywheel) type printer or an HP7220 flatbed plotter.

Statistical analysis is available through the ANALYZE command, which provides access to the following procedures in a "conversational" mode: means and standard deviations, correlation coefficients, several forms of regression, ANOVA, discriminant analysis, factor analysis, cross tabulations, exponential smoothing and forecasting, descriptive statistics, and time series analysis. The number of observations is limited by the amount of memory available.

Special Options. Except for the statistical options, there are no assisted or conversational procedures. All commands may be performed as entered. But normally commands are stored in procedures that are preprocessed by the FOCUS "dialogue manager" at execution time. This scans the procedures for items that should be replaced with values before execution begins. The dialogue manager is a simple procedural language that allows the development of complex, fully automated applications that can isolate the end user from the interactive FOCUS environment altogether, if desired. Another feature that assists in this process is the LET command that allows the application developer to define new language elements relevant to the user in terms of the native language of FOCUS. When the users enter their own "language," it is automatically translated into FOCUS terminology.

Installation, Support, and Costs. FOCUS is distributed world-wide through a number of offices that provide phone support and training seminars. Micro-FOCUS sells for $1595 and costs $275 per year for support and upgrades. Micro-FOCUS runs on the IBM XT and AT, and some IBM PC compatibles, including the TI Professional, the AT&T 6300, and the Zenith 15. The company provides a user newsletter and works closely with a national user group, which meets annually. A 900-page manual is the primary reference document available with the system.

dBASE II

Through a very aggressive marketing effort, in 2 years dBASE III and its predecessor dBASE II have become among the fastest selling microcomputer data base packages on the market. dBASE II currently has a 39 per cent market share for the smaller 8-bit microcomputers. It is currently selling at 2000 copies a month and growing "exponentially." Although touted as a DBMS, dBASE is in fact quite close to a file manager. dBASE provides some nonprocedural, menu-driven features for data entry and display, but it is primarily a high-level, highly structured data capture, storage, and manipulation language similar in flavor to Pascal or C. This data manipulation language incorporates symbolic reference to data items. For most nontrivial applications users write dBASE "Programs" that are interpreted by the dBASE program, which is written in 8080 assembler. The II in the name was attached for marketing purposes. There was no version I.

File Definition. A new file is described by entering the command CREATE, which prompts the user for the data dictionary items to describe each item. The items are: item name, type (character, numeric or yes/no), width, and decimal places. Only seven items or combinations of items may be indexed to speed retrieval and reporting. These indexes are maintained automatically as file updating occurs. Note that the data dictionary contains the minimal description of items and cannot contain data checking, redefinition, or security information. There are no data security provisions available. Furthermore, there are no provisions for the handling of null data items. If the instance of an item is not present, it still occupies space in the file.

Once one or more of these tabular files have been created, they must be physically combined to give the effect of having relational or hierarchical files. The JOIN command takes each record of one file and compares it individually with each record in a second file. If the specified keys match, a record is written to a third file containing a list of items from both sources files. The UPDATE command can copy items from one file into another based on common keys, provided that both files are first sorted on these keys. Also, the clever use of indexed items and storage of redundant data aid in providing simulated relational and hierarchical data structures, although this can require some programming effort because only two files can be open at one time. In particular, it is difficult to handle the complex, sparse hierarchical files generated in clinical research environments. Because each level of a branch must be a separate file in dBASE and only two files may be open at once, the programming verbiage necessary to get around these limits can be very large. dBASE is limited to 1000 characters and 32 items per row in the file or table, 254 characters per item, and 65,535 rows per file or table.

Data Entry. In the simplest case data entry may be performed

298 • CLINICAL APPLICATIONS OF COMPUTERS IN MEDICAL CARE

immediately after entering the data dictionary by answering yes to "INPUT DATA NOW?" after the last item is defined. Full screen editor features are built into the dBASE language and are available during data entry to allow the correction of errors easily. The curser is controlled by the ESDX keys on the keyboard. Records may be added later with the INSERT command. Specific records may be changed with the EDIT command, and the BROWSE command allows the user to scroll up and down through the file, displaying and updating records.

Specially formatted data entry screens may be written using the dBASE II language. Because the command language controls the use of the screen and the data entry sequence, it is possible to show retrieval and entry for two files on the same screen. All data checking statements must be provided as part of the programming of data entry screens. This means that if an item is entered or updated from several different procedures, the data checking statements must be repeated in each case. This can be laborious and error-prone in complex applications.

Retrieval. For simple, quick reports on the video screen or the printer the DISPLAY command can produce an automatically formated report using selected items for a subset of records. A complex boolean expression may be specified for record selection. However, there is no way to save records for further manipulation short of programming.

The REPORT command allows the direct formating of items into specific rows and columns with page headings, totals, and one level of subtotals. A printed item may be an arithmetic expression involving data base items. More complex formating or data summarization may be handled with the dBASE programming language and can involve the development of various intermediate files. The development of reports involving several files (several hierarchical branches and levels) can require much time and effort to bring together all the fields needed. There is no facility beyond the usual method of copying and combining files to select and flag for subsequent use the full data base for selected cases.

Data retrieval speed is improved by the use of indexed items. Sorting should use an additional commercial sorting package for large files.

Analysis. There are no statistical or graphics capabilities in dBASE although Fox & Geller, Inc. (Teaneck, NJ) does sell dGRAPH, which works with dBASE to produce pie charts, bar graphs, and line graphs. A comparably simple statistical package called ABSTAT is available from Anderson Bell. Also, the COPY command can create non-dBASE files for use by other packages.

Special Options. The dBASE programming language allows the use of "macros," which provide the ability to substitute variables into the language at run-time. This, along with the language in general, allows the development of complete, menu-driven applications. Several commercial systems have appeared on the market programmed in dBASE. A file restructuring facility is provided to add and delete items from a file and to easily create new files from old ones. There are no security provisions in the system and only one user may access files at a time.

Installation, Support, and Costs. dBASE is sold for computers running the CP/M and MS-DOS operating systems (including MP/M and CDOS) for $700. It is installed by inserting a diskette and typing dBASE. A function is provided to select the kind of terminal you are using in order to support the full-screen editing.

A 350-page manual is provided in two parts: a tutorial and a reference guide. Software Banc (Arlington, MA) also sells a User's Guide and teaches classes nationally. Ashton-Tate provides phone support, and many dealers also provide support.

As a result of the limitations and the programming nature of the dBASE language, other vendors have developed utilities and program generators such as Quickcode and dUTIL (Fox & Geller), DBPlus (HumanSoft, Arlington, MA), and the dBASE Window (Tylog Systems, Inc., Miami, FL).

dBASE II is available from Ashton-Tate, 9929 West Jefferson Blvd., Culver City, CA 90230.

MEDICAL RECORDS SYSTEMS

Medical records systems such as COSTAR tend to be optimized for the entry and retrieval of individual cases through the use of predefined, patient-centered files in a file manager. Flexibility is sacrificed for speed and hard-coded functionality to deal with a number of administrative and patient care tasks on a per patient basis. Such a sacrifice is getting to be increasingly unnecessary as the processing power of low-cost machines continues to grow. It is also unnecessary in the many group practices and hospital departments consisting of specialists, whose data volume tends to be lower than that for an outpatient clinic.

The computer resources needed for handling large volumes of data on a case by case basis differ from those needed for processing such data on an overall or aggregate basis, as in research. A system's primary file structure will generally be "upright" in the patient record system but "inverted" in the aggregate system. Upright files store data for one patient together, facilitating access to that patient's data. However, such a structure will lead to aggregate query times measured in hours as opposed to minutes and seconds.

There are various schemes for optimizing queries for research uses, usually by keeping the data for one item in one place: all patients' sex together, all patients' blood pressure, and so on. Some systems initially store data in upright files and then move the data to inverted files. Such a two-step process can be cumbersome and time-consuming and may not allow queries on up-to-date information, a problem in patient care.

Predefined medical record systems generally allow the user to specify a list of codes for an item or a choice of coding schemes. They enable the user to choose items from a predefined list to be in the system. However, since they are "canned" file managers, they do not allow one to vary the structure of the data or to specify how items relate to other items. Items can only be placed under those headings when they are predefined. No new headings can be created. This precludes representing much of the real-life characteristics of inpatient data. The only relationships allowed are those predefined.

Large outpatient practices and hospitals not infrequently experience a need to run studies; a solution is to link the patient care Hospital Information System or patient record system to a research-oriented DBMS so that some data can be passed to the research system where it can be augmented under more controlled and flexible conditions. Sometimes this can be accomplished on the same computer. Data that would take hours or overnight to query in the upright files of the patient care system can then be queried much more rapidly.

Finally, it should be noted that full medical records systems tend to be far more expensive to install than research systems. Quite aside from the programming expenses involved, the entire administrative procedures of the medical unit must undergo review to see how the system can accommodate them and how they must be changed to conform to the system. The staff must be trained in the use of the system for a great variety of tasks. The pay-off is potentially great, but so is the investment. DBMSs that allow a more phased implementation may meet more acceptance.

COSTAR

The COSTAR Ambulatory Medical Record System is a file manager operating through a menu-driven dialogue to provide patient records with a built-in structure, patient registration, scheduling, and billing. It was developed at Massachusetts General Hospital and is the most successful to date of the medical records systems.

File Definition. COSTAR has a predefined ENCOUNTER module with a code dictionary embodying the designer's sets of codes for diagnoses, procedures, medications, and so on. Codes can be added to these lists, but the relationship of the data items that carry these coded lists to other data items cannot be modified. Codes can be mapped to other codes such as H-ICDA, ICDA-9, CRVS, or CPT. In addition, COSTAR accepts considerable amounts of free text at different points in the data base.

The COSTAR data model is basically a three-level hierarchy, although in places it descends to four levels.

Data Entry. The built-in data entry programs incorporate on-line help and error checking. There is a REGISTRATION module and a SCHEDULING module.

Retrieval. Numerous reporting options provide rich reporting capabilities tailored to physicians' needs, within the limits of the predefined file structure. There are flow charts for capturing time trends, status reports, and encounter reports. A number of management reports are built into the system such as Densen tables, utilization and membership reports, and revenue analysis reports.

Analysis. COSTAR presently features a medical query language (MQL), a procedural language oriented toward the COSTAR data base. Queries take a long time to run and typically are run overnight. The command set is in English and works easily enough for simple requests, but requires a programmer with more complex queries. There is no step-by-step help dialogue. MQL can be used to set up files for statistical packages.

Special Features. A BILLING and ACCOUNTS RECEIVABLE module works off data captured during the patient care process. A SECURITY module governs access control.

Installation, Support, and Costs. COSTAR itself is in the public domain. A number of vendors have enhanced it and sell licenses. Still more confine themselves to minor enhancements and primarily sell installation and support services. COSTAR is written in MUMPS and requires a MUMPS programmer to install. Because COSTAR is in standard MUMPS, it will run on a variety of microcomputers, including IBM XT/AT, DEC Micro-11, Micro Vax, Motorola 68000, Plexus, AT&T 3B2, Convergent Technology microcomputers, Altos, and many others. A list of COSTAR vendors can be obtained from the MUMPS Users' Group, P.O. Box 37247, Washington DC, 20013.

APPENDIX: EXAMPLES OF SYSTEM INTERACTION

The first example is a procedural language example in BASIC, shown only to give an idea of the details that one must be involved in when working at that level. The second example is a nonprocedural language: the data base definition in SIR. It is intended to show that the user needs to be familiar with the precise command formats and method of specification; there is no on-line documentation. The third example is a dialogue with on-line help, which echoes back the terser nonprocedural form so that users have a chance to learn as they work.

APPENDIX I

A Procedural BASIC Program

The following program asks for a patient number and displays the patient's name. Note the use of such constructs as FOR, which denotes an iteration or repetition of the commands following it. Another command of this type is NEXT. GOSUB is a call to a subroutine, which is another program. These types of commands are typical of procedural languages.

```
05      DIM P$(6), N$(25)
10      PRINT 'ENTER PATIENT NUMBER'
20      INPUT P $
30      REMARK: TEST EACH DIGIT TO SEE IF NUMERIC
40      FOR I = 1 TO 6
50      IF P$(I,I)<"0" GOTO 400
60      IF P$(I,I)>"9" GOTO 400
70      NEXT I
80      REMARK: LINE 1000 IS THE SUBROUTINE TO RETURN
        PATIENT NAME IN N$
90      GOSUB 1000
100     PRINT 'PATIENT NAME IS: ', N$
110     STOP
400     PRINT 'NON-NUMERIC, TRY AGAIN'
410     GOTO 10
```

APPENDIX II

Nonprocedural SIR Data Base Definition

Each command line is typed out precisely as is, and the resulting specification is submitted as a "run." The commands of this language are words like NEW FILE and TASK NAME. They have to be in precise relationship with other elements of the program. Note that they are much more like English than the BASIC program and do not have to include the same level of tedious detail. However, using this language does require familiarity with its syntax and access to a manual.

```
NEW FILE            CLINIC
TASK NAME           CASE DEFINITION
N OF CASE           1000
RECS PER CASE       50
RECTYPE COL         80
CASE ID             PATIENT
COMMON VARS         PATIENT PATTYPE      SEX
MAX REC TYPE        10
```

DOCUMENTS   THE CLINIC DATA BASE CONTAINS CLINICAL
             LABORATORY RESULTS FOR ALL PATIENTS IN
             THE SERUM RHUBARB STUDY. BOTH SUBJECTS
             AND CONTROLS ARE DATA BASE CASES.

TASK NAME   PATIENT ENROLLMENT RECORD
RECORD SCHEMA   1, ENROLL
MAX REC COUNT   1

DATA LIST   (1)
                 /1 PATIENT   1-5   (I)
                    PATTYPE   6   (I)
                    SEX   7   (I)
                    DOB   8-13   (A)
DATE VAR   DOB ('MMDDYY')
VALUE LABEL   PATTYPE   (1) SUBJECT   (2) CONTROL
                 SEX   (1) MALE   (2) FEMALE
ACCEPT REC IF   ((PATIENT LE 4999 AND PATTYPE EQ 1)
                 OR   (PATIENT GE 5000 AND PATTYPE EQ 2)   )
END SCHEMA

APPENDIX III

CDM-Assisted Query System Dialogue

This dialogue features abundant on-line help, which can extend to several levels of detail. Note that this dialogue translates the query request into the terser nonprocedural query language as a learning aid. The final nonprocedural language statement is marked off by [***NON-PROCEDURAL***] to aid the reader.

Data Analysis Option: QD

Query by Dialog
Enter "?" for help, "∧" to exit at any point

Name a heading you want to make a subset of: ?

   Name any heading in your data base. You will then be asked to name one or more subitems on which you will be able to specify conditions. You will be able to save the results of this search, a list of heading occurrences meeting the conditions, in a special file called a "subset," which you can use for displays and analyses.

Name a heading you want to make a subset of: P

Name a subitem of PATIENT: ?

Please name a subitem of the item you want to find occurrences of. You will be asked this question until you provide a data item name: you will then be able to specify a condition on that item, and if you wish, you will be able to specify other items.

After placing all your conditions, you will be asked how you want to combine them with "and," "or," and "not."

To get a list of the subitems for PATIENT, enter "??".

Name a subitem of PATIENT: DOB

What condition should DATE OF BIRTH satisfy?

There are two ways to satisfy a condition:
1) Name a value that DATE OF BIRTH may assume.
2) Specify a two-letter operator (explained below) in capital letters, followed by a space, then by a value. For example, if TEST RESULTS is a simple integer item, you could place the condition "greater than or equal to 30" by entering "GE 30."

If you want to see a list of operators for this item and their meaning, enter "??". You will also get information as to the nature of the item and its allowed values.

What condition should DATE OF BIRTH satisfy?   BT "1/1/60;1/1/0"

– – – > This is condition C1:
DATE OF BIRTH[<AF "1/1/40"> <BF "1/1/50">]

Name a subitem of PATIENT: SEX

What condition should SEX satisfy? M

– – – > This is condition C2:
SEX<EQ "MALE" >

Name a subitem of PATIENT: PO

Ambiguous reference
Do you intend "PO" to mean:
1) PATIENT•HOSPITALIZATION•OPERATION•POSTOP-PROBLEMS
2) PATIENT•HOSPITALIZATION•OPERATION•POSTOP-HYPOTEN-SION-DURATION
3) PATIENT•HOSPITALIZATION•OPERATION•POSTOP-BLOOD-LOSS
0) None of the above

Which? 3

What condition should POSTOP-BLOOD-LOSS satisfy? <u>GT</u> <u>3</u>.2

– – – >This is condition C3:
POSTOP-BLOOD-LOSS<GT "3.2 liters">

Name a subitem of PATIENT: <u><RETURN></u>

What logical condition should C1, C2, C3 satisfy? C1+C2+C3

The query premise for this search is
   [***NONPROCEDURAL***]

PATIENT•[DATE-OF-BIRTH<AF "1/1/60"> <BF "1/1/70"> SEX<EQ M>
   HOSPITALIZATION•OPERATION•POSTOP-BLOOD-LOSS<GT "3.2
   liters">]

Under what name do you wish to save this subset?
<u>YOUNG-MALE-HIGHLOSS</u>

This search will locate all instances of PATIENT for which

   | DATE OF BIRTH satisfies
       | is after or the same as "Jan. 1, 1960"
      and
       | is before "Jan. 1, 1970"
   and
   | SEX is MALE
   and
   | some instance of HOSPITALIZATION satisfies
   | some instance of OPERATION satisfies
   | POSTOP-BLOOD-LOSS is greater than 3.2 liters

OK?   Y//

Glossary

Acoustic coupler: A connection between a modem and a telephone line that allows one to use a standard telephone handset instead of directly connecting to the telephone network.

ANSI (American National Standards Institute): This organization develops data processing standards, which are quite often used as industry guidelines.

Applications program: A computer program that is written to solve a particular problem or serve a specific need, such as word processing or data manipulation.

ASCII: An acronym for the American Standard Code for Information Interchange. This 8-bit code represents up to 128 characters, which are often used in modem-to-modem communications and in many situations in which standardized processing of information is important.

Assembler: See Translator.

Assembly language: A machine-oriented programming language that formulates from mnemonic instructions the specific machine language code that interacts directly with the microprocessor in an applications program.

Backup: The process of creating a duplicate copy of programs or data on the same or different storage media for the purpose of safe-keeping; any resource needed for disaster recovery.

BASIC: An acronym for Beginner's All-Purpose Symbolic Instruction Code. This easy-to-use programming language uses simple English words and is designed for neophytes. As a language, it is widely used by many microcomputers. The many different variations of BASIC are called "dialects."

Batch mode: A method of processing data in which an accumulation of items is grouped together for eventual processing as a single unit. It is a mode that contrasts with "real time" processing in which instructions are immediately processed.

Baud: A unit of transmission speed equal to 1 signal element (usually 1 bit) per second. Traditionally, telephone data transfer is performed at 300 or 1200 baud. Increased baud rates such as 2400 and 9600 are currently available.

Benchmark program: A sample program used to test and compare the performance of different computers or software packages.

Binary notation: Representation of numeric values in the base 2 number system, using only zeroes and ones. Computers use base 2 numbers internally because two states (such as on and off) are easily implemented.

Bit: A contraction for *Bi*nary digi*t*. A single digit of a binary number: 0 or 1.

Bootstrapping: The process of starting an inoperative system by an automatic subroutine in which the first instructions call a series of additional instructions into the computer. The process is so named because of its similarity to pulling oneself up by the boot straps.

Bug: An unintentional error in a computer program. Occasionally it is also used to refer to a hardware defect.

Buffer: A segment of random access memory (which may or may not be an integral part of the central processing unit) reserved for storing information from a specific task (such as printing, disk storage).

Bus: The data bus is the circuit over which electronic data is transmitted within the machine.

Byte: A group of bits (usually 8) that specify a single character in a computer system. Used to assess the storage capacity of a computer because the number of bytes is usually equivalent to the number of characters that can be stored in random access memory.

Canned software: A term for prewritten commercially available software.

Card: An electronic plug-in hardware module that inserts into available slots in the central processing unit. This piece of hardware may perform various functions, ranging from modem communications to graphics output.

Cathode-ray tube (CRT): An electronic vacuum tube that is used to produce the video display. A familiar example is the television picture tube.

Central processing unit (CPU): The circuits in a computer that manipulate data, execute instructions, and control the sequence of operations. It is the computer's main unit (brain) and most vital hardware device.

Character: Any letter, numeric digit, command, or punctuation mark.

Chip: An integrated circuit or circuits on a wafer-thin slice of semiconductor material (usually silicon); the basis for the microcomputer.

COBOL (Common Business-Oriented Language): A computer language designed for general commercial data processing and most often used in the financial industry.

Compiler: See Translator.

Computer language: A defined set of characters, symbols, or words and the rules for combining them into meaningful instructions on a computer. See also Assembly language, BASIC, and COBOL.

Crash: A breakdown or failure in a computer system, resulting in down time and loss of information. Often this is caused by electrical failure or information overload within the computer.

Cursor: An indicator on the video screen that demarcates the position where information will be entered.

Data base: A usually large and continuously updated file of information on a particular subject or subjects designed for easy search and retrieval.

Debug: The process of discovering and removing errors from a computer program.

Digital cassette drive: A peripheral hardware device that utilizes electronic components similar to those in a cassette tape recorder for the purpose of permanently storing digital information on a magnetic cassette tape.

Disk drive: A peripheral hardware device which permanently stores digital information on magnetic disks.

Disk: A round, flat surface, similar in appearance to a phonograph record, which is coated with magnetic particles capable of storing digital data. There are several types of disks, varying in size, capacity, and sturdiness.

Diskette: A small magnetic disk made of flexible Mylar, usually 5¼ inches in diameter or less, also known as a floppy disk. Not to be confused with a hard disk.

Disk pack: A stack of disk platters enclosed in a case designed to be placed in commercial disk drives (usually in mainframe facilities) as a single unit.

Distributed data processing: A process by which all computing tasks are divided between several computers, which communicate with each other to perform a related task(s) in a cooperative manner.

Documentation: All documents, manuals, and diagrams that are associated with the use of a computer or software package. These materials are used to supplement program instructions and explain the use of the software.

Dot matrix printer: A peripheral hardware device that outputs hard copy information. This method of printing uses a matrix of dots to form the outline of the desired character. This is usually an inexpensive form of output.

Down time: Any period when a computer (or other hardware device) is unavailable for use.

Drives: A generic name for hardware devices that have moving mechanical parts that are designed to store data on magnetic disks, either hard or floppy.

EBCDIC: An acronym for Expanded Binary-Coded Decimal Interchange Code. A standardized 8-bit code that represents up to 256 characters and is used especially on IBM systems. This is similar in function to the ASCII.

EDP: An acronym for Electronic Data Processing.

Encoding: The process of converting information to a coded form for easy and compact data storage or transmission.

Field: A subdivision of a record that contains one unit of information of a specific type. An example would be a phone number field in a patient record of a data base.

File: A collection of related records, which usually are stored on magnetic disk or tape. Files may contain data, programs, or both.

File maintenance: The process of modifying the contents of a file to correct errors. This is distinguished from "updating," in which changes are made in a file that reflect real changes in the information recorded in it.

Firmware: Processor instructions that are located in read only memory (ROM). This information may be read at will but not altered. These instructions are a cross between hardware and software because they are actually computer programs that have become part of the computer's hardware.

Floppy disk: See Diskette.

Floating point: A method of mathematical calculation in which the number is represented in a form similar to scientific notation. This is distinguished from integer arithmetic in which fractional values are not allowed.

Format: A predetermined standardized method for performing a computer operation. Also used to describe the manner by which information is physically stored on a peripheral storage device.

FORTRAN (FORmula TRANslator): A computer language which was originally designed for scientific and mathematical use.

Full-duplex: This refers to the ability of a communications system to send and receive information at the same time.

GIGO (Garbage In, Garbage Out): This expresses the concept that unreliable input data produce an unreliable output.

Half-duplex: A communications link that can send or receive data but cannot do both at the same time.

Hard copy: A computer output that is printed on paper or some other permanent medium that can be read with the naked eye.

Hard disk: A random access mass storage device that consists of a continuously rotating circular metal plate. It is accessed by a read/write head that sends and retrieves information.

Hardware: All the tangible components of the computer and its peripheral devices.

Head: The part of a magnetic storage unit that reads and writes information on the magnetic media.

High-level language: A computer programming language that is independent of the processor. A program written in a high-level language must be translated before it can be executed. Examples include BASIC, COBOL, FORTRAN and Pascal.

Instruction: A single machine language level operation or high-level program directive.

Intelligent peripheral: A hardware device that is capable of some limited processing of data by itself independent of the processor to which it is connected.

Interactive mode: A method of data processing that places the user in a form of "conversational" communication with a computer and providing immediate response to user input.

Interface: The point or boundary at which independent systems communicate or interact. In a computer system, this term quite often relates to a hardware device that translates information from one form to another (electrical voltage to a numerical value).

Interpreter: See Translator.

I/O: The abbreviation for input/output.

K: An abbreviation for a binary kilo ($1 \times 2^{10} = 1024$). A kilobyte = 1024 bytes, which is usually rounded to 1000 in normal parlance.

Keyboard: A peripheral input device much like a typewriter keyboard.

Load: The process of entering programs or data into random access memory.

Light pen: A stylus that is capable of sensing light on a video display or of determining the shape of a character for text input to a computer.

Language: See Programming language, High-level language, and assembly language.

Line printer: A type of printer that prints a whole line at a time.

Local area network (LAN): A computer system that consists of several microcomputers connected to a single transmission cable. This network allows for information to be shared among all users on the system while maintaining autonomy and low costs.

LPM: An abreviation for lines per minute; used to describe the output speed of a printer.

Machine language: A set of instructions that are coded and can be read and used directly by the computer without further processing or translation. See also Assembly language.

Mainframe: A large commercial computer. Mainframes are distinguished from microcomputers and minicomputers by relative price, size, computing power, and number of users simultaneously supported.

Mass storage device: A large capacity peripheral hardware device that is used for information storage. See also Digital cassette drive and Disk drive.

Mega: A prefix for an order of magnitude that is 2^{20} or approximately 1 million; most often used to describe memory capacity.

Memory: See Random access memory (RAM) or Read only (ROM).

Microprocessor: A large-scale integrated circuit that performs all the operations in most modern computer systems.

Modem: A contraction of *modulator* and *demodulator*. This device permits computer-to-computer communications over the telephone network. Information is transmitted by altering the frequency of a tone. The lowest frequency of the tone is the baud rate of the communications device and specifies the maximum rate of data transfer.

Monitor: See Video display terminal.

Mouse: A peripheral input device that is particularly useful in selecting information from menu-driven programs and for drawing with the cursor on the video display.

Multiprocessor: Use of multiple processors or computers to handle the processing of a task. One processor always acts as the master and sends instructions to each of the slave processors.

Multitasking: The process of executing more than one software package at a time—for example, through the use of an integrated software package. This software configuration allows more than one task to be performed apparently at the same time; however, the computer performs each task serially.

MUMPS: (Massachusetts General Hospital Utility Programming System): A high-level computer language designed to be physician-friendly. It is being widely used for commercial applications on minicomputers, especially for medical applications.

Network: See Local area network.

Node: A single computer station in a local area network.

Object code: A sequence of instructions (program) in binary form, resulting from either the output of an assembly language program or a compiled high-level language that is able to be executed immediately by the processor without further translation.

Off line: A temporary state of operation for a peripheral device in which it is not under direct control of the central processing unit (CPU). The device can perform operations without affecting the CPU. Likewise, information cannot be sent to or received from the device in this state.

On line: The state of operation for a peripheral device in which it is under the direct control of the central processing unit. This is the exact opposite of off line.

On line processing: See Interactive mode.

Operating system: A software package that is usually provided by the computer manufacturer; designed to control the basic input/output operations of the computer. The operating system handles tasks such as loading and running programs, storing data, and multiprocessing.

Parallel interface (data transmission): A method of transmitting data in which all 8 bits of a byte are transmitted simultaneously. An 8-bit parallel interface must have at least eight electrical lines.

Parity: A software method used to determine whether hardware has correctly sent and received the appropriate information. This is performed by adding an additional bit to the end of a character's ASCII code.

Pascal: A highly structured computer language designed to enhance the teaching of programming as a systematic discipline; named for the seventeenth century mathematician Blaise Pascal.

Password: A unique set of characters or digits that are used to identify a user and provide limited access to electronic files and sensitive information.

Peripheral hardware device: A piece of hardware that is physically separated from the central processing unit and connected via a transmission cable. Examples of a peripheral include printers, disk drives, and video display.

Plotter: A peripheral hardware device that can provide high-resolution graphic hard-copy output. It has the ability to draw continuous lines under computer control.

Printer: A peripheral hardware device that provides a hard-copy output of information. Types of printers available include electrostatic, thermal, dot matrix, letter quality, ink jet, and laser.

Processor: See Central processing unit.

Program: A predetermined set of instructions that direct a computer to perform a specific function or task.

Programming language: A defined set of characters, instructions, and commands and the rules or syntax for combining them into meaningful instructions for the computer's processor. Examples include BASIC, COBOL, and Pascal. A language is often needed to write a program or to execute a program written in a high-level language.

Random access memory (RAM): Internal computer storage that is essential to the central processing unit and allows immediate access to any memory location. The contents of any location may be read or changed at will.

Read only memory (ROM): Internal computer storage that is similar to RAM but different in that the contents of any location can be read but not changed.

Real time processing: A computer term that implies that an operation is performed virtually simultaneously with the event generating the data or person issuing the commands.

Record: A group of one or more fields in a file containing related information about a common subject. A series of records make up a file. For example, a record might contain three fields of information about a particular patient: name, address, telephone number.

Serial interface: A method of transmitting data in which each bit of a byte of information is transmitted sequentially over the same electrical line. At least one line is necessary for this type of transmission.

Slot: A plug-in connector in the central processing unit, in which additional hardware cards may be inserted. This connector is directly wired to the computer's main electronic data bus. See also card.

Software (package): See Program. Contrasts with hardware; all the non-physical "thought processes" of the computer.

Source code (program): A computer program in its original high-level language form before it has been translated into object code.

Spool (spooling): An acronym for Simultaneous Peripheral Output On Line; also refers to input. Spooling is a software feature that allows slow devices in a system to place or receive their information in buffers, therefore not slowing the processor.

Spreadsheet software: A software package that acts as a hybrid between a high-level programming language, data base, calculator, and ledger pad. It has the ability to numerically process data and provide multiple forecasts for such areas as financial planning and trend analysis.

Structured programming: A programming method that advocates the formulation of programs into small modules in creating a software package. This method makes programs easier to write and modify by giving them a highly formal structure; thus, they can be easily modified by the user if the structure is known.

Subroutine: A self-contained section of a program that performs a specific but limited task. Equivalent to a module in a structured program.

System: The hardware (input/output devices, central processing unit, storage), software, and all related components of the computer combined. May also be used to describe all the associated nodes in a local area network.

Systems programs: See Operating system.

Tape drive: See Digital cassette drive.

Tape, magnetic: A continuous ribbon of magnetic-coated material wound on a reel or cassette; used as a mass storage device.

Terminal: An input/output device consisting of a keyboard, communications line, and video display.

Throughput: The productivity of a system based on all aspects of its operation. This may be used as a measure of a system's processing power.

Time-sharing: The use of a single computer for two or more functions or by two or more users during the same period of time. Time-sharing is performed by interspersing in time the actions of the peripheral hardware devices and the central processing unit. Most mainframes are used in this manner.

Translator: A program that converts a sequence of instructions in one computer language to an equivalent sequence of statements or code in another. Compilers, assemblers, programming languages, and interpreters are types of translators.

Turnkey system: A complete computer system for which a single vendor assumes complete responsibility for hardware and software maintenance and installation. Many mainframe time-sharing systems are turnkey systems.

Update: The modification of a file with current information according to a specified procedure.

User Friendly: Indicates that a program was designed for the nonexpert; also implies that a program is easily mastered and prompts the user as to the correct responses and options at any point in the program.

Utilities: Standard software programs or subroutines that are supplied with the computer system. Examples include directory listing, diagnostic hardware, testing software, and file manipulation routines; often acquired with the operating system.

Variable: A symbol whose numeric value changes during program execution.

Video display terminal: A hardware device that outputs data by visual display on a cathode ray tube (similar to a television screen).

Virtual machine: The software method that allows each user in a time-sharing system to interact with the computer as if the computer were dedicated to only that user. This is performed by serially polling the input and output devices connected to each user in rapid but transparent succession.

Virtual peripheral: The same concept as a virtual machine applied to a peripheral hardware device connected to many users.

Word: A basic unit of data in a computer's memory. Often a multiple of the 8-bit byte length (usually 16 bits with microprocessors).

Word processing: A set of automated functions that aid in the production of documents. Software that performs this task allows text editing, formating, storage, and printing.